Springer Wien New York

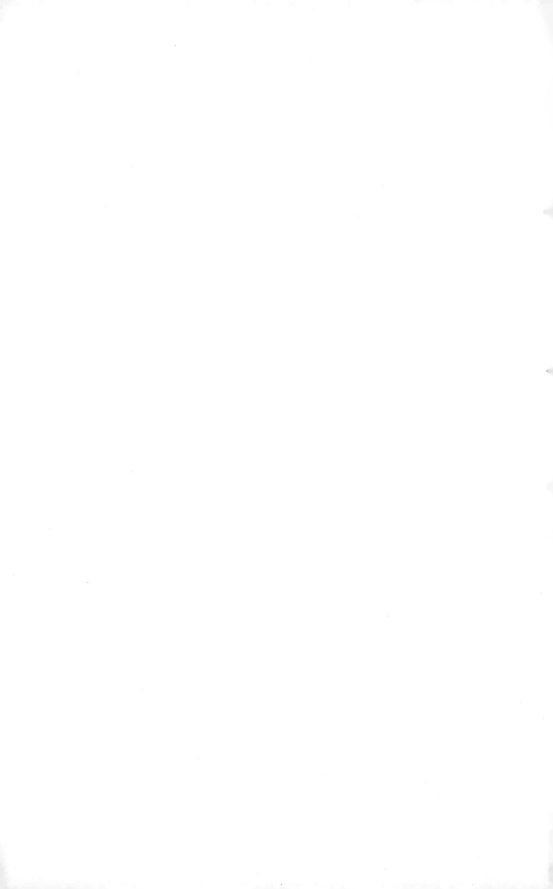

Jozef Rovenský and Juraj Payer (eds.)

Dictionary of Rheumatology

With contributions by
Roy B. Clague, Manfred Herold,
Milan Bayer, Helena Tauchmannová,
Miroslav Ferenčík, Zdenko Killinger

SpringerWienNewYork

Jozef Rovenský
National Institute of Rheumatic Diseases, Piestany, Slovak Republic

Juraj Payer
5th Department of Internal Medicine, Medical Faculty of Comenius University
Faculty Hospital Bratislava-Ruzinov, Slovak Republic

Roy B. Clague – Nobles Hospital, Isle of Man, UK
Manfred Herold – Medical University of Innsbruck, Austria
Milan Bayer – Faculty of Medicine in Hradec Kralove, Charles University Prague, Czech Republic
Helena Tauchmannová – National Institute of Rheumatic Diseases, Piestany, Slovak Republic
Miroslav Ferenčík – Institute of Neuroimmunology, Slovak Academy of Sciences and Institute of Immunology, Faculty of Medicine Comenius Universtiy, Bratislava, Slovak Republic
Zdenko Killinger – 5th Department of Internal Medicine, Medical Faculty of Comenius University Faculty Hospital Bratislava-Ruzinov, Slovak Republic

With financial support by *Bundesministerium für Wissenschaft und Forschung in Wien*, Austria.

Sponsors, who thankfully granted the translation from Slovak into English: *Eli Lilly Slovakia* s.r.o., Bratislava; *Servier Slovensko*, spol. s.r.o., Bratislava; *Novartis Slovakia* s.r.o., Bratislava; *Roche Slovensko*, s.r.o., Bratislava; *sanofi-aventis Pharma Slovakia*, Bratislava.
The printing was sponsored by: *Teva Pharmaceutical*, Bartislava, Slovakia; *Novartis Slovakia* s.r.o., Bratislava; *Mayor of Piešťany*, Slovakia.

Parts of the book were translated from Rovenský et al. "Revmatologický výkladový slovník" GRADA Publishing, 2006 and Payer et al. "Lexikón osteoporózy" SAP, 2007.

Project management, translation and compilation work: Language Sense Ltd. (John Boyd), Bratislava

© 2009 Springer-Verlag/Wien
Printed in Germany
SpringerWienNewYork is a part of Springer Science + Business Media
springer.at

Typesetting: Composition & Design Services, Minsk 220027, Belarus
Printing: Strauss GmbH, 69509 Mörlenbach, Germany
Printed on acid-free and chlorine-free bleached paper
SPIN: 11953708

Library of Congress Control Number: 2008940520

ISBN 978-3-211-68584-6
SpringerWienNewYork

Preface

This dictionary of rheumatology has been prepared as a quick reference source for the clinical, diagnostic and therapeutic aspects of rheumatic disorders and related immunology. Rheumatology is a well-recognised specialty of medicine. Recently, due to many factors (the environment, new viral diseases, genetics, increased life expectancy, improved diagnostic tests) an increase in the incidence and prevalence of rheumatological disorders has been witnessed. Rheumatology has close relationships with a number of medical specialties and health professionals, such as orthopaedic surgery, sports medicine, neurology, immunology, osteoporosis as well as clinical rheumatology nurses, physiotherapists and occupational therapists, so we have endeavoured to collate some basic knowledge from these fields. When compiling this dictionary, we have taken into account the fact that an integral part of prevention and treatment of rheumatological diseases includes rehabilitation. We therefore provided guidelines on how to prevent the onset of functional damage and its progression towards increased disability. We believe this dictionary will serve not only rheumatologists, but also the many related specialists, trainee doctors, health professionals and nurses involved in the management of patients with disorders of the human musculoskeletal system.

The early diagnosis and treatment of rheumatological disorders can help to improve their prognosis and we hope that this modest monograph will contribute to a successful therapeutic management.

Jozef Rovenský
On behalf of the collective authors

α₁-antitrypsin A serum glycoprotein inhibiting proteolytic enzymes, such as trypsin, chymotrypsin and elastase. It also acts as an acute-phase protein. Its serum level rises in inflammatory diseases. The coding gene is located on the 14th chromosome, where it can occur in form of 25 alleles. Some of them code for physiological products (PiMM phenotype), while others are related to pathological states, e.g. PiZZ phenotype, which is often associated with emphysema, cirrhosis, and cholelithiasis, where its serum levels are diminished (α_1-antitrypsin deficiency).

α-fetoprotein An oncofetal antigen that can be found in small concentrations in normal human serum. Its level is high in the fetal serum, where presumably thanks to its immunosuppressive effect, it participates in neonatal immunological tolerance. The α-fetoprotein level is also increased in sera of pregnant women when fetal development is defective (central nervous system defects, immunodeficiency syndromes, gastrointestinal or other abnormalities). An increased serum level can be found in patients with certain neoplastic disorders, especially hepatic cancer and can be used as a marker of hepatocellular carcinoma.

α₁-microglobulin (α₁M) A protein synthesised in the liver and present in blood, serum and urine. Complexes of α_1M with monomeric immunoglobulin A (IgA) participate in renal IgA nephropathy where the serum level of α_2M is also usually increased.

α₂-macroglobulin (α₂M) A serum glycoprotein working as inhibitor of a number of proteases including thrombin, plasmin, kallikrein, trypsin, chymotrypsin, elastase, collagenase and cathepsin B and G. α_2M is produced mainly by macrophages and regulates the proteolytic balance in a number of extra-cellular processes that exert their action mainly in blood coagulation, fibrinolysis and inflammation. α_2M and protease complexes are proteolytically inactive and are eliminated quickly (in minutes) from the circulation. Its serum levels are increased especially in nephrotic syndrome, atopic dermatitis, diabetes mellitus and ataxia-telangiectasia.

Abatacept Abatacept (Orencia®) is an injectable, synthetic (man-made) soluble fusion protein that consists of the extracellular domain of human cytotoxic T-lymphocyte-associated antigen 4 (CTLA-4) linked to the modified Fc portion of human immunoglobulin G1 (IgG1). Abatacept is produced by recombinant DNA technology in a mammalian cell expression system.

Abatacept belongs to a new class of drugs called costimulation modulators, shown to inhibit T cell activation by binding to CD80 and CD86, thereby blocking interaction with CD28. Blockade of this interaction has been shown to inhibit the autoimmune T-Cell activation that has been implicated in the pathogenesis of rheumatoid arthritis Abatacept attaches to a protein on the surface of T-lymphocytes and blocks both the production of new T-lymphocytes and the production of the chemicals that destroy tissue and cause the symptoms and signs of arthritis. Abatacept slows the damage to joints and cartilage and relieves the symptoms and signs of arthritis.

Abatacept is indicated for reducing signs and symptoms, inducing major clinical response, slowing the progression of structural damage, and improving physical function in adult patients with moderately to severely active rheumatoid arthritis who have had an inadequate response to one or more DMARDs, such as methotrexate or TNF antagonists. Abatacept may be used as monotherapy or concomitantly with DMARDs other than

A

TNF antagonists, but has not yet been approved by NICE.

Approval of abatacept was supported by five randomized, double-blind, placebo-controlled clinical trials. In all five studies, subjects received treatments with abatacept or placebo at weeks 0, 2, and 4, then every 4 weeks thereafter. Studies have found that abatacept can reduce the signs and symptoms of rheumatoid arthritis. It can also reverse some signs of joint damage. Abatacept/MTX slowed the progression of structural damage compared to placebo/MTX alone (Furst et al. 2007).

Abatacept is infused over 30 minutes. The initial dose of abatacept is followed by doses two and four weeks later with further doses every 4 weeks thereafter. Patients weighing <60 kg should receive a 500 mg dose, weighing 60–100 kg a 750 mg dose and weighing >100 kg a 1000 mg dose.

The most common side effects of abatacept include: back pain, cough, dizziness, headache, high blood pressure, nausea, rash, upper respiratory tract infection, and urinary tract infection. Administration of abatacept in patients with chronic obstructive pulmonary disease (COPD) has been associated with exacerbation and increased incidence of COPD symptoms. Patients suffering from both rheumatoid arthritis and COPD who elect to have abatacept therapy should monitor symptoms carefully, and in collaboration with their physicians. Concurrent administration of a TNF inhibitor with abatacept has been associated with an increased risk of serious infections and no significant additional efficacy over use of the TNF antagonists alone. Concurrent therapy with abatacept and TNF antagonists is therefore not recommended.

The long-term effects of abatacept aren't yet known, as it hasn't been studied over an extended period.

Abduction Movement of extremities of the body away from the body's midline.

Achilles tendon The common insertion of soleus and both gastrocnemii muscles tendons. It inserts on the posterior side of calca-

neus, separated from it by the Achilles bursa. Tendonitis can be part of the clinical picture of spondyloarthritis, especially ankylosing spondylitis. It can remain thickened (by fibrosis) after the inflammation has subsided and nodules may be palpable.

Achillodynia Pain of the Achilles tendon, especially of its insertion, most frequently after a trauma or sporting overload.

Achondroplasia and hypochondroplasia An autosomal dominant hereditary syndrome characterized by a small stature with short extremities, in most cases caused by a mutation of the fibroblast growth factor receptor-3 (FGFR-3). It belongs to the most frequent dysplasias with an incidence of 1 to 15.000–77.000 births, depending on race. The mutation of FGFR-3 results in a defect of chondrocyte proliferation in the growth cartilage of long bones.

Clinical symptoms and signs: Some children have breathing difficulties/obstructive sleep apnoea, episodes of cyanosis or chronic respiratory insufficiency. Specific developmental abnormalities lead to the above-mentioned clinical picture: Hypoplasia of the middle part of the face with a tendency of obstruction of the upper airways; dysplastic changes of the craniovertebral junction with a tendency towards stenosis of the foramen magnum and compression of medulla oblongata; constriction of the chest. The condition can lead to a picture of "respiratory distress syndrome in achondroplasia". Problems can be divided into three groups. The mildest type is accompanied only by obstructive sleep apnoea (most probably related to hypertrophy of adenotonsillar tissue); a more severe course includes episodes of apnoea and upper airway obstruction persisting even after adenotonsillectomy, often accompanied by the formation of hydrocephalus; severe distress progressing to cardio respiratory failure with oxygen dependency, eventually with coincidental gastroesophageal reflux.

Acquired immunodeficiency syndrome An infectious disease due to the HIV retrovirus (human immunodeficiency virus). Two types of virus exist: HIV-1 and HIV-2. Both cause serious immune system defects. The present pandemics are predominantly due to HIV-1, which is more pathogenic. It is transmitted by homosexual or heterosexual intercourse, transfusion of infected blood and its derivates, IV drug administrations using infected needles, organ transplant from an infected donor, or from an infected mother during labour or breast-feeding.

HIV infects cells that possess differential antigen CD4 on their surface (particularly T lymphocytes and macrophages). Non-specific symptoms occur at an early stage after infection. Subfebrile temperatures, weakness, sweating, arthralgias, myalgia, headache, diarrhoea, lymphadenopathy and also certain neurological symptoms may occur. Such symptoms last for several days to two weeks. In the majority of infected individuals, these symptoms may not be apparent. Approximately two weeks after virus transmission, the viral antigens (p24, gp41) can be detected in the blood of the infected individual. Later on these antigens disappear and antibodies against certain HIV antigens (anti-p24 and anti-gp41) can be detected in the blood of the infected individual at two to three months, which is diagnostic confirmation of infection. The disease now often enters a latent period without any clinical symptoms, except for possible lymphadenopathy. Such a period may last up to 12 years and it terminates by activation of the disease, which in untreated cases, leads to death in 6 to 30 months.

Activation of the disease is manifested by decreasing antibodies against the HIV antigens (anti-p24) and concurrent reoccurrence of these antigens in the blood. Such an event is referred to as seroconversion. The number of T lymphocytes in peripheral blood decreases. If the number of T lymphocytes is less the 0.2×10^9/l, then the infected individual is considered to have severe AIDS, even though the patient may be asymptomatic. AIDS symptoms include infections due to normal, non-pathogenic micro-organisms (pneumonia due to *Pneumocystis carinii* – in 50% of all patients) and certain malignancies

with rapid course (Kaposi sarcoma – approximately 1/3 of all patients). Dementia and changes of psychomotor functions, which are very likely due to direct HIV infection of glial cells in the brain, occur in approximately 2/3 of all patients. The typical clinical picture of AIDS does not develop in certain patients; however, these patients suffer from a group of symptoms referred to as ARC (AIDS related complex) in which infections and tumours are not present. ARC may or may not progress to full blown AIDS.

The diagnosis of AIDS consists of serological assessment, immunological assessment (determination of CD4⁺-lymphocytes, or the CD4⁺/CD8⁺ ratio in peripheral blood), clinical assessment and relevant medical history. Contemporary treatment is only partial and generally it allows inhibition of HIV replication in infected cells (azidothymidine, zidovudine) and thereby prolongs the period free of any clinical symptoms. However, after development of the symptoms, treatment cannot cure the disease.

ACR classification criteria for diagnosis of rheumatoid arthritis 1987 → see Rheumatoid arthritis (RA) – classification criteria

Action potential Electrical activity in the nerve axon or muscle fibre according to the "all or nothing" type, when the membrane potential polarity ceases or is restored abruptly.

Acupuncture (AC) Used in rheumatology for pain relief. Metallic needles are inserted into specific body points by rotation movement. Acupuncture should induce a balance between "yang" (spirit) and "yin" (blood) principles that run in 14 meridians comprising 361 acupuncture points. AC has been considered as a form of neuromodulation. Its effects have been explained by the gate theory of pain relief, and also by a presumption that the insertion of the needle acts as a noxa, inducing the production of endogenous opiate-like substances (opioids). The locations of acupuncture points often overlap myofascial trigger points and painful muscle points.

A

Electro-acupuncture refers to the stimulation of the acupuncture points with needles plugged into a source of electrical current or by the application of small electrodes on those points. Similarly, laserpuncture and magnetopuncture is used.

Acupressure refers to a method when acupuncture points are influenced by pressure from the fingers or rounded sticks.

Acute febrile neutrophilic dermatosis (Sweet's syndrome)
A rare disease of unknown aetiology characterised by marked inflammatory neutrophilic skin infiltrates.

Symptoms and signs:
- painful nodules and red-violet maculae on the skin of the shoulders, torso or head; ulceration usually doesn't occur,
- lesions generally heal without scarring,
- concomitant high fever,
- leukocytes with polymorph nuclear predominance,
- tendency to relapse.

Acute phase proteins (APPs)
Glycoprotein mediators whose production is significantly modified after activation of the inflammatory response or any other kind of tissue damage. That is why they are also referred to as acute-phase (of inflammation) reactants. They are produced mainly by hepatocytes, but also by monocytes, endothelial cells, fibroblasts and other cells. They are divided into positive and negative APPs. The concentration of positive APPs increases in the course of inflammation, whilst the concentration of negative APPs decreases. Albumin is an example for a negative APP. The increase of the major APPs can be greater than a thousand fold, while the concentration of other positive APPs increases only by less than three fold. C-reactive protein (CRP) and serum amyloid A (SAA) are the most strongly reactive positive APPs in humans. Their main biological functions include direct neutralisation of inflammatory reactions, minimising the damage due to inflammation, involvement in reparatory mechanisms and regeneration of damaged tissues. TNF-α, IL-1, IL-6, IL-11 and other cytokines stimulate the transcription of genes encoding APPs, whereas glucocorticoids and insulin inhibit the transcription.

Acute phase reactants
→ see Acute phase proteins

Acute prolapse of cervical intervertebral disc
Protrusion of the intervertebral disc with intact annulus fibrosus and prolapse of the intervertebral disc with nucleus pulposus prolapse through the perforated annulus fibrosus are the consequence of degenerative changes in intervertebral disc tissues. Prolapse of the disc is usually directed posteriorly through a weak dorsal longitudinal ligament.

Symptoms and signs: Medial protrusion of the disc can cause compression of the spinal cord and lead to development of spastic paraparesis, dorsal column syndrome and urinary bladder dysfunction. More frequently posterolateral prolapse of the disc causes isolated compression of the corresponding spinal nerve. In most patients the symptoms include pain projecting into corresponding dermatome, movement limitation of the cervical spine and spasm of the paravertebral muscles. Initially the neck pain can be provoked by ambulation and later manifests itself by a typical radicular syndrome.

Acute shoulder pain
Pain caused by irritation of the phrenic nerve and recognised as shoulder pain (Eiselsberg´s phenomenon; first described by the Viennese surgeon Anton von Eiselsberg, Vienna, 1860–1939). This includes pain in angina pectoris, myocardial infarction, gall bladder disorders, trauma of the spleen, neoplasms, diseases of thyroid gland, pleuritis. Also bursitis calcarea, impingement syndrome of one of the rotator cuff tendons, most frequently the supraspinatus muscle, may radiate to the shoulder.

Acute shoulder pain without movement limitation may be caused by radicular syndrome of C5, herpes zoster (shingles), diseases of the bones around the shoulder, Paget-Schroetter syndrome, subclavian, axillary or brachial vein thrombophlebitis leading to livid oedema of the hand.

Limitation of active movement (passive movements are unlimited) is caused by complete disruption of the rotator cuff usually following trauma, overload, mechanical friction or trauma to the rotator tendons with break up or rupture. Commonly the supraspinatus muscle tendon is affected. In the case of complete rupture, active abduction to the extent of 0 to 30 degrees is impossible and the anterior tip of the acromion is tender upon palpation. Sooner or later the supraspinatus muscle atrophies. In some cases, the X-ray shows calcification in the supraspinatus muscle tendon. Ultrasound or magnetic resonance imaging can confirm disruption of the tendon.

Treatment includes bed rest, extremity positioning, analgesics, physiotherapy and surgical reconstruction.

Adduction Movement of extremities of the body towards the midline.

Adenosine deaminase (ADA) An enzyme in humans and mammals catalysing the deamination of adenosine and deoxyadenosine to inosine and deoxyinosine, respectively. In the case of deficiency, the metabolism of DNA is impaired, resulting in severe disruption of T-lymphocyte function (adenosine deaminase deficiency).

Adhesion Abnormal union of parts that are normally separate. Increased tissue adhesion, caused in rheumatology most frequently by inflammation, is expressed by limited reciprocal movement of tissues.

Adhesive capsulitis (frozen shoulder) This is characterised by pain and gradual progressive limitation in shoulder movements due to contraction of the glenohumeral capsule. There is often partial or complete resolution over months to years. It is commonest in later life and can be associated with neurodystrophy, for example in the "shoulder-hand" syndrome, following strokes, metabolic disorders (especially insulin-dependent diabetes mellitus) etc.

Adhesive molecules Glycoproteins or lectins taking part in interactions between immune system cells, especially during colonisation of primary and secondary lymphatic organs and within inflammatory reactions. They belong to several families, such as selectins, integrins, members of the immunoglobulin super family (ICAM-1, VCAM-1, PECAM) and cadherins.

Adjuvant A supplemental agent that increases the effect of the main drug. In immunology, it is an agent of organic or inorganic origin that is capable of potentiating the immune response to a concomitantly administered antigen (e.g.: Freund's adjuvant).

Adson's test Test to examine for impingement of the subclavian artery. During the examination, the patient is upright with the upper extremity extended to 40 degrees and his/her head rotated to the examined side. When inspiring and elevating the chin, there is a diminution of the radial pulse on the side of the extended upper extremity, which indicates evidence of impingement of the subclavian artery.

Agammaglobulinaemia A condition in which the total serum immunoglobulin level in the individual is lower than 1g/L (immunodeficiency). It is caused by genetically conditioned insufficient production of immunoglobulins. There are two forms: Bruton's or Swiss type. Bruton's type is congenital, sex-linked agammaglobulinaemia in boys. The clinical picture is dominated by pyogenic infections. No antibodies are produced after vaccination.

Treatment: Infusion of intravenous preparations of Ig (IVIg).

The Swiss type of idiopathic agammaglobulinaemia with lymphopenia is a severe combined immunodeficiency (SCID). The clinical picture is dominated by systemic fungal infections, mainly candidiasis, together with bacterial infections such as in Bruton's type. The mere repletion of immunoglobulins is rarely therapeutically successful, so bone marrow transplantation should be considered (immunoglobulin deficiency).

Agonist The principal acting muscle (prime mover) responsible for the movement in the required direction. The antagonist acts in the opposite direction to the agonist. The synergist co-acts in the direction of the agonist.

Albers-Schönberg Disease → see Osteopetrosis

Alendronate A bisphosphonate licensed for the treatment and prevention of osteoporotic fractures (vertebral and nonvertebral) in postmenopausal women, patients with glucocorticoid-induced osteoporosis and men with osteoporosis. The drug is taken on an empty stomach washed down with a cup of water in an upright posture and remaining upright for the next 30 minutes. It is taken in a dose of 70 mg once weekly or (rarely nowadays) 10 mg daily. Calcium and Vitamin D supplements are normally prescribed concurrently to aid its effect.

Alexander technique → see Exercise techniques

Algodystrophic syndrome (ADS) ADS is characterised as a complex of symptoms elicited by a nociceptive stimulus.

Symptoms and signs: The clinical picture is characterised by severe burning pain, autonomonic vasomotor dysfunction, skin changes and subsequent locomotor malfunction of the affected extremity. Radiographically, it is characterised by regional osteoporosis in the affected area.

ADS – synonyms: algoneurodystrophy, reflex sympathetic dystrophy, Sudeck's atrophy, complex regional pain syndrome (CRPS), shoulder–hand syndrome, causalgia. The complex of symptoms includes regional pain, vasomotor disturbances, skin changes and sensory disturbances. Any region on the upper and lower extremities may be affected.

The development of ADS can be divided into:
- *acute phase* This begins usually 10 days after an injury. It is characterised by intensive, dull, roughly circumscribed pain, oedema with reddening to cyanosis of the skin that is glossy and sweaty. The aim of physical therapy is to improve local blood perfusion without increased afferentation from the affected region. Diadynamic currents and pulse ultrasound are advisable or interferential currents in analgesic doses (Transcutaneous Nerve Stimulator). Vacuum-compressive therapy (cautiously), passive positioning of the extremity, and active exercise of the fingers.
- *dystrophic phase* This begins 2 to 4 weeks after the injury or damage. The skin goes pale, the oedema decreases and a spotty or diffuse osteoporosis of the whole affected region occurs on the X-ray image. In this stage Basset currents or vacuum/compressive treatment is advisable. Passive exercise of the extremity, beginning with antigravity exercises.
- *atrophic phase* This is characterised by persisting trophic changes in the skin and dermis, limitation of passive and active movements up to ankylosis. Functional changes in this stage are very difficult to influence; application of pulse, low-frequency magnetotherapy or distance electrotherapy (Basset currents) may be applied. Intensive locomotor treatment, exercise in a sling, hydrokinesiotherapy, thermotherapy.

Prevention of ADS: early active mobilisation of the affected extremity focusing on functional training.

Algometry (evaluation of pain threshold)
- Instrumental measurement of the pressure on a joint or muscle already causing pain. Using the Phyaction device (ultrasound + mid-frequency currents) one can, according to current density and ultrasound frequency, localise a painful trigger point. Using thermovision, it is possible to localise tender or trigger points on the skin surface.
- thermal by measuring thermal stimulus endurance
- different types of visual analogue scales (VAS; on a vector from 0 to 10, or 100 with plus values on the right side and minus values on the left) horizontally and vertically

- verbal e.g. Likert 5-degree scale
- pain evaluation using questionnaire systems
- Melsack's questionnaire where pain can be expressed by 78 words divided into 4 groups. Furthermore, the questionnaire contains 3 indexes with a degree scale from 1 to 5:
  - NWC – number of words chosen,
  - PRI – pain rating index,
  - PPI – present pain intensity.

The evaluation of pain is an integral part of each evaluation system in rheumatology, e.g. HAQ, RADAI, WOMAC, Lequesne index, AIMS and others.

Alkalising agents Compounds used in cytostatic treatment. They act as agents alkalising DNA, thereby blocking cell division, which is why they are used in the treatment of neoplasms. Rarely some of them are used as immunosuppressants (cyclophosphamide).

Alkaptonuria and ochronosis Alkaptonuria is a rare inborn (autosomal recessive) error of the metabolism of aromatic amino acids phenylalanine and tyrosine where, due to a defective activity of the enzyme called homogentisic acid oxidase, there is no cleavage of homogentisic acid (alkapton) causing accumulation in the body and excretion in urine. Its polymer – ochronotic pigment – impregnates the bradytrophic tissues.

Symptoms and signs:
- presence of homogentisic acid in the urine (turns dark when left standing),
- visible, black-grey pigmentation on eyes and ears,
- degenerative changes of locomotor organs, especially the spine.

Allodynia Pain elicited by a stimulus normally insufficient to cause pain.

Allopurinol Acts as an inhibitor of xanthine oxidase. The recommended starting dose is 100 mg daily, with many patients requiring a dose of 300 to 400 mg daily, while with others a dose of 100 mg a day is enough. 100 mg and 300 mg tablets are available.

Indications for hypouricaemic treatment initiation:
- recurrent acute gout attacks,
- occurrence of complications of hyperuricemia and gout,
- development of tophi,
- involvement of kidneys,
- patients with a uric acid level persistently >700 μmol/L who have already experienced an attack, because they have a higher risk of developing complications.

Alphacalcidol (1-alpha-hydroxycholecalciferol) is indicated in the treatment of the postmenopausal osteoporosis and osteoporosis in patients with severe renal insufficiency. Alphacalcidol is rapidly metabolised in the liver to calcitriol. Its principal mechanism of action is to increase the circulating 1,25-dihydroxycholecalciferol level, thus increasing the absorption of calcium and phosphate from the intestine. It is important in disorders where the hydroxylation process of vitamin D in the kidneys is disturbed, as in chronic renal diseases.

Amyloid A family of fibrillar proteins depositing in different tissues in primary and secondary amyloidosis. Their molecules have a typical folded leaf structure (anti-parallel β-structure). Chemically they are composed of the two different types AL (amyloid light) and AA (amyloid associated). The amyloid AL fibres consist of light-chain immunoglobulins or their fragments, whereas amyloid AA consists of non-immunoglobulin fibroproteins. The precursor of amyloid A is a serum amyloid P (SAP) which belongs to an important group of acute phase proteins and is an integral part of high-density lipoproteins (HDL). Besides these two forms AL and AA, amyloid deposits comprise to a lesser extent the amyloid P (AP) component, whose precursor is serum amyloid P.

Deposition of amyloid can result from an inflammatory, hereditary or neoplastic origin. Primary (genetically predisposed) amyloidosis is rare. Secondary and reactive amyloidosis is occasionally the consequence of a number of chronic and recurrent diseases, e.g. leprosy, tuberculosis, bronchiestasis, systemic lupus erythematosus, juvenile idiopathic arthritis and rheumatoid arthritis. It is characterised by extracellular deposition of insoluble protein fibres in a number of tissues, including spleen, liver, kidneys and lymphatic nodes, leading eventually to death. In the liver, the vessels of the portal system are most affected; sometimes, in the advanced stage, the space of Disse is filled with amyloid. In the myocardium, the amyloid is deposited in the vessels and basal membranes of cardiomyocytes, whilst in kidneys it is deposited in the mesangial loop and in the advanced stage in the perimeter of the glomeruli. Primary systemic amyloidosis is caused by the overproduction and insufficient elimination of light-chain immunoglobulins (mainly lambda) and occurs in multiple myeloma (approximately 20% of myelomas). Secondary amyloidosis is caused by deficient elimination of acute phase protein cleavage products and accompanies chronic autoimmune and systemic inflammatory processes. The deposits consist of 85–90% of amyloid A and 10–15% of amyloid P. It is therefore referred to as amyloidosis AA. The AP component can be found also in other forms of amyloid plaques, including those present in the brain in Alzheimer's disease. Amyloidosis AL with fibrillar deposits formed by light-chain immunoglobulins occurs frequently in multiple myeloma or Waldenström's macroglobulinemia. Usually it affects the heart, gastrointestinal and respiratory systems, peripheral nerves and the tongue. Amyloidosis can also occur due to age.

Symptoms and signs:
- latent course,
- prominent weakness, dyspnoea, oedema, weight loss, orthostatic collapse, macroglossia,
- subsequently there are signs of nephrotic syndrome, cardiomyopathy, speech disorders and polyneuropathy.

Anabolic steroids Anabolic steroids having a generalised anabolic effect, but are no longer recommended in treating osteoporosis because of their adverse effects (virilisation, hepatopathy, unfavourable influence on the metabolism of lipids, etc.). Theoretically it can be used in elderly women with low bone turnover. In male osteoporosis secondary to hypogonadism, testosterone derivatives are the treatment of choice.

Anaesthesia dolorosa Severe spontaneous pain occurring in an anaesthetised region.

Analgesia Painful stimulus does not elicit pain. It can be linked to a change of perception of other modalities.

ANCA Autoantibodies against the cytoplasm of neutrophils (Antineutrophil cytoplasmic antibodies). ANCA participate in the pathogenesis of systemic vasculitides and glomerulonephritis. These antibodies are directed against several enzymes or other proteins located, predominantly, in the azurophilic granules of neutrophils. Using the indirect immunfluorescence method, it is possible to differentiate three types of ANCA during a reaction with the neutrophils:
1. Diffuse fine granular cytoplasmic fluorescence (cANCA) can be found in most cases of Wegener's granulomatosis, microscopic polyarteritis and glomerulonephritis. Proteinase-3 is the specific antigen.
2. Perinuclear fluorescence is caused by pANCA which is shown in cases of microscopic polyarteritis, crescent and segmental necrotizing glomerulonephritis and in Churg-Strauss syndrome. These are antibodies against myeloperoxidase (MPO), but also against elastase, cathepsin G, lactoferrin and others.
3. Atypical ANCA display nuclear fluorescence and certain atypical cytoplasmic patterns. The above-mentioned enzymes, and also other as yet unidentified proteins, are their antigens.

Ankylosing hyperostosis → see Diffuse Idiopathic Skeletal Hyperostosis (DISH; ankylosing hyperostosis; Forestier's disease)

Ankylosing spondylitis (AS; Bechterev's disease) A chronic systemic inflammatory disorder belonging to the group of seronegative spondylarthritides affecting predominantly the axial skeleton, sacroiliac, apophyseal and costovertebral joints of the spine. Much of the pathology occurs at the entheses. Secondary metaplasia of the inflamed tissue of anterior and lateral borders of the vertebrae causes a gradual ossification of the peripheral part of fibrous annulus of the intervertebral disc and adjacent ligaments. Occasionally, peripheral joints are also affected. The shoulder and hip joints are affected in up to 50%, with other joints affected in about 20%. Extraspinal organ involvement such as iritis and aortal valve disease is less frequent than in rheumatoid arthritis, but inflammatory bowel disease can occur in 5–10% of patients. Pulmonary fibrosis, amyloidosis and neurological signs of compression can be observed in late disease.

Symptoms and signs:
- pain with stiffness in the back of inflammatory nature,
- movement limitation of the spine in all three planes,
- a trend towards development of spinal deformity,
- occasionally, peripheral arthritis, mostly of hip and shoulder joints, and joints of the lower extremities,
- extraspinal organ manifestations (ocular, skin, mucosal, cardiovascular, pulmonary, neurological, IgA-nephropathy and amyloidosis),
- radiological presence of sacroileitis, syndesmophytes and peripheral enthesiopathy,
- high association with HLA-B27 antigen.

Anorexia nervosa A disorder characterised by low body weight (BMI usually under 17.5) with an intense wish to remain thin, amenorrhoea and relative hypercorticism. It most commonly affects adolescents. All these factors cause a significantly decreased bone density in women with anorexia nervosa.

Antibodies Immunoglobulins produced by plasma cells that originate from B lymphocytes after specific antigen stimulation. They play two major roles in the humoral immune system. The first is antibody specificity, the essence of which represents the recognition and binding to complementary antigen determinants (recognising function). The second role includes specific biological functions, which are referred to as effector functions. These represent the ability to bind to specific Fc-receptors of various cells, to activate complement, to transfer through the placenta etc. All of these activities are induced by interaction with specific antigen but different parts of immunoglobulin than the binding side are responsible for these functions. Antibodies are present in serum and other body fluids, or inside the producing cells. They can be divided depending on their structure (different classes of immunoglobulins), how they are produced (conventional and monoclonal antibodies) or depending on their properties (anti-idiotypic, cytophilic, cytotoxic etc.).

Antibodies against cyclic citrullinated peptides (Anti-CCP antibodies; anti-citrullinated peptide antibodies, ACPA)

Anti-CCP antibodies (ACPA) have a high specificity and sensitivity for rheumatoid arthritis (RA). They belong to the IgG class and have more than 56% sensitivity and more than 90% specificity for RA, depending on the assay kit used. They are directed against peptides and proteins, which possess the unusual, non-standard amino acid citrulline. Citrullinated proteins develop during enzymatic post-translation enzymatic deimination of arginine residues catalysed by peptidylarginine deiminases in the presence of Ca^{2+}. Such post-translational modification of proteins leads to loss of the positive charge of arginine residues with subsequent modification of antigenicity of the proteins. Antiperinuclear factor, antikeratin antibodies (both directed against citrullinated filaggrin), anti-Sa antibodies (against citrullinated vimentin) and cyclic citrullinated peptide antibodies (anti-CCP) are among the best-known citrullinated reactive antibodies associated with RA. Recently, it has been shown that the basic component of the antigenic epitope of filag-

A

grin and vimentin is citrulline. The formation of citrullinated antigens is a dynamic process that takes place in inflamed synovia in the presence of peptidylarginine deiminases (PADs). Five subtypes (PAD 1, 2, 3, 4 and 6) are known. Expression of PAD4 isotype with increased enzymatic activity is typical for RA. Anti-CP antibodies (ACPA) are produced in the area of inflammation and pannus, probably by plasma cells and B cells.

Apart from high specificity, antibodies against citrullinated peptides are typically present in the very early stage of RA. Their presence is associated with the more active and severe forms of the disease. A combination of these antibodies with rheumatoid factor increases the specificity and positive predictive value of these markers, and enables early intervention. Currently, ELISA methods are used to assess antibodies against citrullinated peptides and cyclic citrullinated peptide antibodies (anti-CCP). Measurement of ACPA is now the most frequent assay in clinical practice.

Antibodies against Ku antigen Ku antigen is a heterodimer of two peptides consisting of units with MW= 70 kDa and MW = 80 kDa, which are present in the nucleus and nucleolus. Ku protein is a component of DNA-dependent protein kinase. Ku antigen binds the enzyme to DNA and helps in DNA repair. Anti-Ku antibodies were first found in patients with scleroderma-polymyositis overlap syndrome in Japan. Apart from Japan, these antibodies are frequently found in patients with systemic lupus erythematosus or mixed connective tissue disease. In addition, such antibodies have been found in some patients (23%) with primary pulmonary hypertension. Anti-Ku antibodies induce macular fluorescence of the nucleus with nucleolar fluorescence when cells are in the G1 phase of the cell cycle.

Antibodies against U1RNP and Sm antigen Antibodies present in systemic lupus erythematosus (SLE) directed against small nuclear ribonucleoprotein particles (smRNP). They are usually autoantibodies against proteins complexed with small nuclear RNA. Anti-Sm antibodies (antibodies against Sm antigen or Smith antigen named in honour of the first patient with SLE where anti-Sm antibodies were found) are very specific to SLE. However, their sensitivity is low (10 to 30% of patients with SLE). Anti-Sm antibodies are almost always accompanied by the presence of anti-U1RNP antibodies, a contrary relationship does not apply.

The clinical correlation of anti-Sm is not significant, some studies report a more frequent presence in central nervous system disease, nephritis, lung disease, pericarditis and their correlation with disease activity. In 1972, Sharp described antibodies against an extractable nuclear antigen (subsequently defined as U1RNP) and its association with mixed connective tissue disease (MCTD, Sharp's syndrome; first described 1972 by Gordon C. Sharp, American physician) (Sharp et al. 1972). Antibody against U1RNP is also found in SLE but usually with low titres. Interestingly, many of the features of MCTD, particularly fibrosing alveolitis, myositis, arthritis and Raynaud's phenomenon, were found in these patients.

Anticardiolipin antibodies → see Antiphospholipid syndrome (APS)

Anticentromere antibodies → see Systemic sclerosis (SSc)

Anti-citrullinated peptide antibodies (ACPA) → see Antibodies against cyclic citrullinated peptides

Anti-dsDNA antibodies Anti-DNA antibodies form a heterogenous group directed against different antigen determinants of DNA. Several groups are differentiated:
- Antibodies reacting only with the double stranded DNA (dsDNA). These antibodies form the majority. 65% patient sera with systemic lupus erythematosus (SLE) react with dsDNA.
- Antibodies cross-reacting with dsDNA and ssDNA (single stranded DNA). These antibodies are the most frequent in SLE.

- Antibodies reacting solely with ssDNA.
- Antibodies reacting with Z conformational DNA (Z-DNA).

Clinical importance of anti-dsDNA antibodies:
- high levels of anti-dsDNA antibodies are associated especially with SLE,
- circulating anti-dsDNA can be found in IgM, IgG and sometimes IgA classes,
- IgG antibodies are more significant than IgM; their presence correlates with the activity of the disease and severity of glomerulonephritis,
- this correlation to glomerulonephritis can be found mainly with complement fixating and activating antibodies especially IgG anti-DNA,
- IgG antibodies occur in four subgroups with prevalence of IgG1 and IgG3,
- single-shot assessment of anti-dsDNA is highly diagnostic, though for determining prognosis longitudinal follow-up is recommended. In most cases a rise in anti-dsDNA levels indicates an exacerbation of the SLE.

Mechanism of renal impairment by anti-dsDNA antibodies in SLE:
- anti-dsDNA bind to histone complexes and DNA having affinity to heparin sulphate of glomerular basement membrane,
- anti-dsDNA with the ability to cross-react with several other antigens like A- and D-peptides of small nuclear RNP or ribosomal P-protein, can have a direct impairing influence on renal cells by penetration into cytoplasm and nucleus or by binding to the cell surface with subsequent binding of the complement and cytolysis.

Antigen presentation Modification of antigen into a form that can be recognised by T lymphocytes and thus activate the immune response. Currently, most of the available information relates to the presentation of protein antigens. The presentation of exogenous and endogenous protein antigens differs slightly. In the exogenous pathway of antigen presentation, the antigen must first be phagocytosed by antigen presenting cells (APC) where its further transformation takes place.

This is a complicated process in the course of which its molecule is fragmented within endosomes of APC to immunogenic fragments (peptides containing usually 12 to 20 amino acids), which bind to a certain location (binding channel) in the molecule of MHC (HLA class II in humans) products (antigens). This complex is transferred to the surface of APC and recognised by T helper lymphocytes. The T_H lymphocyte through its antigen receptor (TCR) recognises only complexes in which immunogenic peptide is firmly bound in the binding channel of HLA class II molecules. The T_H lymphocyte does not recognise free or weakly bound peptide fragments and this is the basis of the specificity of the subsequent immune response. The binding of immunogenic peptide to TCR is the first signal to 'attract the attention' of the specific T_H cell clone. For their activation and initiation of the immune response, T_H lymphocytes must also obtain the second (confirming, co-stimulating) signal, which mediates interaction of co-stimulation molecules (e.g. CD28 on the surface of T lymphocyte and CD80 on the surface of APC).

Antigens originating from cells infected by viruses or antigens associated with malignancies are subject to an endogenous pathway of presentation. Moreover, in this case, the antigen is first degraded in the cytoplasm of the affected (target) cell in an organelle referred to as proteasome. Thereby immunogenic peptides, containing mainly 8 to 9 amino acid units, are formed and these peptides bind to synthesised HLA class I molecules. This complex is transferred to the surface of the cell where it is recognised by cytotoxic T lymphocytes, which initiate lysis of the 'target' cell. The capability of T_H lymphocytes to recognise immunogenic peptide incorporated only into HLA class II molecules and T_C lymphocytes only into HLA class I molecules is referred to as immunologic restriction. A significant majority of antigens undergo such a presentation. The exceptions are certain polysaccharide antigens, which can be recognised directly by B lymphocytes without T_H lymphocytes, and superantigens that non-specifically activate a large number of T_H lympho-

A

cyte clones. Other exceptions are glycolipid and lipid antigens that are presented by CD1 molecules instead of HLA molecules.

Antigen targets of antinuclear antibodies (ANA) in the cell (antibodies against intranuclear antigens)
- chromatin – essential components of the chromatin are DNA, histones and non-histone nuclear proteins,
- nuclear membrane and pores,
- nucleolus,
- RNA complex with the proteins (ribonucleoproteins; RNP),
- matrix-fibrillar skeleton of the nucleus,
- different components of cytoplasm, e.g. enzymes, ribosomes or RNP.

Antihistone antibodies and antinucleosome antibodies
Histones are alkaline nuclear proteins containing a great amount of positively charged aminoacids (lysine, arginine). They are present in eucaryotic cells associated with DNA. There are five main types of histones – H1, H2A, H2B, H3 and H4. Histones rich in H3 and H4 form a tetramere, binding lysine-rich dimers of H2A-H2B on both sides. These histones form a central core encircled by two threads of a 146-nucleotide long segment of DNA. This structure is called a nucleosome and individual nucleosomes are interconnected by a segment of DNA with a bound H1 histone.

Anti-idiotypic antibodies
Antibodies directed against idiotypic determinants of immunoglobulins (immunoglobulins, idiotypes). Antigenic determinants created by the combining site of an antibody (= immunglobulin) are called idiotypes and antibodies directed against these idiotypes are anti-idiotypic antibodies.

Anti-immunoglobulin antibodies
Antibodies directed against antigenic determinants, which are present on the surface of immunoglobulin molecules. Basically they can be divided into anti-isotypic, anti-allotypic or anti-idiotypic antibodies. Antibodies against isotypic determinants define the competence

of antibodies to particular classes and subclasses of immunoglobulins, and are utilised in the diagnostic assessment of their concentrations in various immunochemical methods.

Anti-Jo-1 antibodies → see Antisynthetase syndrome

Anti-La antibodies → see Anti-SSA/Ro and anti-SSB/La antibodies

Antimalarial drugs
Misleading nomenclature for drugs used in rheumatology as not all preparations applied for the treatment of malaria are used in rheumatology as well. It applies only to quinoline derivates, namely, only the two 4-aminoquinoline derivates chloroquine and hydroxychloroquine that differ from each other only by substitution of the hydroxyethyl group for the ethyl one on the tertiary nitrogen atom on the lateral chloroquine chain.

Mechanism of action in autoimmune diseases

The exact mechanism of action of antimalarial drugs is unknown. Possible mechanisms are shown in table 1. Probably intensive accumulation of chloroquine in the intracellular lysosomal system of lymphocytes, fibroblasts and polymorphonuclear cells is needed. This, in consequence, affects differ-

Table 1. Mechanism of action of antimalarial drugs in autoimmune diseases

Accumulation in lysosomes

• affects antigen processing,
• decreases antibody formation,
• decreases activity of NK cells,
• decreased release of IL-1, IL-2 and TNF-α,
• prevention of receptor-dependent lysosomal endocytosis
  – decreases receptor formation at lower density,
  – decreases influenza and adenoviral receptor internalisation,
• in Plasmodium malariae infection
  – decreases activity of lysosomal acidic proteases and so the degradation of haemoglobin-invaded erythrocytes.

ent functions of cellular functions, such as protein glycosylation, membrane lipid digestion and cell receptor development, which can be influenced by alkalisation of normally acidic lysosomal pH, or by influencing the elimination and function of acidic proteases. Antimalarial drugs further inhibit multiple functions of phagocytes, including the release of reactive oxygen species. Antimalarial drugs can also influence the antigen processing ability of the monocyte-macrophage system, thus inhibiting the function of lymphocytes. The release of interleukin-1 is also inhibited.

Further action of antimalarial drugs – decrease in lipidemia, anti-platelet aggregation effects, hypoglycemic effects

The decrease in platelet aggregation with antimalarial drugs has been known for some time. Unlike the similar effect of salicylates, no prolongation of bleeding time has been observed in antimalarial drugs. This led Charnley, (Johnson et al. 1977, 1979) otherwise a pioneer in total hip joint replacements, to use antimalarial drugs as a prophylactic treatment against deep venous thromboses after implantation of hip joint prostheses. A study was carried out involving 10,000 patients who were administered 600 – 800 mg of hydroxychloroquine per day 1 to 2 weeks after surgery; a significant drop in the rate of thrombotic complications was observed. Retrospective and prospective studies showed a lower incidence of venous, as well as arterial, thrombotic complications in patients with systemic lupus erythematosus (SLE) treated with antimalarial drugs (Petri et al. 1994). Even in the group of patients at high risk with the presence of antiphospholipid antibodies, there was a decrease in the rate of thrombembolic events. In a study spread over 9 years, in a group of 54 patients treated with hydroxychloroquine, there were only 2 (4%) thrombembolic events, whereas in the group without hydroxychloroquine this figure was 20% (Petri et al. 1992).

In studies, it was also shown that antimalarial drugs decreased the total cholesterol, LDL-cholesterol and triglycerides by 10 to 15% in patients treated over the long term (Wallace 1990). This is indirectly related to a possible decrease in steroid dose in these patients. Antimalarial drugs increase the number of LDL-receptors and decrease the cholesterol synthesis in the liver. The hypoglycaemic effect of antimalarial drugs has not been completely explained so far; it is likely to be due to an increase in insulin binding to its receptor.

A combination of corticosteroid-sparing effect, hypoglycemic effect, lipid-lowering effect and anti-platelet aggregation effect, leads to an overall decrease in cardiovascular events with antimalarial drugs.

Pharmacokinetics: Chloroquine and hydroxychloroquine are rapidly absorbed after oral administration. The bioavailability varies between 75% and 90%. The average time needed for absorption of 50% of the preparation is 4.3 hours.

The biological half-life of antimalarial drugs is very long, up to 40 days, which means a steady state is reached in 3 to 4 months. Antimalarials accumulate predominantly in the acidic environment of lysosomes. This explains their high accumulation in the liver that is rich in lysosomes, and low accumulation in muscle, which have a low amount of lysosomes. A significant accumulation can also occur in ocular tissues, especially those containing melanin. The majority of the absorbed drug is excreted in urine in an unaltered state; only 1/3 of the drug is metabolised through removing of ethyl group on the terminal amino ethyl group of the lateral chain. The therapeutically effective serum concentration of chloroquine is thought to be in the range 700 to 1200 ng/mL, but this has not been entirely confirmed.

Dosage: The recommended daily dose of chloroquine is 250 mg/day. The therapeutic effect of antimalarial drugs takes up to 3 months of continuous daily administration. In the course of treatment it is essential to have regular eye checks, including ophthalmic examination, visual acuity and colour vision (every 12 months). In patients over 60 years of age, it is advisable to have an ophthalmic assessment prior to initiating treatment because of the stronger probability of developing degenerative changes, especially with coincident disorders (arterial hypertension and diabetes mellitus). In recent years, hydroxychloroquine has been favoured more than chloroquine as it has a safer profile with far less ocular toxicity. It is commenced at 200 mg twice a day, then reduced to 200 mg daily after 3 months if effective. It is now often combined with methotrexate in moderate to severe rheumatoid arthritis.

Clinical efficacy: The results of long-term controlled clinical trials performed over the last 40 years have shown that chloroquine and hydroxychloroquine are effective in mild rheumatoid arthritis (RA). When administered they have demonstrably better efficacy compared to placebo and can decrease the clinical activity of the inflammatory process measured. Antimalarial drugs decrease the activity of acute phase reactants, but have failed to slow the rate of erosive progress on X-rays in clinical trials. Its efficacy is comparable to D-penicillamine, but lower than sulphasalazine and intra-muscular administration of gold compounds. Antimalarial drugs are indicated in rheumatoid arthritis with mild clinical activity, especially in cases without unfavourable prognostic signs.

Furthermore, antimalarial drugs are used in juvenile idiopathic arthritis, SLE and psoriatic arthritis.

Adverse effects related to treatment with chloroquine and hydroxychloroquine:
- *gastrointestinal:* anorexia, nausea, vomiting, epigastric pain, spasms, diarrhoea and weight loss
- *skin:* rashes, pruritus, pigmentations of the skin and nails, photosensitivity, exacerbation of psoriasis,
- *neurological:* headache, drowsiness, insomnia, irritability, tinnitus, proximal myopathy, myasthenic syndrome, polyneuropathy, lowered threshold for seizures,
- *haematological:* toxic granulation of leukocytes, leukopenia, agranulocytosis, aplastic anaemia,
- *ocular:* accommodation disturbances, diplopia, corneal deposits, retinopathy,
- *other:* arrhythmia, cardiomyopathy, porphyria.

Anti-Mi-2 → see Idiopathic inflammatory myopathies (IIM)

Antineutrophil cytoplasmic antibodies → see ANCA

Anti-nuclear antibodies (ANA) Antinuclear antibodies (ANAs) were initially discovered in the 1940s using the lupus erythematosus (LE) cell test, but have now been replaced by serum testing for ANA. They are a useful and initial cost-effective screening test for patients suspected of having a systemic autoimmune disease. However, false positive ANAs (can be found in women and in elderly patients, but usually in low titer so results have to be interpreted with the clinical picture. ANA is positive in most patients with SLE (>95%), most patients with MCTD (90%), and commonly (>50%) found in patients with pauciarticular juvenile idiopathic arthritis, Sjögren's syndrome and polymyositis/dermatomyositis. It is also present in the serum of some patients with rheumatoid arthritis (40%), other autoimmune diseases (autoimmune hepatitis, autoimmune thyroid disease), and idiopathic pulmonary hypertension. Nowadays, more specific antibody testing can confirm a particular connective tissue disease (e.g. anti-dsDNA for SLE, anti-histone antibodies for drug-induced lupus, anti-Scl-70 for scleroderma, etc.)

Anti-PCNA/cyclin antibodies (proliferating cell nuclear antigen) DNA-polymerase delta associated protein with a molecular weight of 36 kDa. The antibodies are highly specific for systemic lupus erythematosus, but they are rare (approximately in 6%). One suggestion is that anti-PCNA positive patients more frequently have diffuse proliferative glomerulonephritis and lymphadenopathy. Positive immunofluorescence of the nuclei occurs only in rapidly dividing cells because the amount of PCNA rises proportionally to synthesis and cell growth.

Antiphospholipid syndrome (APS) A syndrome with the following:
symptoms and signs: Venous or arterial thrombosis, or both, often multiple, repeated

miscarriages and pregnancy failures and moderate thrombocytopenia; all with the presence of lupus anticoagulant (LA), elevated aCL (anticardiolipin antibodies), or both.

Diagnostic criteria of primary/secondary APS:
- clinical signs: venous thrombosis, arterial thrombosis, repeated miscarriages (pregnancy failures),
- laboratory findings: thrombocytopenia, IgG-aCL (moderate/high levels), IgM-aCL (moderate/high levels), and positive test for LA.

Diagnostic criteria for APS: one clinical sign including thrombocytopenia and the presence of aCL (>20 GPL units) or presence of LA; evidence of antiphospholipid antibodies (aPL) on two occasions at least six weeks apart; up to 5-year follow-up of the patient to eliminate systemic lupus erythematosus (SLE) or other autoimmune disease.

In principle we distinguish primary APS, i.e. it is impossible to show evidence of other concomitant autoimmune disorder, especially SLE, over at least 5 years; and secondary APS when the patient, besides APS, also suffers from SLE or drug induced lupus, or another autoimmune disorder.

Some authors broaden out the possible disorders, likely related to the presence of aPL, into two basic groups:
1. Disorders elicited by aPL without a direct connection to thrombosis
   - *neurological:* Guillain-Barre syndrome, transversal myelitis, chorea, migraine,
   - *obstetric:* preeclamptic toxemia and eclampsia, postpartum serositis,
   - *other:* non-thrombogenic (idiopathic) pulmonary hypertension, avascular necrosis of the bone.
2. Disorders elicited by aPL with a direct connection to thrombotic vascular signs
   - veins:
   limbs: thrombophlebitis,
   liver:
   – major vessels: Budd-Chiari syndrome,
   – hepatomegaly, increased concentration of enzymes,
   adrenal glands: Addison's disease, adrenal insufficiency,

lungs: pulmonary embolism, thromboembolic pulmonary hypertension,
skin: livedo reticularis, skin nodules, chronic venous ulcers, superficial purpura resembling a vasculitis,
eyes: venous thrombosis of the retina
- arteries:
limbs: ischaemia, gangrene,
brain:
– major vessels: acute stroke, transient ischaemic attack,
– minor vessels: acute ischaemic encephalopathy, multi-infarct dementia,
heart:
– major vessels: myocardial infarction,
– minor vessels: acute – circulatory collapse, cardiac arrest,
   chronic – cardiomyopathy, arrhythmia, bradycardia,
kidneys:
– major vessels: renal artery thrombosis,
– minor: thrombotic renal microangiopathy,
liver: infarction of the liver,
aorta:
– upper part: aortic arch syndrome,
– abdominal part: claudication,
skin: gangrene of the fingers,
eyes: thrombosis of arteries and arterioles of the retina,
endocardium, valves:
– acute: vegetations, "pseudoinfectious endocarditis",
– chronic: valvular dysfunction (regurgitation, stenosis),
Sneddon's syndrome – coincidence of stroke, hypertension and livedo reticularis.

A proposal of new classification criteria of APS (Sapporo, 1998):

Antiphospholipid antibodies – the presence of aPL (aCL or LA) demonstrated at least twice at least 6 weeks apart with one or more clinical signs.

Clinical symptoms and signs:
- arterial or venous thrombosis (or both) demonstrated radiographically, by ultrasound or histologically,

A

- three or more consecutive miscarriages (up to 10th week) unexplained by other reasons, or one or more deaths of morphologically normal foetus after the 10th week of pregnancy, or one or more still births after the 34th week of pregnancy accompanied by serious pre-eclampsia or placental insufficiency,
- two or more episodes of reversible cerebral ischaemia,
- occurrence of multiple sclerosis like syndrome or otherwise unexplainable focal neurological deficit.

Additional features, no criteria:
- thrombocytopenia below 100,000/mm^3,
- haemolytic anaemia with reticulocytosis and positive Coombs test,
- otherwise unexplainable transversal myelopathy,
- livedo reticularis,
- otherwise unexplainable thickening of mitral or aortal valve and regurgitation demonstrated on echocardiography,
- unexplained chorea observed by a physician,
- migraine lasting one year with concomitant presence of aPL in the serum.

Anti-Ro antibodies → see Anti-SSA/Ro and anti-SSB/La antibodies

Anti-SRP antibodies → see Idiopathic inflammatory myopathies (IIM)

Anti-SSA/Ro and anti-SSB/La antibodies Anti-La antibodies occur practically together with anti-SSA/Ro antibodies, but not vice versa as in the case of the relation between anti-Sm and anti-U1RNP antibodies. Anti-SSA/Ro can be found in primary Sjögren's syndrome and systemic lupus erythematosus (SLE). There are two Ro antigen peptides (Ro60 and Ro52) differing from one another according to molecular weight. The bond with Ro60 and Ro52 is in some cases distinct in SLE and systemic sclerosis (SSc). Approximately 40% of patients with SSc who are anti-Ro positive have antibody only to Ro52, and 20% of sera from SLE patients to only Ro60. Other patients in both groups

have antibodies to both Ro peptides, which is why this difference doesn't have much clinical significance.

The presence of anti-SSA/Ro and anti-SSB/La antibodies is clinically significant because of their association with several SLE subtypes: subacute cutaneous lupus, neonatal lupus and SLE in C2 and C4 deficiencies. Likewise, there exists an association between patients with pneumonitis and renal disturbance with the presence of anti-SSA/Ro antibodies in the serum.

There are certain differences among patients with only anti-SSA/Ro or in combination with anti-SSB/La.

Characteristics of patients with anti-SSA/Ro and anti-SSB/La antibodies

Anti-SSA/Ro	*Anti-SSA/Ro + Anti-SSB/La*
more frequent HLA-DR2	more frequent HLA-DR3
young patients	SLE in elderly
frequent homozygotes for C2 and C4 deficiencies	no relation with complement deficiency

Association between the presence of anti-SSA/Ro or anti-SSB/La and congenital heart block

The risk of congenital heart block is probably highest when the mother's serum contains a combination of anti-SSA/Ro and anti-SSB/La, and in the case of antibodies against Ro52 antigen.

Anti-SSB/La antibodies → see Anti-SSA/Ro and anti-SSB/La antibodies

Antisynthetase syndrome Myositis and interstitial pulmonary fibrosis with fever, arthritis, Raynaud's phenomenon and thickened, fissured radial margins of index fingers on both hands (the so called car mechanics' hands). Typically, serum antibodies against cytoplasmic enzymes are present (aminoacyl-tRNA synthetases), e.g. anti-Jo-1.

Apoptosis Programmed cell death in multicellular organisms. It can be regarded as the opposite of mitosis. Multicellular organisms keep their integrity not only based on the

A

ability to form new cells as a replacement for those worn-down and withered, but also by regulated apoptosis. This is an active process going on by continuously eliminating unwanted and unnecessary cells. It is applied, for example, in disposing of those T-lymphocytes that are able to react with self antigens and so cause an autoimmune response. It is, however, a common biological event and not unique to the immune system. Apoptosis is regulated by growth factors, several cytokines and oncogenes. Cells undergoing apoptosis are mainly proliferating ones that failed to get the necessary signalling ensured by growth factors during their development, or on the contrary, got an apoptotic signalling. The signalling is often produced by TNF, lymphotoxin or Fas-ligand. In the cell, the apoptotic signalling causes water loss and an increase in intracellular ionized calcium concentration. This leads to chromatin condensation and activation of the endonucleases that split the DNA to 50 – 300 kb fragments, leading to cell death and its disintegration into smaller fragments ingested by surrounding phagocytes without the development of an inflammatory reaction. Proteolytic enzymes mainly the so called caspases participate in this process. The second mechanism of terminating cells in a multicellular organism is necrosis. It is, however, morphologically and by its mechanism, distinct form apoptosis.

APS → see Antiphospholipid syndrome (APS)

ARA Diagnostic criteria of SLE → see Systemic lupus erythematosus (SLE)

Arachidonic acid A polyunsaturated fatty acid found in the phospholipids of cell membranes from which it is released by the activity of phospholipases A_2 or C. The free arachidonic acid has a short half-life and rapidly metabolised by either cyclooxygenase or lipoxygenase. In the cyclooxygenase pathway, prostaglandins, prostacyclin and thromboxane occur, while the lipoxygenase pathway produces leukotrienes or lipoxins.

Arthritis associated with erythema nodosum in the course of infection
Erythema nodosum (EN) is characterised by painful nodular subcutaneous infiltrates due to an inflammation of the subcutaneous adipose tissue. Its onset may be associated with the use of certain drugs (penicillin, sulphonamides, contraceptives, etc.), sarcoidosis, ulcerative colitis, Crohn's disease, systemic lupus erythematosus, neoplasms, but most frequently it is associated with infection. Pathogenically it is most probably a hypersensitive reaction to a trigger factor.

Clinical picture: The red nodules are 1–10 cm in size; they take the form of subcutaneous prominent infiltrates and are usually painful. They are localised most frequently on the lower extremities. They are generally of time-limited duration and often spontaneously resolve in 6 to 8 weeks. In approximately half of cases, joints (arthralgia, arthritis) are affected. Acute arthropathy in EN can be easily distinguished from chronic arthropathy in sarcoidosis with EN. In some cases the occurrence of EN can be regarded as the symptom of a clinically well-defined disease (e.g. post-Yersinia reactive arthritis).

Arthritis impact measurement scale (AIMS) → see Instruments of assessing (health status measurements, outcome measurement)

Arthritis in brucellosis Infectious arthritis caused by Brucella (B) melitensis, B. abortus, B. suis and B. canis.

Symptoms and signs: Brucellosis can be accompanied by arthralgia at any stage of the disease. Besides other symptoms and signs, arthritis of peripheral joints can occur and the sacroiliac joints and the spine can be affected. Rarely osteomyelitis develops.

Arthritis in chronic sarcoidosis In prolonged disease, a polyarthritis similar to rheumatoid arthritis (RA) develops in 30–40% of afflicted people. The course of the disease is relapsing and remitting, and the most affected joints are the knees, ankles, wrists and (symmetrically) small joints of the hand (MCP, PIP). Dactylitis can occur.

Laboratory diagnostics: Attention should be drawn to a high erythrocyte sedimentation rate, eosinophilia, positive latex-fixation test (that's why this disease could be confused with RA), hypergammaglobulinaemia and negative tuberculin test (Kveim test is no longer performed due to risk of transmitting viruses such as Creuztfeld disease). A histological picture is also characteristic (noncaseating granulomas).

Arthrogryposis multiplex congenita

This disease belongs to the congenital muscular syndromes. It is characterised by muscle weakness and fibrosis leading to joint contractures.

Clinical symptoms: Significant symmetrically deformed limbs in fixed flexion positions with reduced movement are typical. The knees and hips are flexed in most cases, and furthermore the hip joints are abducted. Affected limbs are usually shortened. Crepitus is audible during movement of the affected limbs. Shortening of muscles and tendons of unknown neurogenic or myogenic aetiology is the cause of limb deformity. The muscle of the affected extremities is very hypoplastic. Other abnormalities such as syndactyly, cleft palate and pigment defects are frequently associated with the disease.

Arthropathy in the course of inflammatory bowel diseases

Arthropathy can be a systemic complication of regional enteritis (Crohn's disease) or ulcerative colitis. Most frequently it is a peripheral arthritis; with sacroileitis occurring less often. The incidence of arthropathy in the course of inflammatory bowel disease is estimated at about 7.5 to 21%. The occurrence of sacroileitis is associated predominantly with the presence of HLA-B27 antigen; there is no known association of HLA with peripheral joint involvement.

Symptoms and signs: Erythema nodosum, but also pyoderma gangrenosum, can be important extraarticular manifestations. The course of the peripheral arthritis mirrors the severity of underlying bowel disease; but has no influence on the progression of changes in the axial skeleton

Arthropathy in ochronosis

This is principally a degenerative process of known aetiology with a profound tendency to disability. The core of clinical signs and symptoms in ochronotic arthropathy affect the spine. Symptoms begin at the end of the 3rd decade of life. The male to female ratio is 2:1.

Objective signs include flattening of the thoracic kyphosis and lumbar lordosis, a mild rigidity with a tendency to worsening. Gradually in the advanced stages, an unevenness of the contours of the spine appears with irregular prominence of spinous processes and complete ankylosis of the whole lumbar and thoracic spine. The cervical part of the spine preserves its mobility for quite a long time despite considerable radiographic changes. In the advanced stages, extension and rotation movements are limited, with the head in a flexed position. Due to the degenerative changes in the intervertebral discs, the intervertebral spaces narrow down causing a marked decrease in body height over 20 years.

Radiographic examination of the spine shows characteristic calcification of the intervertebral discs. Osteolytic and hyperplastic changes and secondary new bone formation occurs on the vertebral bodies. Osteophytes, and sporadically massive bone bridging of the ankylosing hyperostosis type are formed.

Arthropathy in thyroid disease

Autoimmune thyroid diseases include Hashimoto's thyroiditis and Graves' disease. These diseases can be associated with other rheumatic disorders, such as rheumatoid arthritis, Sjögren's syndrome, systemic sclerosis, polymyalgia rheumatica, giant cell arteritis and relapsing polychondritis. These disorders are often interconnected and have a close relation to HLA-B8 and HLA-DR3 haplotypes. The presence of rheumatoid factor and anti dsDNA antibodies is often seen in autoimmune thyroiditis. Autoimmune diseases of the thyroid gland develop in patients with systemic lupus erythematosus (SLE), which is often accompanied by the occurrence of antibodies against the thyroid gland. Autoimmune thyroiditis has been reported in Sjögren's syndrome. Polymyalgia rheumatica or giant cell arteritis can be related to the development of autoimmune disease of the thyroid gland. The occurrence of Hashimoto's thyroiditis with rheumatoid arthritis, SLE or other connective tissue diseases has also been reported. On the other hand, Hashimoto's thyroiditis alone can be characterised by a clinical picture of inflammatory polyarthritis not responding to thyroid hormone replacement, which can be erosive with the development of nodules.

Hyperthyroidism
The following rheumatic syndromes occur in hyperthyroidism:
- thyroid acropachy,
- proximal myopathy,
- osteoporosis.

Hypothyroidism
In hypothyroidism, we often see an arthropathy resembling rheumatoid arthritis, articular chondrocalcinosis or synovitis of the flexors of the hand. There may be carpal tunnel syndrome and a proximal myopathy with muscle hypertrophy..

The following rheumatic syndromes occur in hypothyroidism:
- arthropathies,
- carpal tunnel syndrome,
- myopathies.

Arthroscopic joint washout and cartilage
Arthroscopic washout of a joint helps to remove small fragments of cartilage that irritate synovia. The washout can also be combined with arthroscopic debridement of the cartilage ('shaving'). There is evidence that this combined approach provides pain relief and improves the joint function but does not improve cartilage turnover.

A number of microsurgical arthroscopic techniques have been developed in an attempt to improve cartilage turnover, e.g. small holes are drilled into the subchondral circulation to stimulate the growth of fibrocartilaginous tissue into subchondral bone. Spongialisation, which is resection of the whole subchondral bone disc in chondromalacia patellae, also improves outcomes.

The other method of improving cartilage turnover is to use cartilaginous auto- or al-lotransplants. This technique is particularly used in young individuals after intra-articular trauma. The area of damage is covered by numerous autologous small transplants (mosaic plasty) or by precisely turned and closely inserted osteochondral transplants to the area of the damaged cartilage.

Frozen allogenic transplants are also used, but they are associated with the risk of immunological rejection. Periosteal and perichondral tissue is also used to cover defects of the cartilage. The main problem with these techniques is the fixation of the transplants to the area of the defect and their frequent calcification. More recently, as part of tissue engineering, autologous cells, which are obtained by small biopsy, e.g. from nasal cartilage, are implanted directly into the subchondral bone.

Articular cartilage → see Hyaline cartilage

Aseptic necrosis of the navicular bone
→ see Köhler's disease

Atopic reactions Anaphylactic reactions occurring in atopic individuals (atopy). Atopic individuals have a genetic predisposition to the development of allergic diseases of hypersensitivity, such as bronchial asthma, allergic rhinitis, urticaria, eczema, certain gastrointestinal disorders, etc. Atopy is a genetically conditioned feature, whereas anaphylaxis is a reaction that occurs more frequently in atopic individuals than in common individuals.

Atrophy A decrease in cell volume and restriction of cell functioning. Atrophy is often seen in regions with insufficient vascular supply or chronic inflammation. It can be a consequence of decreased skeletal muscle activity and can be regarded as an adaptive response to stress, whereby the cells decrease their volume, restrict different functions which leads to a decrease in energy consumption. As soon as the conditions in the affected region normalize, the atrophied cells restore their function and increase their volume. Their specific functions, such as protein synthesis or contractile muscle strength, also normalise.

Inactivity-induced atrophy

This most common atrophy is subsequent to decreased requirements for a function, e.g. immobilisation of the limb after a fracture or in long-term confinement. Atrophy of muscle cells and decrease in muscle strength occurs. Restoring the activity leads to normalisation of the volume, function and strength of the muscle.

Insufficient oxygen supply

A disturbance of blood supply to the tissues ends with ischaemia. Total ischaemia with interruption of oxygen supply to tissues leads to cell death. A partial ischaemia or incomplete occlusion of the vessel or places with inadequately formed collateral circulation leads to chronic restriction of oxygen supply and as a consequence the life expectancy of the cells is shortened. This process can be seen in regions of borderline ischaemia, e.g. necrosis (infarction) of heart, brain and kidneys.

Malnutrition

Starvation or malnutrition associated with a chronic disease leads to cell atrophy, mainly in skeletal muscles. It is presumed that the cell atrophy is caused by a partial ischaemia leading to undernutrition of the tissues.

Interruption of trophic signalling

The function of a number of cells depends on a signal transmitted by chemical mediators (e.g. endocrine system or neuromuscular transmission). Elimination of the sources of signalling (hormonal, transmission, etc.) decreases the requirements of cells of certain organs like adrenal glands, thyroid gland, skeletal muscles and so on. This can happen in the case of endocrine gland removal or muscle denervation.

Persistent cell damage

This is caused most often by a chronic inflammation associated with prolonged viral or bacterial infection. It's not clear whether an irritant agent, inflammatory process or both cause the cell damage. In any case, the cells at the place of chronic inflammation often atrophy. Physical damage, e.g. permanent pressure in an unsuitable locality, also induces atrophy.

Cell ageing

A process, which is independent of disease. The main cause of ageing of cells, especially those not replicating (heart, brain), is atrophy of such cells. The volume of all parenchymal organs in the body decreases with age. The volume of important organs decreases in old age and in the very elderly a decrease in volume of the heart can also be seen – senile atrophy.

Auranofin → see Gold salts

Auto-antibodies
Antibodies, whose formation is induced by auto-antigens.

Auto-antibodies assessed in systemic lupus erythematosus (SLE) – other
In approximately 30% of patients with SLE there are antibodies against the hnRNP (heterogenic nuclear) A1 protein. Clinically, it correlates with the occurrence of Raynaud's phenomenon and disturbance of oesophagus motility. The antibodies against the RA-33 antigen (hnRNP-A2) were originally regarded as specific to rheumatoid arthritis. They have been observed also in patients with mixed connective tissue disease (MCTD) and SLE. In these cases they often appear together with anti-snRNP antibodies. The nuclear membrane contains laminins A, B and C, serving partly as a structural component of the membrane and partly as a foot holding of the chromosomes in the cells during interphase. The antibodies against these structures induce a peripheral or marginal fluorescence on the nucleus of Hep-2 cells; it was presumed that anti-dsDNA antibodies were the main cause. Anti-laminin antibodies were reported in systemic connective tissue diseases including SLE, where they are likely to be associated with the presence of lupoid or chronic active hepatitis.

There were antibodies against heat shock proteins hsp90 (5–50% of SLE patients), ribonuclease P (25%), ubiquitine (80%), RNA-polymerase II (9–14%) or interferon gamma inducible protein p16 (29%) found in SLE. The diagnostic and clinical importance of all the mentioned antibodies is still not clear. In

30% of SLE patients, the antibodies belonging to p-ANCA, i.e. antibodies against neutrophil cytoplasm were demonstrated. To be specific, there are antibodies against elastase that occur most frequently in drug-induced lupus.

Autoimmune diseases They occur as a consequence of the overproduction of antibodies or autoreactive T-lymphocytes inducing a state of autoaggression, i.e. harm to one's own tissue and its structure. The presence of a small number of antibodies doesn't necessarily mean it is a pathological process. To prove this it should be demonstrated that: 1) certain antibodies are formed regularly only in the case of one specific disease, 2) the autoantigen inducing their formation can, after immunisation, provoke the development of the same pathological process in an experimental animal model, and that 3) this experimental disease can be transmitted via the serum or lymphocytes to a non-immunised animal (Witebsky's criteria). The autoimmune disorders may impair several organs (systemic) or only one specific organ (organ-specific).

Systemic autoimmune disorders include, for example, systemic lupus erythematosus, rheumatoid arthritis, Sjögren's syndrome and systemic sclerosis.

Organ-specific autoimmune disorders may impair:
- *endocrine system:* Addison's disease, Graves' disease, Hashimoto's disease, juvenile diabetes mellitus,
- *haematopoetic system:* autoimmune haemolytic anaemia, autoimmune neutropenia, paroxysmal cold haemoglobinuria,
- *gastrointestinal organs:* ulcerative colitis, Crohn's disease, chronic active hepatitis, primary biliary cirrhosis,
- *neuromuscular system:* myasthenia gravis, multiple sclerosis,
- *skin:* pemphigus vulgaris,
- *cardiopulmonary system:* rheumatic fever,
- *genitourinary system:* IgA-nephropathy, idiopathic membrane nephropathy.

Autoimmune haemolytic anaemia It is caused by antibodies against erythrocyte an-

tigens that after binding to a corresponding antigen activate complement and thereby cause haemolysis. Most of these anaemias can be divided into warm and cold antibody anaemia. Warm antibody haemolytic anaemia is caused by IgG antibodies against Rh-antigens and the optimal reaction temperature is 37°C. Cold antibodies are aimed at antigens H and I, belonging to the IgM isotype, and an optimal interaction with erythrocytes occurs at 4°C, but it is positive also at 25°C and 31°C.

Autoimmune hepatitis This is referred to as chronic active hepatitis. It affects mostly young women who present with fever, arthralgia, jaundice and skin eruptions. The inflammatory changes can be seen predominantly in the periportal region where the infiltrating T_H1-lymphocytes and other cells damage the hepatocytes. The disease is associated with HLA-A1, HLA-B8, HLA-DR3 and HLA-DR4 antigens, and a familial predisposition has been observed. There are antibodies against the smooth muscles, actin and hepatocyte membranes. Autoantibodies against hepatocytes do not have a pathogenic role. A polyclonal hypergammaglobulinaemia is present, mostly of the IgG class, and to a lesser extent the IgM and IgA class. The disorder is associated with other immunopathological conditions such as systemic lupus erythematosus, Sjögren's syndrome, autoimmune thyroiditis, insulin-dependent diabetes mellitus etc.

Autoimmune neutropenia This is caused by increased destruction of neutrophils or by suppression of myeloid cell growth by autoantibodies not always detectable in the serum. It occurs as a primary condition or secondary to other autoimmune disorders. Patients suffer form recurrent infections or can be asymptomatic.

Autoimmunity Usually an immunopathological process with disregulated immune response to autoantigens (self antigens). This response is inhibited in physiological states or has only a regulatory purpose, so its products cause no harm to one's own tissue and cells containing relevant autoantigens on their surface. The harmful autoimmune reactions appear in an overreaction of the immune system caused by disturbances in immune homeostasis (the balance between stimulating and inhibiting factors), and then they are referred to as autoaggressive reactions. They induce autoimmune diseases.

Autonomic nervous system (ANS) The autonomic part of the nervous system which maintains homeostasis in the body and harmonises activity of the visceral organs, mostly without the conscious participation of the individual. It is divided into the sympathetic and parasympathetic nervous system.

Autotolerance The ability of the body not to stimulate immunocompetent cells into an immune response to potential antigens that are components of one's own tissues and cells.

Avascular necrosis of the lunate bone
→ see Kienbock disease

Axon The prolonged sprout of the nerve cell transmitting impulses from the cell body. It can vary between 1 mm long or longer than 1 m in length.

Azathioprine A nitroimidazole derivative of 6-mercaptopurine, a purine antagonist. It inhibits DNA synthesis, and so is used in the treatment of acute leukaemia and as an immunosuppressant for B-cell and T-cell response. It decreases the number of circulating NK-cells, neutrophils and monocytes. It is used in the treatment of various autoimmune disorders (systemic lupus erythematosus, Sjögren's syndrome and rheumatoid arthritis).

Azathioprine and 6-mercaptopurine belong to purine analogues. Currently, neither aza-

thioprine nor 6-mercaptopurine is the drug of first choice in the treatment of rheumatoid arthritis (RA) but they both remain a valuable therapeutic option for RA when complicated by vasculitis, glomerulonephritis or when other DMARDs are not tolerated.

Dosage: Azathioprine in RA is administered orally in a daily dose from 1.5 to 2.5 mg/kg (75 to 200 mg daily). Its full effects take a couple of months. It is necessary to monitor the blood count and liver function tests during treatment: every 14 days for the first two months, and subsequently every 6–8 weeks. The occurrence of leukopenia is an indication for withdrawal of treatment.

Clinical efficiency: Several clinical trials show the comparable clinical efficiency of azathioprine with antimalarials, penicillamine, parenteral gold, cyclophosphamide and cyclosporin, but less when compared to methotrexate in RA.

The therapeutic efficiency and toxicity of azathioprine are dose dependent increase proportionally to the administered dose. However, patients with a genetic deficiency of thiopurine methyltransferase (TPMT) are at increased risk of severe myelosuppression and liver toxicity, so studies are looking at the efficacy of measuring the TMPT genotype and/or enzyme activity in patients prior to treatment (Szumlanski et al. 1992). Azathioprine is well tolerated in pregnancy and is not associated with congenital malformations in humans. In spite of data showing that only very small amounts transfer into breast milk, its administration during breast-feeding is not recommended.

Adverse effects: Gastrointestinal symptoms such as nausea and vomiting, leukopenia and increased liver transaminases. Clinical symptoms resolve after withdrawal of treatment. Long-term treatment with azathioprine is associated with a higher risk of malignancies, particularly haematopoietic and lymphoreticular malignancies.

B

Baker's cyst A palpable resistance or swelling in the popliteal fossa, often communicating with the joint cavity of the knee. It develops by enlargement of the gastrocnemius and semimembranosus muscles bursae. It is a frequent finding in arthritides and in osteoarthrosis. A ruptured cyst mimics the signs of deep venous thrombosis of the calf.

Ballottement of the patella This is a clinical sign of increased fluid within the knee joint (synovitis, haemarthrosis). It is examined by placing the palm of the hand on the patella, pushing caudally and eliciting pressure on the patella with the fingers of the other hand; when the fluid is increased, a wobbling of the patella as in pushing on a balloon is felt.

Balneophototherapy → see Tomesa (balneophototherapy)

Balneotherapy (BT) The use of natural healing sources (thermal springs, peloids, mineral waters) for healing purposes. The term "complex BT" refers to the additional use of other forms of physical therapy (thermotherapy, aquatherapy, electrotherapy, massages), and above all therapeutic rehabilitation. In rheumatic disorders, health resorts (spas) with sulphur (S^{2-}) content or with radon content in the natural healing sources are recommended, together with complex treatment, in particular high-quality rehabilitation

Bare lymphocytes syndrome Autosomal recessive primary immunodeficiency. The fundamental of the syndrome is the absence of class I or II HLA antigens, or the absence of both classes of HLA antigens on the surface of lymphocytes causing inefficient or defective cooperation between immunocompetent cells. This leads to an increased risk of infection from various infective agents. Patients with this syndrome suffer from opportunistic and recurrent infections, chronic diarrhoea and eventually aplastic anaemia. Laboratory findings include decreased levels of immunoglobulins, impaired specific immune responses; decreased numbers of T lymphocytes (particularly CD4$^+$) but the numbers of B lymphocytes are normal or slightly increased.

Barthel's index A clinical assessment tool used to measure the activities of daily living and mobility (functioning) of a patient. It is commonly used in evaluating functioning in different disorders, mainly neurological (multiple sclerosis, stroke).

Bartter's syndrome A group of disorders with an autosomal recessive type of inheritance characterised by disturbance or absence of salt transport in the thick ascending limb of the loop of Henle. The consequence is a loss of salts in the urine, a drop in blood pressure, hypokalaemic, hypochloraemic metabolic alkalosis and hypercalciuria with a variable degree of risk of developing urine stones. At present there are 5 defined genes whose mutation causes BS (types I–V). In the prenatal form of the syndrome there is, among other things, an overproduction of prostaglandin E leading to hypercalcaemia and increased bone resorption.

Basilar impression This occurs rarely as an isolated congenital anomaly. Usually it is associated with other inborn defects, such as incomplete fusion of posterior arch of the atlas, Klippel-Feil deformity, atlanto-axial dislocation, as well as foramen magnum stenosis. It accompanies disorders related to ossifluence, such as Paget's disease, osteomalacia, and osteogenesis imperfecta. The weight of the head working on a soft cranial base causes

B

invagination of the axis through the foramen magnum. A basilar impression induced by trauma usually has fatal consequences.

Bassett's current A pulsatile, monophasic, sinus, 72 Hz current used to stimulate bone formation. It facilitates the influx of Ca^{2+} ions into cells. Selectively it acts on osteoblast sensitivity towards parathormone and so increases the rate of bone tissue formation. Usage: non-healing fractures, pseudoarthroses, osteoporosis.

Bath ankylosing spondylitis indices (BAS-indices) → see Instruments of assessing (health status measurements, outcome measurement)

Bechterev's disease → see Ankylosing spondylitis

Behçet's disease A vasculitis which affects skin, mucosa, eyes and the central nervous system. Significant clinical signs include recurrent mouth ulcers appearing at least three times a year plus at least two of the following signs: recurrent genital ulcers, ocular signs (uveitis, retinal vasculitis), cutaneous signs (erythema nodosum, pseudofolliculitis, papulopustulous lesions or acneiform morphae and patergic phenomenon read by a physician). Behçet's disease is most prevalent (and more virulent) in the Mediterranean region, Middle East, and Far East, with an estimated prevalence of 1 case per 100.000 persons.

Beighton criteria → see Hypermobility syndrome (HMS), Beighton-Horan score

Beighton-Horan score The assessment of the degree of joint hypermobility consists of five manoeuvres:
1. passive hyperextension of the 5th MCP (metacarpophalangeal) joint over 90°,
2. passive backwards belong of the thumb to the volar side of the forearm,
3. hyperextension of the elbows over 10°,
4. hyperextension of the knees 10°,
5. anteflexion without bending the knees, the palms rest on the floor.

The manoeuvres are rated bilaterally; bilateral involvement with 2 points, the anteflexion with one point. Hypermobility has a score of 4 and more points; a generalized hypermobility has a score of 9. Hypermobility is assessed also by the test of Janda.

Bence-Jones proteins (BJ-proteins) A monoclonal globulin protein found in blood or urine, consisting of identical light chains of immunoglobulins (kappa or lambda), which are produced in the course of multiple myeloma and malignant transformation of plasma cells (gammopathy). Their daily secretion increases depending on disease intensity. They precipitate when heated to 40–60°C and redissolve at 90–100°C. According to their low molecular weight BJ-proteins are completely eliminated by kidneys. BJ-proteins can first be detected in urine. BJ-protein in serum is only found if renal function rate is disturbed or BJ-protein formation is greater than the clearance rate.

Bicipital Tendinitis This is due to degenerative changes of the long head of the biceps tendon, which may evoke tenosynovitis, subluxation or luxation and partial or total tendon rupture. Pain over the anterior shoulder area, pain provoked by pressure applied to the biceps tendon, and sometimes on movement of the tendon are typical.

Bisphosphonates These are synthetic analogues of pyrophosphates that are resistant to the action of endogenous pyrophosphatases. They have a high affinity for the bone mineral of the skeletal surface and exert an inhibitory effect on several catalytic enzymes, of which the most important is farnesyl diphosphate synthetase (FPPS), thus interfering with the mevalonate pathway of cholesterol formation. An insufficient prenylation results with a consequent dysfunction leading to apoptosis of osteoclasts. Osteoabsorption slows and, depending on the type of bisphosphonate, leads to disturbed remodelling, and prolongation of secondary mineralisation. The following are bisphosphonates used in the treatment of osteoporosis: alendronate, ibandronate, risedronate, and zoledronate, with pamidronate, clodronate and etidronate used in some countries.

Bioengineering technologies These techniques represent the possibility of repairing tissue defects such as in cartilage. It may, for example, lead to the successful transplantation of autologous chondrocytes, allogenic chondrocytes, perichondral grafts and biodegradable membranes.

Biolamp – bioptrone lamp The effect (biostimulation) is based on the use of polarised light, but unlike a laser it is not monochromatic, nor coherent. In rheumatology used to treat painful conditions of soft tissue structures (tendinitis, epicondylitis, and bursitis). It has practically no contraindications, but care must be taken not to expose to the eyes.

Biologic drugs (BD) The research of BD (short form of biotechnological produced drugs, also called biologics or biologicals) today is concentrating on the inhibition of a number of functional antigens of B- and T-cells, and adhesive molecules, but the best results are currently obtained by treatments influencing the activity of pro-inflammatory cytokines. Of these, especially tumour necrosis factor-alpha (TNF-α) and interleukin-1 (IL-1), are associated with destruction of the joints, erosions and development of deformities. The inhibition of TNF-α is rather well developed and there are several agents such as etanercept, adalimumab and infliximab that have been used in the treatment of severe forms of rheumatoid arthritis (RA), either individually or in combination with methotrexate. Etanercept is a recombinant soluble receptor protein for TNF-α, which was found to have better efficacy in clinical trials with RA in combination with methotrexate than methotrexate alone. Adalimumab is a fully humanised monoclonal antibody against TNF-α and is administered subcutaneously. It has good efficacy in treating RA with or without concomitant methotrexate. Infliximab is a chimeric monoclonal antibody against TNF-α containing 75% human protein and 25% murine protein; it is administered intravenously. The combination of infliximab and methotrexate has a significantly higher efficacy in suppressing clinical activity in resistant forms of RA than methotrexate alone. Treatment with these antibodies is associated with an increased incidence of septic complications, especially mycobacterial infection. Despite their high clinical efficacy, they are currently reserved for RA not responding well to monotherapy or combined treatment with disease modifying anti-rheumatic drugs (DMARDs). Recently, they have been indicated in early aggressive forms of RA.

Most of these agents are now licensed for the treatment of severe juvenile idiopathic arthritis, and severely active and resistant forms of ankylosing spondylitis and psoriatic arthritis. As TNF-α undoubtedly participates in the development of osteoporotic changes in chronic inflammations, the agents improve bone mineral density in these patients.

Many newer biologic drugs have been or are being developed. Rituximab is a B cell depleting monoclonal anti-CD20 antibody, licensed for severe SLE and RA. Anakinra is an IL-1 agonist, but appears less potent than TNF inhibitors in rheumatoid arthritis. Abatacept is a soluble fusion protein causing co-stimulation blockade by blocking CD28, but is not yet licensed for clinical use. Other biologic drugs are in development to block other cytokines such as IL-6 (Tocilizumab), and many more.

Bioptrone lamp → see Biolamp – bioptrone lamp

Birefringence (Double refraction) **Birefringence**, or **double refraction**, is the decomposition of a ray of light into two rays when it passes through certain types of material depending on the polarisation of the light. Through a double refracting material a line is seen as two parallel lines. Bifurcation of a beam of light occurs during refraction into an optically anisotropic environment. Both beams are linearly polarised and proceed in different directions. All crystals except the cubic system are characterised by their birefringence. The optical axis of the crystal is a bisector leading through an arbitrary point of the crystal in the direction in which birefringence does not occur. The plane containing the optic axis and the beam is the principal plane of the crystal. An ordinary beam is polarised on the plane of the principal section and an exceptional beam is polarised in the plane perpendicular to the principal section. Birefringence does not occur with single axis crystals which only have a single direction beam. Crystals with two such directions are referred to as double-axis crystals. In most single-axis transparent crystals, the intensity of the ordinary and exceptional beams are the same.

The crystals are particles characterised by a well-organised arrangement of their molecules. They have, in general, three optic axes that are identical to the length, width and depth of the particle. For the majority of materials, the most significant descriptions of light are the length and width, and the refraction indices of these two axes are approximately the same. Such materials are isotropic. The majority of crystals have unequal refraction indexes in their longer axis compared to the shorter one. Such material is referred to as anisotropic and demonstrates the properties of birefringence.

Polarisation of light through birefringence

In an optically isotropic environment the light radiates in all directions at the same velocity, but the crystals of certain substances are anisotropic in terms of light propagation. The velocity of light is different in different directions. When the light strikes on such a crystal, birefringence occurs. The beam of light is divided at the interface of the crystal into two beams: ordinary and exceptional beams. Both beams are linearly polarised. Polarised light is used in the investigation of optically active substances; it does not differ from natural light. To determine the orientation of the plane of polarised light, a device called the analyser is needed. The analyser complements the polarisation instrument and transmits light only with a certain orientation of the oscillation plane. The principle of the function of an analyser and polariser can be explained by a simple observation. If the slit of the polariser and analyser are parallel, the light goes through it. If the slits are not parallel, the light does not go through and the analyser is dark.

The polarising microscope is equipped with a polarisation device that enables the study of phenomena that are undetectable in normal unpolarised light. Generally the study can be divided into observation of light passing through and reflected light. Using the polarisation device in the polarising microscope, one can also observe changes in the colour of crystals. The colour is determined by the rate of light absorption. When the absorption is weak across the whole range of the visible spectrum, the material is glassy. When any part of the spectrum is absorbed, only that part of the spectrum that was not absorbed is seen by the eye. This phenomenon is seen in polarised light where the crystal appears variably coloured. The crystals of sodium urate (negatively) and calcium pyrophosphate (positively) can be clearly distinguished by their different birefringence using the polarisation device.

Bobath method

In adults it arises from three principles:
1. inhibition of developmentally lower locomotor reflexes and facilitation of greater postural reactions,
2. processing of superior postural reactions, hence improvement in targeted movement,
3. influence of central motor control from the periphery.

The Bobath method is also used as therapy for children with cerebral palsy.

Body mass index (BMI)

A measure of a person's body weight scaled for their height. BMI is calculated as dividing the body weight (kg) by height in meters squared (m^2).

Bone and Joint Decade – 2000–2010

The Decade is a global world campaign focusing the attention of the public on taking care of people with bone and joint disorders. Supported by the UN and World Health Organisation (WHO), the idea of the Decade developed on the basis of a consensus of experts led by Prof L. Lidgren at a meeting in Lund in 1998. The Decade was officially launched on the January 13, 2000 in the WHO headquarters in Geneva in the presence of the UN Secretary General Kofi Annan.

A stimulus for this initiative had been the great success of "The Decade of the Brain" in the years 1990–2000 and a fact that research in the field of musculoskeletal disorders in the recent decades led to high expectations that the start of a new millennium would mean a significant improvement of the patient care. The priorities of the Decade included: joint diseases, osteoporosis, spinal disorders, severe traumas and inherited diseases of the locomotor system. The aims of this initiative have been to increase public awareness of the growing burden of the musculoskeletal disorders on society, promoting cost effective prevention and treatment strategies through research, improvement in the quality of life of these patients by implementing novel treatment procedures, encourage patients to a more active approach in decision-making processes related to their healthcare.

Reaching these aims demands a broad cooperation of the public administration authorities, media, and scientific, professional and lay communities. Towards the end of 2005, fifty-nine governments have entered the Decade. The worldwide campaign is coordinated by a controlling committee based in Lund. There is a national action network (NAN) in each country whose activities are coordinated by a national coordinator.

Bone Densitometry
A bone densitometry scan measures the density of bone using various methods.

Types of densitometry:
a) Peripheral densitometry:
- single-energy X-ray absorptiometry (SXA) – forearm,
- dual-energy X-ray absorptiometry (DXA) – forearm,

- quantitative ultrasound (QUS)-heel, tibia,
- peripheral quantitative computerised tomography,
b) Central densitometry (DXA):
- standard measured areas:
  – proximal femur and lumbar spine,
- complementary measurements:
  – lateral lumbar spine,
  – whole-body densitometry,
  – densitometry in patients after joint prosthesis implantation,
  – morphometric measurements in the lateral projection,
c) Quantitative computerised tomography QCT – measurement in the spinal region.

At present, DXA (previously DEXA) measurements in the lumbar spine in the AP projection and in the area of proximal femur are considered the gold standard. The principle of DXA measurements is a detection of a difference in the weakening of X-rays passing through the measured bone and surrounding soft tissue. Appropriate software in the computer then evaluates the measured difference of X-ray weakening and gives the results as T- and Z-score, respectively, or in percentage.

Bone Mineral Density Measurement – evaluation
The results of a bone mineral density (BMD) scan is normally expressed as a the T-score, reflecting the number of standard deviations (SD) above or below the average BMD in a group of individuals of the same gender at the time of reaching the peak bone mineral density (normally 25–35 years of age).

The Z-score reflects the number of SD's above or below the average bone mineral density of a healthy population of the same gender, age and ethnicity.

The WHO classification of osteoporosis in postmenopausal women is based mainly on the results of the T-score.

In interpreting the results, it is necessary to take into account the following:
1. the error of measurement, especially in older patients with prominent degenerative changes within the spine and/or vertebral fractures, patients with ectopic cal-

B

cification in the scanned area (aorta, lymph nodes) or remnants of contrast (barium) medium after a gastrointestinal tract examination (false negative finding).

2. site of measurement (lower density in regions where trabecular bone, which has a more rapid bone turnover, dominates),

3. the method of measurement used and the database of normal values for that device and population.

Osteopenia measured at one site (for example measurement in the area with cortical bone dominance – forearm, femoral neck) does not exclude osteoporosis at another site.

Bone Mineral Density Measurement – indications

The indications vary between different countries, and are regularly reviewed. Some variation occurs depending on the availability of BMD machines. Indications for a scan include:

a) oestrogen deficiency: premature menopause (< 45 years of age), prolonged secondary amenorrhoea (> 1 year), or primary hypogonadism,

b) corticoid treatment with prednisone at a dose of 5mg daily or more assuming the duration will be more than 3 months,

c) family history of a hip fracture,

d) low body mass index (BMI < 19 kg/m^2),

e) all disorders associated with osteoporosis: anorexia nervosa, malabsorption, primary hyperparathyroidism, diffuse connective tissue disorders, rheumatoid arthritis, chronic inflammatory bowel diseases, post-transplant syndrome, chronic renal insufficiency, hyperthyroidism, prolonged immobilisation, Cushing syndrome, chronic hepatopathies, myeloproliferative disorders, genetic disorders and other metabolic bone disorders,

f) osteopenia on plain radiographs or a finding of vertebral deformity,

g) fracture of the hip, vertebra, or forearm after an inadequate trauma,

h) significant loss of height or thoracic kyphosis,

i) monitoring of antiresorptive treatment,

j) prolonged use of certain drugs (heparin, anticonvulsants).

Bone Mineral Density Measurement – individual areas

At present, any part of the body skeleton can be measured. In practice, however, only those sections for which we possess a database of normative data and are clinically relevant are measured. These are the following areas: L1 to L4 in PA and lateral projections, proximal femur, region of the great trochanter of the femur, femoral neck, Ward's triangle, distal forearm and the area called 1/3 forearm, heel and whole body density.

The spinal region (in PA projection) and proximal femur are considered the gold standard in BMD measurement, and according to the WHO criteria are suitable for establishing the diagnosis of osteoporosis. These areas are the best for predicting the risk of fractures. Low bone mineral density established at any skeletal site, however, is associated with an increased risk of fractures in general. Normal bone mineral density or osteopenia found at one skeletal site does not exclude the presence of osteoporosis at another site. There is a significant correlation between sites that are measured most frequently. The differences between individual areas are caused by the different proportional representation of trabecular and cortical bone at the measured areas, various velocity of bone loss in the individual sections of the skeleton as well as the presence of coincident changes in the measured area (osteophytes, calcifications in the surrounding tissue, etc.). The bone turnover in trabecular bone is markedly higher than in cortical bone, therefore there is a more accelerated bone loss in trabecular bone in the postmenopausal period. The BMD measurement in regions with dominance of trabecular bone is therefore more sensitive and capable of detecting the postmenopausal bone loss earlier than the BMD measurement in regions with a dominance of cortical bone. In evaluating the results of a measurement, the sensitivity and specificity of the method of measurement used for that area should be known.

Bone Mineral Density Measurement – least significant change (LSC)

The minimally significant change of the bone mineral density scan. It is therefore important to ensure good quality control by measurement of a standard phantom. It enables evaluation as to whether the measured change of density is significant. LSC depends on the accuracy of the device, the experience of the operator and the measured segment. It should be determined at each densitometry session and for each segment measured. The measured change in bone mineral density, if lower than the determined LSC in the same session and segment of the skeleton, should be judged as insignificant. See the entry "error of measurement".

Bone Mineral Density Measurement – measurement errors The error of measurement should be taken into account when interpreting the BMD result. There are 2 parameters to be distinguished:

Accuracy of measurement is the difference between the measured value and the true density of the measured bone.

Precision or reproducibility of measurement indicates the difference between two or more measurements of the same portion of the skeleton. It is therefore important to check quality control by repeated measurement of a standard. It is necessary to declare whether the measured change is statistically significant when interpreting follow up measurements. A parameter, called Least Significant Change (LSC), represents the minimally significant change in measurement of the difference between two BMD scans.

Bone Mineral Density Measurement – repeat The following two factors should be considered when considering a repeat BMD scan:
• The assumed bone loss velocity per year,
• The reproducibility bias of the measurement by the densitometer being used (precision).
A BMD scan should only be repeated if the presumed change of BMD is expected to be greater than the minimally significant change value established within the given department and measured area of the skeleton.

Generally, a statistically significant change in the spinal region may be considered if there is a change of more than approximately 3%.

Assuming the annual loss of bone mass of 1–3%, the period between two measurements should be at least 1–2 years. The majority of authors recommend a 2- to 3-year interval. However, there are conditions where the annual bone loss is substantially greater – osteoporosis with a high bone turnover and the concomitant presence of several risk factors in the postmenopausal woman. In these cases, it is possible to detect a statistically significant change in bone density in a shorter time period. For example, in glucocorticoid-treated patients, it is recommended to repeat the bone densitometry scan 6 months after the initiation of treatment. The same applies for patients with long-term immobility. On the other hand, in patients with already documented favourable response to the antiresorptive treatment, the scan may be repeated after 2 or more years.

Bone Mineral Density (BMD) Scans → see Bone Mineral Density Measurement

Bone remodelling There exists constant bone transformation – remodelling throughout life. The constant renewing and repairing of impaired bone guarantees optimal bone function. Bone remodelling proceeds in 4 main phases – activation, resorption, reversal phase and new formation. During the activation phase, osteoclasts appear at the site of future resorption, and then through the osteolytic enzymes absorb the original bone thereby forming the so-called Howship's lacunae. After this phase lasting approximately 7 days, the reversal phase starts and lasts 5 to 15 days. During the next osteoformation phase, lasting 1 to 3 months, the resorption lacunae gradually fill in with osteoid produced by osteoblasts. The completion of bone mineralisation is done by deposition of hydroxyapatite crystals into the osteoid. There is a dynamic balance – coupling between the osteoresorption and osteoformation processes.

During bone resorption, the degradation products of collagen and lysosomal enzymes

B

of the osteoclasts are released into the circulation, measurement of which can be used in the assessment of bone resorption (a marker of osteoresorption). Similarly, during the process of osteoformation, the bone specific isoenzymes of alkaline phosphatase and osteocalcin that are considered as markers of osteoblastic activity are released into the circulation. Evaluation of the plasma levels of these individual markers of bone remodelling provides indirect information of the velocity of bone turnover. Increased velocity of bone turnover may predict the risk of an osteoporotic fracture, which is independent of bone mineral density.

The velocity of bone turnover is substantially greater in trabecular bone. The site of bone remodelling is on bone surfaces which are abundant in trabecular bone. Up to 25% of trabecular bone is renewed annually, while in the case of cortical bone, it is only 2–3% per year. Total bone loss is therefore more rapid and greater in bones with predominance of trabecular bone. This has implications in decision-making about the sites of bone mineral density measurement and its evaluation in the early diagnosis of osteoporosis.

Bone scan → see Nuclear Scintigraphy of the skeleton (bone scintigraphy or bone scan)

Bone (skeletal) Scintigraphy The role of bone scintigraphy lies mainly in the assessment of the velocity of bone turnover at different sites of the skeleton. It has a high sensitivity but a relatively low specificity. The pathological finding of increased bone activity in certain regions of the skeleton established by scintigraphy therefore needs a differential diagnostic solution using alternative imaging techniques and suitable laboratory investigations.

Bone specific isoenzyme of alkaline phosphatase The total serum alkaline phosphatase is less specific for bone. The human serum contains various alkaline phosphatase isoenzymes: bone, liver, intestinal

and placental (during pregnancy). The intestinal and placental forms are relatively easily separable; telling apart the bone and liver specific isoenzymes causes greater problems. Various laboratory methods have been assessed for the selective assessment of bone specific alkaline phosphatase; however none of them has a sufficient sensitivity, specificity and reliability necessary for routine application. Newer methods using monoclonal antibodies bind a small number of liver specific isoenzymes (5–15%) as well as bone specific isoenzymes.

The level of bone specific isoenzyme of alkaline phosphatase is significantly increased in hyperphosphataemia and decreased in hypophosphataemia. It increases in hyperthyroidism, primary hyperparathyroidism and chronic renal insufficiency. In Paget's disease, it correlates with the activity of the bone disease. In postmenopausal women, the activity of bone specific isoenzyme increases and decreases with the effective antiresorptive treatment.

Bouchard's nodes → see Osteoarthritis – hands (Heberden and Bouchard type)

Bragard's sign If the Lassegue test does not cause pain on the examined side, the examination should be appended by performing dorsiflexion of the ankle (Bragard's sign). If pain is provoked by this manoeuvre, a radicular irritation is suspected.

Brittle Bone Disease → see Osteogenesis Imperfecta (Brittle Bone Disease)

Brodie abscess → see Osteomyelitis

Brunkow's method The basic principal of the method arises from the hypothesis that the way to normal movement is blocked somewhere. The aim is to remove the blockade and restore the interrupted connection. After complete dissociation of the false connection in the central nervous system, the way to initiate normal movement is free.

Bursae Structures resembling vesicles filled with synovial fluid. They are positioned in regions with increased friction between muscles, tendons and bones.

Bursitis – iliopectineal bursitis An inflammation on the biggest bursa in the body located under the iliopsoas muscle and anterior side of the joint capsule. It often communicates with the hip joint cavity and may be an accompanying phenomenon of coxitis. When enlarged it may be palpable in the groin.

Bursitis – ischiogluteal bursitis Affection of the bursa located between the ischial tuberosity and gluteus maximus muscle causing pain mainly in the sitting position. It is frequent particularly in professional truck drivers and tractor operators, obviously as a consequence of irritation during sitting.

Bursitis – olecranon bursitis It starts most frequently after a trauma or microtrauma (miner's elbow). Often it occurs in the course of rheumatoid arthritis, gout and chondrocalcinosis (crystals can be found in the aspirated fluid).

Bursitis – subacromial (subdeltoid) bursitis Involvement of the bursa located in the space between the deltoid muscle and shoulder joint capsule. The pain is manifested predominantly on abduction (facial hygiene, dressing, undressing). The involvement of the bursa induces an inflammation of lesser bursae around the shoulder (coracoid b., supraspinatus b., coracobrachial b., etc.) Affection of these bursae is a sign of the so called "rotator cuff syndrome", humeroscapular periarthritis and frozen shoulder syndrome.

Bursitis – trochanteric bursitis The bursa lies between the major trochanter and gluteus maximus and tensor fasciae latae muscles, in the region of the fascia lata and iliotibial tract junction. Its affection provokes severe pain, mainly over the greater trochanter. Movement in the hip joint need not be limited. It often forms calcification (X-ray examination is necessary).

B

C

C1 A component of complement (C), consisting of three subunits, C1q, C1r and C1s. In the classical pathway of activating C, the subunit C1q binds to an immune complex containing an IgM or IgG antibody, which is a signal for the creation of the macromolecular complex C1q-C1r-C1s stabilised by Ca^{2+} ion and initiation of the whole complement cascade.

C1-inhibitor This is a regulatory glycoprotein of the complement system that binds to C1r and C1s, thereby blocking their activity (C1). What's more, it facilitates the dissociation of the active C1 component complex and hampers further activation of complement. A hereditary angioedema develops in the C1-inhibitor deficiency.

C2 A component of the complement system. It is split into C2a and C2b fragments by the C14b enzyme, which is formed after activation of C1 and C4 components. The C2b fragment is a serine protease which participates in further complement activation. The C4b2b complex is formed, which serves as C3-converting enzyme of the classical pathway.

C3 A component of the complement system that plays a central role in all pathways of complement activation. Two polypeptide chains form this glycoprotein. Its molecule has a unique thiolester bond whose hydrolysis is fundamental for the alternative pathway of complement activation. With the action of C3-converting enzymes it is cleaved to C3a and C3b fragments. The C3a fragment belongs to anaphylatoxins, while the C3b fragment can become either a component of C5-converting enzymes or can acquire an opsonising function. The C3b fragment participates in immunoadherence reactions through its CR1 to CR4 receptors localised mainly on professional phagocytes and certain other cells.

C3a receptor A binding receptor for C3a fragment. It is localised on neutrophils (stimulating aggregation, the release of lysosomal content and the formation of reactive oxygen species), macrophages (activation, stimulation of IL-1 secretion) and mast cells (stimulating the release of anaphylaxis mediators).

C3-convertases Enzymes cleaving C3 into C3a and C3b fragments. There are two enzymes: C3-convertase of the classical pathway – C4b-C2a complex and C3-convertase of the alternative pathway – C3bBb complex.

C4 A component of the complement system cleaved by C1s of the activated C1 component into C4a and C4b fragments. The C4a fragment belongs to anaphylatoxins, while the C4b fragment is a component of a C3-converting enzyme of the classical pathway (C4b2b). C4 and C2 deficiency is often associated with systemic lupus erythematosus or glomerulonephritis.

C4bp A protein binding C4b fragment, regulatory molecule of the complement system. It regulates the activity of C4b fragment.

C5 A glycoprotein composed of two polypeptide chains. The C5-converting enzymes cleave it into C5a and C5b fragments. The C5a fragment has anaphylatoxic (anaphylatoxins) and chemotactic activities towards professional phagocytes. The C5b fragment couples with the C6 component, thereby creating a membrane-attacking complex (complement, MAC). A very rare C5 deficiency manifests in increased sensitivity to *Neisseria*-induced infections.

C5a receptor A receptor specifically binding the C5a fragment. It is localised on mast cells and basophils (anaphylaxis), professional phagocytes (chemotaxy, release of the content of granules, stimulation of reactive oxygen species production) and thrombocytes (stimulation of the aggregation and release of the content of granules).

C6 A component of the complement system that is a part of the membrane-attacking complex (complement, MAC).

C7 A component of the complement system that is a part of the membrane-attacking complex.

C8 A component of the complement system that is a part of the membrane-attacking complex.

C9 A component of the complement system that is a typical perforin. After binding to the C5b678 complex it polymerises and so creates a definitive structure of membrane-attacking complex, which enables the formation of a number of holes in the cytoplasmic membrane of target cells, and consequently, its lysis.

Calcaneal Spur A spur under the heel bone, which occurs particularly in older individuals, and may cause pain during walking (plantar fasciitis). Treatment is based on the use of a special relieving insert.

Calcific Tendinitis Deposition of calcium in tendons, often leading to inflammation. Symptoms include chronic and relapsing pain. Acute painful inflammation develops when the calcification infiltrates the subacromial bursa referred to as bursitis calcarea.

Calcifying tendinopathies, enthesopathies and periarthritis Calcific tendinitis, bursitis or enthesitis are characterised by the presence of hydroxyapatite microcrystals (calcium phosphate) at the point of the damaged tendon and its insertion, which may penetrate into the adjacent bursa in the form of crystals. In calcifying periarthritis, the crystals accumulate in the periarticular fibrous tissue.

Calcineurin A protein phosphatase specific for serine and threonine. It is an enzyme that eliminates the phosphate groups binding the above mentioned amino acids from proteins. This dephosphorylation of the proteins has a significant regulatory effect on their biological activities. In T-lymphocytes, calcineurin stimulates the transcription factor NF-AT, which activates the promotor region of the gene coding for IL-2. The immunosuppressive agents cyclosporin A and tacrolimus fuse in lymphocytes in the presence of immunophillins and the resulting complex inhibits calcineurin. This leads to an IL-2 deficiency and blocks T-lymphocyte activity.

Calcitonin It is a polypeptide belonging to inhibitors of osteoclastic resorption of the bone. Calcitonin receptors are found on osteoclasts. They inhibit its activity and decrease the number of osteoclasts. The plasma level of calcitonin decreases with age, but it is not considered an important factor in the pathogenesis of osteoporosis. Calcitonin was the first antiresorptive agent. Salmon calcitonin in the form of a nasal spray at a dose 200 IU reduces the risk of vertebral fractures. Particularly when given subcutaneously, it has good painkilling effects for bone pain related to osteoporotic vertebral fractures.

Calcitriol Several studies have confirmed the high prevalence of vitamin D deficiency in the European population (Ovesen et al. 2003). An important portion of 1,25-dihydroxy vitamin D3 deficiency is caused by chronic hepatic and renal disorders as well as drugs influencing the metabolism of vitamin D or its clearance. In recent years the active metabolites of vitamin D3 (no need for an endogenous hydroxylation in the liver or kidneys) are increasingly used in the treatment of osteoporosis. The beneficial effect of calcitriol in the treatment of primary, as well as secondary, osteoporosis has been demonstrated by certain studies. (Payer et al. 2007)

The calcitriol deficiency has several causes and can be subdivided as follows:
- type I – primary deficiency due to low food intake or low sunlight exposure,
- type II – insufficient effect of 1,25(OH)2D3 due to decreased production in the kidneys or increased resistance in the target organs

(decreased concentration of the receptors in the bowels due to ageing).

Hypocalcaemia results, followed by an increased level of PTH and the development of senile osteoporosis. Treatment of the deficit depends on its cause. While type I may be treated by the inactive form of vitamin D, type II needs treatment with the active form of calcitriol. Type I also responds to treatment with calcitriol, while it is impossible to treat the type II with the inactive vitamin D. In practice the differentiation between these two types is not simple and combinations of both types are frequent

Calcium oxalate calcification A calcification process caused by calcium oxalate microcrystals. It is a sign of hyperoxalemia occurring due to disturbance of the internal environment, especially in dialysis patients.

Calcium requirements in diet An adequate supply of calcium in the diet is essential for the achievement of adequate bone stock in the premenopausal period. Calcium inhibits the release of parathormone and increases the levels of endogenous calcitonin, thereby suppressing osteoresorption. The calorific value and fat content of recommended food should be taken into account when making recommendations (cheese, milk, yoghurts, fish and vegetables).

A daily calcium intake of up to 2000–2500 mg is considered safe. It is hazardous only in patients with nephrolithiasis and increased absorption of calcium from the intestine. Higher doses are usually unnecessary and may have adverse effects (constipation, renal stones). If the patient does not ingest enough calcium in the diet (intolerance of milk products, high fat content in the ingested products, etc.), then there are a number of calcium preparations available.

Calcium-Sensing Receptor (CaSR) A protein (MW 120 kDa) that can be found on the surface of the cells of a number of organs (parathyroid gland, thyroid gland, renal tubules, bone, pancreas, keratinocytes, gastrointestinal mucous membrane, salivary glands and placenta). CaSR belongs to G-protein associated receptors. The gene coding for CaSR has been localized on the long arm of the 3rd chromosome. A rise of extracellular Ca^{2+} concentration leads to decreased secretion of PTH via the CaSR, and on the other hand, a drop of Ca^{2+} causes an increase of PTH secretion and increased proliferation of parathyroid gland cells. CaSR also influences the secretion of calcitonin, but to a much smaller extent than the PTH secretion. Inactivation mutations of CaSR do not react to increased concentration of Ca^{2+}, and therefore the secretion of PTH is not inhibited. Inactivation mutations in heterozygotes lead to the development of familial hypocalcuric hypercalcaemia (FHH) and in homozygotes to severe neonatal hyperparathyroidism. In activation mutations, the

Table 2. Optimal daily supply of calcium (mg)

	Age	Dose in mg
Children	0 – 6 months	400
	6 – 12 months	600
	1 – 5 years	800
	6 – 10 years	800 – 1200
Adolescents	11 – 24 years	1200 – 1500
Men	25 – 65 years	1000
	over 65 years	1500
Women	from 25 years to menopause	1000
	postmenopausal, using HRT	1000
	postmenopausal, without HRT	1200 – 1500
	older than 65 years, pregnant, breast-feeding	1200 – 1500

receptor reacts to physiological concentrations of Ca^{2+} with a decrease in PTH secretion. Autosomal dominant hypocalcaemia and idiopathic hypercalciuria with nephrolithiasis have been reported the clinical features of activation mutations of CaSR. Newly-developed preparations affecting CaSR are divided into calcimimetics and calcilytics.

Caplan's syndrome → see Rheumatoid pneumoconiosis (Caplan's syndrome)

Capsular pattern With certain joints (shoulder, hip, etc.), involvement of the capsule in the course of a pathological process such as osteoathrosis, always appears to limit the range of passive movements within that joint in a specific pattern. Cyriax (Dr. James Cyriax, 1905–1985, Orthopaedic Surgeon in England) referred to this evolutional sequence of movement pattern typical for the given joint "capsular pattern". In the shoulder joint it begins with limitation of external rotation, then abduction and ends with limitation of internal rotation. In the hip joint it begins with internal rotation, followed by abduction, and ending with external rotation.

Carpal tunnel syndrome (CTS) This is the most frequently occurring peripheral nerve compression syndrome. It accounts for 20% of all compression syndromes and is the cause of 50% of all cases of brachyalgia. It is twice as frequent in women than men and usually occurs after the age of 50. The dominant hand is affected more frequently and in the case of bilateral impairment, more serious lesions affect the dominant site.

Clinical symptoms: The most frequent symptom of CTS is nocturnal paraesthetic brachyalgia. Patients wake up in the night experiencing paraesthesiae and a subjective feeling of finger oedema; however, there are no objective signs of the oedema. The pain may radiate up to the elbow and shoulder. Massage, change of the position of upper limb or 'shaking' the hand may provide relief. The feeling of clumsy fingers and finger paraesthesiae gradually subsides in the morning.

Caspases Cysteine aspartate-specific proteases are enzymes cleaving the polypeptide chain between the aspartic acid and any other amino acid using a cysteine residue. They have a fundamental role at the start of cellular apoptosis, in inflammatory reactions (mainly in the nervous tissue) and in the proteolytic conversion of inactive cytokine precursors, such as pro-interleukin-1β, which is converted by caspase 1 (termed also ICE–IL-1β converting enzyme) to an active IL-1β. Currently, 10 different caspases are known, termed caspase 1 to 10. Caspases 1, 4 and 5 participate mainly in inflammatory responses, while caspases 2, 3 and 10 play an exclusive role in initiating apoptosis.

"Knock-out" mice that lack the gene coding for caspase 1 are unable to produce IL-1, have significantly reduced levels of IFN-γ and are resistant to the endotoxin shock induced by lipopolysaccharide. Mice without the gene coding for caspase 3 lack the ability to eliminate neurons impaired by apoptosis, which leads to a number of abnormalities especially in brain tissue. The caspases are synthesised in the form of enzymatically inactive precursor proteins. Their conversion to active forms is accomplished following contact of the Fas receptor with Fas ligand, TNF-α with its receptor, via activity of granzyme B (granzymes) and perforins released from cytotoxic T-lymphocytes and NK-cells (which is the essence of their cytotoxic effect) or by autoproteolysis. The proteolytic reactions made by caspases result in interruption of the cell cycle, elimination of homeostatic and reparation mechanisms, initiation of the separation of individual cells from its surrounding tissue, disintegration of structural components of the cell and the labelling of dying cells for ingestion by macrophages. The activity of caspases is controlled by several natural or synthetic inhibitors.

CaSR (Calcium sensing receptor) modulators Newly developed preparations influencing CaSR are divided into calcimimetics and calcilytics. The calcimimetics activate CaSR thereby inhibiting the secretion of PTH. Currently, cinacalcet is the only avail-

C

able calcimimetic drug used mainly in the treatment of secondary hyperparathyroidism in patients with chronic renal disease. The calcilytics are CaSR antagonists inhibiting CaSR thereby stimulating the secretion of PTH. At present, NPS 2143 is the only representative of calcilytics. The calcilytics are regarded as a possible future alternative for the treatment of postmenopausal osteoporosis, because of a presumed osteoformation effect due to a regular, repeated and mild increase of PTH secretion. Ca SR modulators are regarded as prospective preparations for the treatment of disturbances of phosphate-calcium metabolism.

Cauda Equina syndrome (CES) A potentially serious neurological disease causing saddle anaesthesia, bilateral weakness of the calf muscles, Achilles tendon areflexia, dysfunction of the ano-vesico-genital area with impairment of sphincters and impotence, as well as polyradicular pain of lumbar and sacral nerve roots. The syndrome is most frequently caused by herniation of an intervertebral disc into sacral roots of the spine, rarely by malignancies or by a late form of ankylosing spondylitis. Chronic compression of the cauda has an indistinct course, which can be manifested only by ano-vesicular sphincters impairment and radicular pain in the lower extremities. The diagnosis of CES in patients suffering from lumbar pain requires urgent surgical intervention.

Causalgia A burning pain sensation after a painful stimulus. It is elicited by damage to the sympathetic nervous system. The sensation is localised to the area of innervation of the injured nerve or its surrounding environment. It is linked to autonomic changes (trophic, vascular).

CD (cluster of differentiation) The CD system is a group of surface attributes (antigens) on cells according to which it is possible to establish the type, the differentiation and developmental stage of the cell, or certain other characteristics

CD2 (LFA-2) This transmembrane glycoprotein is localised especially on thymocytes and adult T-lymphocytes. It is a receptor adsorbing sheep erythrocytes, and so creates the basis for various rosette tests for determining T-cell counts. The adhesive molecule LFA-3 is a natural ligand for CD2.

CD3 This is a complex molecule composed of five polypeptide chains – members of the immunoglobulin superfamily – linked with antigen receptors of T-cells (TCR). It is a typical marker for all adult T-lymphocytes. CD3 transmits the signal from TCR into the cell.

CD4 A glycoprotein belonging to the immunoglobulin superfamily is a typical surface marker for T-helper (T_H) lymphocytes. In much lower counts, it also appears on the surface of macrophages, monocytes, dendritic cells, cells of Langerhans and several others. It participates in the presentation of exogenous antigens by antigen-presenting cells in the form of a complex with MHC class II of HLA antigens. It serves as a receptor for HIV infection, leading to AIDS.

CD5 A single-chain glycoprotein localised on B-lymphocytes, as well as on T-lymphocytes. B-cells can be divided into the two subsets CD5+ and CD5- depending on the presence or absence of CD5. The CD5+-cells produce natural antibodies, primarily of IgM isotype, enforcing the elimination of ill-conditioned or unnecessary inherent antigens and cell structures. An increased CD5+-cell count has been found in certain autoimmune disorders (juvenile diabetes mellitus, Hashimoto's thyroiditis, and systemic lupus erythematosus). The cause for the increased autoantibody formation can be due to the fact that CD5+-cells produce IL-10, which inhibits the activity of T_H1-cells, shifting the T_H1/T_H2 balance towards increased activity of T_H2-cells and thus increased autoantibody formation. The CD72 is the ligand for CD5.

CD8 A transmembrane glycoprotein which is a member of the immunoglobulin superfamily and a typical surface sign of cytotoxic

(T$_C$) T-lymphocytes. They participate in recognising antigens on the surface of the target cells, where they are present in the form of a complex of immunogenic peptides with MHC class I HLA antigens.

CD11 This is a family of three different glycoproteins forming α-chains (CD11a, CD11b and CD11c), which together with an identical β-chain (characterised by differentiation antigen CD18) create three heterodimeric molecules of leukoadhesive integrins: LFA-1 (CD11a/CD18), Mac-1 or CR3 (CD11b/CD18), and gp150,95 or CR4 (CD11c/CD18). They participate mainly in adhesive interactions between leukocytes and endothelial cells during initiation of inflammatory reactions. Their ligands (anti-receptors) on the endothelial cells are inter-cellular adhesive molecules ICAM-1 (CD54) and ICAM-2 (CD102).

CD15 An adhesive polysaccharide antigen referred to as Lewis' antigen X. It is localised on the surface of neutrophils and other leukocytes. Via weak adhesive reactions with selectins E and P (selectins) on the surface of endothelial cells, it creates a background for the "rolling" of leukocytes over the endothelium (in inflammation).

CD16 A differentiation antigen having the function of a low-affinity Fc-receptor for IgG (FcγRIII). It is localised on the surface of neutrophils, macrophages, eosinophils and NK-cells. It facilitates the phagocytosis of particles opsonised by IgG antibodies and participates in ADCC (antibody-dependent cellular cytotoxicity) reactions. It is regarded a typical feature of NK-cells.

CD19 An antigen found on the surface of all B-lymphocytes (characteristic feature of B-cells).

CD20 A non-glycosylated phosphoprotein expressed on the surface of all mature B cells. Its function is unknown. It is a useful marker in B cell lymphomas, hairy cell leukaemia and B cell chronic lymphatic leukaemia. It is the target for the monoclonal antibody (rituximab) in the treatment of lymphoma, and B cell mediated diseases such as systemic lupus erythematosus and rheumatoid arthritis.

CD21 An antigen found on the surface of all B-lymphocytes (characteristic feature of B-cells) and follicular dendritic cells. It functions as the receptor for the C3d fragment of the complement (CR2), as well as a receptor for the Epstein-Barr virus.

CD22 A typical surface antigen found on all B-lymphocytes (characteristic feature of B-cells). It is lost during transformation of a B-lymphocyte to a plasma cell (secreting antibodies).

CD25 A single-chain glycoprotein creating the α-chain of the receptor for interleukin 2 (IL-2R). It is localised on activated T- and B-lymphocytes and macrophages.

CD28 This glycoprotein homo-dimer can be found on T-lymphocytes and serves as a co-stimulatory molecule whose ligand is the CD80 (B7) antigen on antigen presenting cells and B-lymphocytes. The CD28-CD80 interaction provides the lymphocytes with a second co-stimulatory signal that is fundamental for their activation.

CD31 This is an adhesive molecule referred to also as PECAM-1 (platelet/endothelial cell adhesion molecule). It is localised on the surface of granulocytes, monocytes, macrophages, B-lymphocytes, NK-cells and endothelial cells. It is of cardinal importance in trans-endothelial migration of leukocytes to the focus of inflammation.

CD35 An antigen representing CR1, the receptor for C3b and C4b fragments of complement. It can be found on a number of cells including neutrophils, eosinophils, monocytes, B-cells and erythrocytes. It plays an important role in eliminating circulating immune complexes.

CD40 A co-stimulatory molecule localised on the surface of B-lymphocytes. The CD40L molecule, found on the surface of T-helper lymphocytes, is the ligand of CD40. The CD40-CD40L interaction provides the B-cell with a second signal necessary for its transformation to an antibody synthesising plasma cell.

CD44 A transmembrane molecule found on the surface of leukocytes, erythrocytes and thrombocytes. It functions as a receptor for hyaluronic acid. Through the CD44 molecule the cell can bind to the intercellular substance and accomplish other adhesive reactions, especially those between leukocytes and endothelial cells, during initiation of the inflammatory reaction, but also during nidation of cancer cells in the course of a metastatic process. In line with the above mentioned increased expression of CD44 is found on metastasising cells or, for example, on epithelial cells in patients with bronchial asthma.

CD45 This membrane glycoprotein is found in a great number of copies on all haematopoietic cells except erythrocytes and thrombocytes. It exists in at least eight isoforms where the CD45RA molecule is typical for memory and activated T-cells. The individual isoforms differ in molecular weight, but they all possess a cytoplasmatic component with protein tyrosine phosphatase activity. Through its effect, the tyrosine units of membrane glycoproteins can de-phosphorylate and so modulate the transmission of activating signals into the cell.

CD46 Regulatory factor of the complement system MCP (membrane co-factor protein) found on the surface of haematopoietic and other cells. It regulates the activation of complement via cleavage of the C3b component thereby preventing the activation of other complement components in its proximity. Its presence on trophoblast cells contributes to mother's tolerance to the foetus. This has been proven by clinical experience where women lacking the CD46 molecule on their trophoblast cells suffer miscarriages. Another regulatory factor of complement, DAF (CD55) acts in a similar way.

CD50 The intercellular adhesive molecule ICAM-3, which is a ligand for LFA-1 (CD11), belongs to the immunoglobulin superfamily and is found mainly on differentiated leukocytes.

CD54 The intercellular adhesive molecule ICAM-1, whose ligand is LFA-1 (CD11), is localised mainly on endothelial cells and follicular dendritic cells. It is also a receptor for rhinovirus.

CD55 A single-chain glycoprotein bound to phosphatidylinositol and found on the surface of haematopoietic and other cells, where it functions as a regulator of the complement system (DAF, CD46).

CD56 This adhesive molecule is the basic differentiation antigen of NK-cells. It can be found also on neurons (N-CAM).

CD58 A single-chain adhesive glycoprotein mainly found on haematopoietic and other cells. It is also referred to as LFA-3 (leukocyte function antigen 3) and is a ligand for the CD2 antigen.

CD62 A family of adhesive molecules (selectins) that includes three members: CD62E – E-selectin (found especially on endothelial cells), CD62L – L-selectin (found on the surface of granulocytes and lymphocytes) and CD62P – P-selectin (found on endothelial cells and thrombocytes).

CD64 A single-chain glycoprotein with a function for the high-affinity Fc-receptor for IgG (Fc$_\gamma$RI). It is localized on macrophages and monocytes.

CD66 A family of at least five antigens that are found on neutrophils (CD66a), eventually on all granulocytes (CD66b), and certain cancer cells. For instance, CD66c is a typical antigen of neutrophils and colorectal carcinoma cells, and CD66e which is also referred to as a carcinoembryonic antigen (CEA).

CD72 A heterodimeric glycoprotein, which is a typical feature of B-lymphocytes and is a ligand for CD5.

CD79 A group of two transmembrane glycoproteins that are components of the antigen receptor of B-lymphocytes (antigen receptors). The CD79a represents an Igα chain (having been referred to as MB1), while the CD79b represents Igβ chain (B29). They are localised on the surface of all adult B-lymphocytes.

CD80 A co-stimulatory molecule found on the surface of antigen presenting cells, including B-lymphocytes. Its ligand is CD28.

CD88 An antigen on granulocytes, mast cells, macrophages and smooth muscle cells. It is a receptor for anaphylatoxin C5a.

CD102 An adhesive molecule belonging to the immunoglobulin superfamily and is found on endothelial cells, lymphocytes and monocytes. It is also referred to as ICAM-2. Its anti-receptor on the leukocytes is the integrin LFA-1 (CD11).

CD106 A vascular cell adhesive molecule (VCAM-1) that is found on the cells of vascular endothelium and during the transendothelial migration of leukocytes it reacts with VLA-4 (CD49d/CD29) molecules on their surface (inflammation).

CD115 An antigen present on monocytes, macrophages and on the placenta. It acts as the receptor for macrophage colony stimulating factor (M-CSFR).

CD116 An antigen present on monocytes, macrophages, neutrophils, eosinophils, fibroblasts and endothelial cells. It acts as a receptor for granulocyte and macrophage colony stimulating factor (GM-CSFR).

CD117 An antigen present on the progenitor cells of bone marrow. It acts as the receptor for stem cell growth factor (SCFR), also referred to as c-kit.

CD119 An antigen on the macrophages, monocytes, B-cells and epithelial cells. It is a receptor for interferon gamma (IFN-γR).

CD120 It is found on a number of cells in two isoforms. Both isoforms, CD120a and CD120b, are receptors for tumour necrotising factors (TNFRI, TNFRII). Each of them can bind TNF-α or TNF-β.

CD121 An antigen occurring in two isoforms. Both represent the receptors for IL-1. The CD121a represents IL-1RI and is localised on T-lymphocytes, thymocytes, endothelial cells and fibroblasts. The CD121b represents IL-1RII and is localised on B-cells, macrophages and monocytes.

CD122 This antigen on T- and B-lymphocytes, NK cells and monocytes possesses the function of β-chain of the receptor for IL-2.

CD124 This antigen on B- and T-lymphocytes and endothelial cells has receptor function for IL-4 (IL-4R).

CD125 An antigen mainly found on eosinophils and basophils with the function of α-chain of the receptor for IL-5.

CD128 This antigen on neutrophils, basophils and certain subpopulations of T-lymphocytes has receptor function for IL-8 (IL-8R).

CDR The hypervariable regions of immunoglobulin chains. They are the integral components of binding sites for antibodies (immunoglobulins, structure).

CEA (carcinoembryonic antigen) It is present in foetal endodermic tissue and can be expressed on the surface of neoplastic cells, especially in colorectal carcinoma (oncofoetal antigens).

CentiMorgan (cM) A unit used in genetics for genome mapping. It represents the distance between two gene loci on the DNA molecule that have a 1% recombinant frequency.

Certolizumab Certolizumab (CDP-870; Cimzia®) is a new agent that employs a novel strategy to neutralise TNF-α, namely the prokaryotic expression of TNF-α-specific Fab antibody fragments, coupled to polyethylene glycol. Certolizumab pegol is the first anti TNF treatment which has been coupled to polyethylene glycol ('PEGylated'). This process slows the body's clearance of the active compound from the blood, thereby prolonging its active period and possibly also resulting in differential accumulation in inflamed tissue over normal tissue. Certolizumab pegol works by targeting TNF-α in inflamed tissue, reducing symptoms and disease progression in RA. The molecule is Fc-free, which means that the Fc region of the antibody, found in conventional anti-TNFs, has been removed. Although it has now been shown in RAPID 1 that the Fc region is not required for efficacy in RA, it does have functions which could potentially be detrimental, including Fc mediated cytotoxicity and transport across the placenta. Therefore, it is hoped that pegylated certolizumab will last longer and have fewer adverse effects.

Pegylated certolizumab adds significant benefit in reducing the signs and symptoms of RA in combination with methotrexate, compared to using methotrexate alone. This represents a significant advance in the treatment of RA.

In a phase III study, 59% of patients receiving certolizumab pegol 200 mg plus methotrexate, and 61% of patients receiving certolizumab pegol 400 mg plus methotrexate every two weeks achieved a 20% improvement in symptoms (ACR 20 response) after 24 weeks' treatment. Only 14% of patients receiving methotrexate alone achieved an ACR 20 response over the same period, highlighting the superiority of the treatment combination at both doses of certolizumab pegol in patients refractory to methotrexate.

The majority of adverse events were mild to moderate and discontinuation due to AEs was low at 4.3%, 5.7% and 1.5% for certolizumab pegol 200 mg, 400 mg and placebo respectively. Early studies in rheumatoid arthritis have shown promise, though more studies

are needed (Emery et al. 2008, Landewé et al. 2008).

Chaining of functional defects Configuration of functional defects that develop as a result of incorrect involvement of functional muscle chains in evolutionary kinesiology (mechanism of gait, breathing, swallowing and grasp).

Charcot's joint (neuropathic arthropathy) The term Charcot's joint refers to progressive destructive changes in joints with a typical clinical and radiological picture as a consequence of sensory trophic neuropathy.

Clinical symptoms and signs: Charcot's joint(s) is mainly a mono-articular or oligo-articular arthropathy. The affected joint is swollen and grossly deformed due to apposition of the bone and soft-tissue swelling. Later joint instability can occur. There is a marked disparity between the prominent objective signs and the minimal subjective complaints of the patient (painless joint). X-rays show a mixture of destruction and heterotropic new bone formation. The severity of the articular changes and their distribution depend on the underlying condition that produced the development of trophic neuropathy and its duration. A variety of injuries and diseases can damage the nerve supply to the joints. In tabes dorsalis and leprosy, the large joints of the lower extremities are predominantly affected, in diabetes mellitus the joints of the feet are more frequently involved and in syringomyelia, the large joints of the upper extremities (the shoulder in 80% of cases) are affected. Progression of the arthropathy can be slow and may be associated with sub-acute attacks of arthritis with significant swelling and warming developing over several hours.

Chemokines A superfamily of more than 40 small proteins (with molecular weights between 8 and 11 kDa) that belong to cytokines. They act in concentrations of 1–100 pg/mL via specific receptors mainly as chemotactic factors for various leukocytes from where their term arises (chemotactic cytokines). They are produced by practically all cells and the pro-

duction is induced by infectious agents, exogenous irritants and many cytokines. They exert important inflammatory and regulatory activities especially on haematopoietic cells and the exchange of lymphocytes between the circulation and the lymphatic organs. The chemokines are regarded as second-degree proinflammatory cytokines because they are less pleiotropic than first-degree cytokines (IL-1, IL-6, TNF-α, etc.). They are also referred to as intercrines. This term was created in an effort to distinguish between these two groups of proinflammatory cytokines that are structurally and genetically unrelated. Individual polypeptides of the chemokine superfamily can be divided into four subfamilies depending on the spacing of their first two cysteine residues; juxta-positioned (-C-C-), separated by one (-C-X-C-), three other intervening amino acids (-C-X-X-X-C-), or one pair of cysteines (-C-).

The -C-X-C- subfamily is also termed α-chemokines or CXC-chemokines and its genes are located on human chromosome 4; the -C-C- subfamily is also known as β-chemokines or CC-chemokines and its genes are located on chromosome 17. The α-chemokines include IL-8, neutrophil-activating protein-2 (NAP-2), and platelet factor-4 (PF-4) that in particular are chemotactic and activating factors of neutrophils. The β-chemokines exert chemotactic activity predominantly on monocytes and macrophages, but also on eosinophils, basophils, lymphocytes and NK-cells. The CC chemokines include monocyte chemotactic protein (MCP-1 to MCP-5), macrophage inflammatory protein (MIP-1 and MIP-3), CCL5 (previously called Regulated upon Activation, Normal T-cell Expressed, and Activation; abbreviated RANTES), and eotaxin – a specifically effective chemotaxin for eosinophils. The C-chemokine subfamily has only one member to date – lymphotactin, which is a chemotactic factor for lymphocytes and NK-cells, but not for neutrophils and macrophages. Also the CXXXC-chemokines have only one member – neurotactin produced by microglial cells and belonging to neurokines (cytokines acting primarily on brain tissue). According to the newast nomenclature CXC chemakines are termed as CXCL and similarly CCL, CX_3CL and CL where the letter "L" means ligand to distinguish it from CXCR, CCR, CX_3CR and CR where "R" means receptor.

CXC chemokines act via 5 known receptors that are classified as CXCR1 to CXCR5. For CC chemokines there are 10 known receptors (CCR1 to CCR10); for neurotactin only one receptor has been identified to date (CX_3CR1). These receptors can be found on various cells and also participate in other activities in addition to inflammation. For example, CXCR4 is a co-receptor for HIV-1 and plays an important role in the pathogenesis of AIDS. Experiments on mice have shown that CCR2, whose ligand is MIP-1, plays a crucial role in the initiation of atherosclerosis.

Chemotactic factors Substances regulating the directed movement of cells (chemotaxy). They are abbreviated as chemotaxins. Both endogenous and exogenous chemotaxins are recognised. The group of endogenous chemotaxins includes chemokines and several other cytokines, certain prostanoids and the fragments of certain proteins (for example fibrin or fibronectin). Typical representatives of exogenous chemotaxins are certain bacterial oligopeptides containing N-formylmethionine (for example N-formyl-methionyl-leucyl-phenylalanine).

Chemotaxis The active movement of phagocytes or cells in a general direction (positive chemotaxy) or opposite direction (negative chemotaxy) related to the concentration gradient of the chemotactic factor. Chemotaxis is the stimulated and directed migration of cells.

Chimeric antibodies These are antibodies in which one part of the molecule (variable domain) originates from one animal species and the other part (constant domain) from another animal species. Humanised antibodies are an example of such antibodies.

Chloroquine → see Antimalarial drugs

Cholinergic crisis → see Myasthenia gravis

Chondrocalcinosis (CCA; chondrocalcinosis articularis) An induced disturbance (rarely genetic) of articular cartilage, presumably proteoglycans, with local overproduction of inorganic pyrophosphate leading to its crystallisation. Microcrystals of calcium pyrophosphate dehydrate (CPPD) form a picture of pyrophosphate calcification of the weakened cartilages of the joints that clinically manifests as episodes of crystalline induced arthritis, and leads to the development of secondary osteoarthritis. It can be associated with hypothyroidism, hyperparathyroidism, haemochromatosis and acromegaly.

Symptoms and signs: Recurrent attacks of acute or sub-acute arthritis (pseudogout) (mostly of large joints, especially the knees and shoulders) in the elderly with a non-specific inflammatory response. Over time, it can lead to secondary osteoarthritis and eventual destructive arthropathy.

Diagnosis The clinical picture may be typical, especially with large shoulder joint effusions. Radiographs show linear calcification on the surface of articular cartilage or in the triangular ligament at the wrist. Joint aspiration may be inflammatory or haemorrhagic, with polarised microscopy confirming positively bifringent rhomboid shaped crystals.

Treatment There is no curative treatment, but episodes of acute and subacute arthritis are treated by joint aspiration and steroid injection. Sometimes, NSAID's or low dose steroids are required in patients with continuing symptoms of joint pain and stiffness.

Chondroitin sulphate A macromolecular substance which is a physiological component of articular cartilage. The administration of chondroitin sulphate has a favourable influence on the metabolism of chondrocytes. It is administered in the form of granules or capsules. The recommended dosage regimen is 2 capsules (1 capsule containing 400 mg) twice a day or 1 sachet (800 mg) twice a day for the first 14 days, then 1 capsule twice a day or 1 sachet daily for the next 3 months, then a 3-month pause followed by 3 months of treatment. It is used in the treatment of osteoarthrosis

Chondromatosis → see Synovial chondromatosis

Christmas disease → see Musculoskeletal complication in rare inherited haemorrhagic diatheses

Chromatography A physiochemical separation technique used for analytical and preparative and for analytical purposed. The principle exploits the differences in the affinity of different components (liquid or gaseous) between two non-miscible phases, of which one is mobile and the other stationary (immobilised). Depending on the nature of the mobile phase, liquid chromatography (LC) and gas chromatography (GC) are distinguished. There are different mechanisms of separation to include adsorption, distribution, ion exchange, affinity (immunoaffinity), gel permeation (molecular screen), gas and high performance liquid chromatography (HPLC; columns with small round particles and higher mechanical endurance, high pressure). The method of washing out components of the sample distinguishes between elution, frontal and size exclusion chromatographies; according to the geometrical organisation of the chromatographic apparatus (bed shape). By using chromatography techniques it is possible to determine or isolate various substances including antigens, haptens and antibodies.

Chronic fatigue syndrome (CFS) A disorder characterised by idiopathic (isolated) permanent fatigue that has a precisely defined onset, does not subside after rest, greatly limits the daily activities of the patient compared to the status before the onset, and is inappropriate to the amount of exertion. Its aetiology is unknown, but it is hypothesised that infections (especially viral), a primary immune system defect, disturbance of hypothalamic–pituitary–adrenal axis and neuropsychiatric factors can play an aetiopathogenic role. Immunologically, there are abnormalities in lymphocyte count and function, mainly NK-cells; elevated levels of certain cytokines and autoantibodies may be observed. There are no specific diagnostic laboratory tests for the diagnosis of CFS. A diagnosis is often only made by exclusion of known illnesses such as infections, neurological and psychiatric diseases. The diagnosis of primary CFS is often very difficult as it can be easily confused with a chronic state of fatigue secondary to various diseases.

Chronic hepatitis → see Hepatitis

Churg-Strauss syndrome (CSS) A syndrome characterised pathologically by a necrotising vasculitis with extravascular necrotising granulomas and eosinophilic infiltrates in the vessel walls and perivascular tissues.

Clinical symptoms and signs: The most important manifestations are asthma (often longstanding), allergic rhinitis, systemic symptoms and multisystem manifestations like transient pulmonary infiltrates, mononeuritis multiplex, and rashes (often palpable purpura). The heart is often affected (with a higher mortality), but gastrointestinal and renal involvement are rare. There is a marked peripheral blood eosinophilia that can reach up to 50% of leukocytes; some patients have high levels of serum IgE and up to 65% of patients are p-ANCA (anti-MPO) positive. A biopsy of affected tissue shows necrotising extravascular granulomas with eosinophils and necrotising vasculitis. Corticosteroids are the treatment of choice (prednisone in doses 40–60mg/day) with the addition of cyclophosphamide or azathioprine if there is an incomplete response. The prognosis has improved with 5 years survival at 70%.

CINCA syndrome CINCA is a rare, but serious, rheumatic disease that affects newborns and children in early childhood characterised by the appearance of chronic exanthema, recurrent joint inflammation and central nervous system disease. The nomenclature CINCA is derived from the English names of its common features, taking the first letter of each: Chronic, Infantile, Neurological, Cutaneous, Articular.

Clinical symptoms: The chronic exanthema is a maculopapular urticaria, rarely associated with pruritus. The trigger for urticaria can be solar radiation. The arthritis is symmetrical and always affects knee joints. Arthritis of hip joints, shoulders and the vertebral column has never been reported. Important symptoms of central nervous system disease are due to a chronic meningitis include headaches, vomiting and convulsions; mental retardation development is very frequent. Other organ impairments include oedema of optic nerve papilla, chorioretinitis, uveitis, optic nerve atrophy, sight defects and even blindness. Serious growth retardation, which is not due to hormonal disturbance, is a generalised sign of CINCA. Mutations of the CIAS1 gene have recently been described.

CJD → see Creutzfeldt-Jakob disease (CJD)

Clinical examination algorithm in rheumatology
1. *history* A good history of onset, duration, localisation, character and subsequent course of the rheumatic pain are particularly significant.
2. *inspection* Observation of changes in joint contour (flattening, coarsening, disfiguration), swelling, oedema, colour of the skin, joint deformities, muscle atrophy, rheumatoid nodules, nodes, tophi, etc.
3. *palpation* The extent of palpable tenderness, skin temperature, joint effusion, crepitation (coarse, soft, snowy), bursal swelling, painful insertions, zones and points of hyperalgesia as in fibromyalgia, trigger points, myogeloses etc.
4. *examination of joint movement* Both active and passive ranges of movement in affected joints are recorded, with restrictions in the movement pattern of individual joints caused by pain, inflammation, or structural changes. Joint laxity/instability is also noted. Muscle strength/weakness is assessed against gravity and resistance.

Club foot (pes equinovarus) This deformity is a birth defect characterised by a plantar flexion of the foot, varus position of the heel and adduction of the metatarsus. It is corrected by wearing special orthopaedic footwear in which pressure is applied to the three fundamental points in the opposite direction to the described deformities.

Cluster of differentiation → see CD (cluster of differentiation)

Codmann's exercises These are intended to relieve the corrugated joint capsule in the affected shoulder joint. They consist of a swinging movement of the shoulder joint either in a supine position with the upper extremity loosely hanging over the edge of the table, or in ante-flexion with both arms loosely hanging. The axial tension on the shoulder can be increased by gradually increasing weight. They are used as the first active exercises in shoulder pain syndrome.

Coeliac disease (Sprue) A genetically determined disorder characterised by an immunopathological reaction against certain prolamins (the proteinous fraction of grains; gliadin in wheat, secalin in rye, hordein in barley, avenin in oat; only rice and corn are considered safe) with consequent damage to the intestinal mucosa. There is loss of villi, hyperplasia of the crypts and increased turnover of enterocytes resulting in a reduced absorption surface and increased mucosal permeability with the development of a malabsorption syndrome. Typical gastrointestinal symptoms and signs (profuse diarrhoea and failure to thrive) are found only in young children after weaning; later extra-intestinal symptoms and signs (growth disturbance, delayed puberty, arthralgia, dysthymia, damaged tooth enamel, osteopenia or osteoporosis, anaemia, etc.) dominate or can be the only clinical symptomatology. Thus only a small number of patients are accurately and timely diagnosed. A high prevalence (1:100 to 300 of a Caucasian population) occurs. The most severe complication in untreated patients is an increased risk of intestinal tumours (especially lymphomas) in late middle-aged persons. There are serum IgA anti-endomysial antibodies and serum IgA antibodies against tissue transglutaminase. A definitive diagnosis is demonstrated by histological and histochemical analysis of the biopsy specimen of the duodenum, usually by gastroscopy. The only curative treatment is a life-long gluten-free diet

COL1A1 gene polymorphism A (G-T) polymorphism in the collagen gene COL1A1 (located on the long arm of chromosome 17) coding for a binding site of the transcription factor Sp1 influences the transcription of COL1A1 gene for type I collagen and induces changes in the properties of the produced collagen. The binding affinity of the polymorphous allele "s" for the transcription factor Sp1 increases which leads to the synthesis of larger amounts of the $\alpha_1(I)$ chain compared to the $\alpha_2(I)$ chain. A ratio of these two chains in the collagen type I is 2,3 in "Ss" heterozygotes and 2 in "SS" homozygotes. This abnormal ratio of α chains in the collagen of "Ss" heterozygotes is associated with a predisposition to osteoporotic fractures. A slight association between the "s" allele incidence and a lower BMD, and conversely an increased association with fractures shows that this polymorphism mainly affects the bone strength independent of the BMD.

Collagen type II defects Articular cartilage collagens are types II, IX, X and XI. Type II collagen is the principal molecular component and consists of three identical polypeptide chains. The gene for its production is localised on chromosome 12. Mutations of this gene lead to various diseases as achondrogenesis type II, hypochondrogenesis, Kniest's dysplasia, and most spondyloepiphyseal dysplasias.

Colony-stimulating growth factors Glycoprotein cytokines regulating proliferation and maturation of haematopoietic progenitor cells as well as the functional activity of mature cells. The best-characterised growth factors are CSF regulating the production of granulocytes and macrophages. There are four of them: macrophage M-CSF, granulocyte G-CSF, granulocyte-macrophage GM-CSF and multi-CSF (IL-3). Some of them are now available in a recombinant form, especially GM-CSF which has been applied in the immunotherapy of tumours and certain immunodeficiencies.

Combination Disease Modifying Anti-Rheumatic Drug (DMARD) therapy

Recent clinical experience shows that joint inflammation in rheumatoid arthritis (RA) can be better suppressed by a combination of DMARDs, if one alone fails. At present, however, it is impossible to explicitly state whether combination DMARD therapy should be given as initial therapy in RA.

Combination of DMARDs
- *with documented efficacy:*
  methotrexate + antimalarials,
  methotrexate + antimalarials + sulfasalazine,
  methotrexate + cyclosporin,
  sulfasalazine + methotrexate,
  sulfasalazine + cyclosporin,
  methotrexate + etanercept,
  methotrexate + infliximab,
- *with probable efficacy:*
  methotrexate + injectible gold,
  sulfasalazine + antimalarials,
- *with unconfirmed efficacy:*
  injectible gold + antimalarials,
  antimalarials + cyclosporin,
  methotrexate + azathioprine,
  penicillamine + antimalarials.

Combined B- and T-cell deficiency

Defects in the function of B- and T-cells appear with subsequent insufficiency of humoral and specific cellular immunity, and sometimes phagocytosis. Typical examples are severe combined immunodeficiency (SCID), ataxia-telangiectasia and Wiskott-Aldrich syndrome.

Complement (C)

A set of over 30 different executive and regulatory glycoproteins, some of which can be found in the blood serum and others on the cell surface, where they form various receptors. Complement exists in serum in an inactive state and may be activated by four pathways – classical, alternative, lectin pathway, and by the production of the membrane attacking complex (MAC), which is a common continuation of all three aforementioned activation pathways and is directly responsible for the impairment and lysis of target cells (cells on whose surface the complement has been activated).

Constituents of complement reacting in the classical pathway are components termed as C1, C2, C3 and C4, whereby the C1 component has three subunits C1, C1r and C1s. These components, except for C1q, also participate in the lectin complement activation pathway, while the components C5b, C6, C7, C8 and C9 together form the membrane attacking complex. Factors B and D and the C3 component are constituents of the alternative pathway, which is also controlled by factors P (properdine), H and I. The other regulatory glycoproteins are named according to their function, for example C1-INH (C1-inhibitor), C4-bp (C4b-binding protein) and MCP (membrane co-factor protein); or they rank among receptors specifically binding only fragments of certain components, for example, C3b and iC3b fragments bind to receptors CR1 to CR4, the C5a fragment binds to C5aR, and so on. The individual components are gradually activated by a cascade mechanism. The activation of one component is followed by the occurrence of usually an active proteolytic enzyme, which cleaves the next component into two fragments, one of which is a protease cleaving the next one, etc. Certain fragments are not proteolytic enzymes, but possess the function of cofactors or various bioregulatory substances.

Complement – biological activities

The complement system has executive and regulatory functions involving the complex of its terminal components (MAC), individual fragments of the first components and of certain factors, as well as a number of receptors on the surface of diverse cells and humoral regulators. In a view of the macroorganism, the activity can be either beneficial or harmful. The basis of beneficial activity is mainly protection against pathogenic microorganisms and heterogeneous cells, then participation in inflammatory reactions and regulation of the immune response. Harmful activity (impairment of one's own cells and tissues) is expressed in certain immunopathological reactions, especially in those induced by circulating immune complexes and cytotoxic autoantibodies (immunopathology). The main biological activities of complement include cytotoxic and cytolytic reactions (MAC being responsible for them), the production of anaphylatoxins, C5a, C3a and C4a, opsonins (C3b, iC3b and C4b fragments) and chemotactic factors (C5a, $C5a_{deArg}$, and Ba fragments).

Complement – genetics
Immunogenetics relating to the localisation, structure and regulation of genes coding for individual components of the complement system. The genes for the majority of glycoproteins of the complement system demonstrate two main forms of genetic variability:

- *absence of a proper gene or existence of zero alleles in the corresponding locus in certain individuals in the population* The zero allele is coding for a non-functional protein or does not transcribe into a protein product at all. Thus a certain deficiency develops that may manifest in various autoimmune or infectious disorders (complement deficiency).
- *existence of a complement protein polymorphism* To date, the incidence of polymorphic forms has been found not only in the majority of components and factors of complement, but also in certain complement regulators such as C4-bp (C4-binding protein) and CR1 (C3b receptor). The determination of these polymorphic forms (allotypic variants) has a significant meaning in the genetic characterisation of the individual and in population studies (Moreland et al. 2004).

Complement (MAC)
An abbreviation for membrane attacking complex. Penetration of the cytoplasmic membrane and lysis of heterologous erythrocytes can be undertaken by the complex C5b678 alone, whilst lysis of nuclear animal cells and gramnegative bacteria can be accomplished only by the complex $C5b678(9)_n$. The C9 component, being a typical perforin, plays a decisive role and the MAC contains 6 to 18 of C9 monomers. The whole complex forms hollow tubules that are built into the cytoplasmic membrane of the target cells, thereby producing holes through which ions, water and other low-molecular weight substances may flow uncontrolled, as the osmotic pressure inside the cell is higher than in its environment. This leads to cell oedema, splitting of its cytoplasmic membrane and then to cell lysis.

Complement receptors
These are present on the surface of various cells and specifically recognise and bind fragments of certain components and fragments of the complement system. They can be divided into two groups:
1. CR1 to CR4 whose ligands are C3b and fragments derived from C3b
2. Receptors for other components of complement, such as receptor for C1q (C1R), anaphylatoxins (C5aR) of factor H (HR).

Complex BT
→ see Balneotherapy (BT)

Complex regional pain syndrome of the shoulder (CRPS; humeroscapular periarthropathy; painful shoulder)
A common term for various lesions of the periarticular structures of the shoulder joint. Most frequently, they are tendinopathies of the rotator cuff tendons, or together with calcium accumulation (calcific tendinitis), then bursitis (most frequently subacromial bursitis), rotator cuff rupture and lesions of the tendon of the long head of biceps. Differentiation of the pain aetiology and localisation of the lesion are essential for effective therapy. See algodystrophy syndrome (ADS).

Complotypes
Polymorphic genes coding for C2 and C4 components of the complement and factor B which are inherited as a single unit, thus as one haplotype. They are located in the HLA complex region on the short arm of the sixth chromosome. There is

a close relationship between complotypes and HLA haplotypes, indicating that certain HLA haplotypes are always related to certain complotypes.

Computed Axial Tomography → see Computed Tomography (CT; Computed Axial Tomography, CAT scan)

Computed Tomography (CT; Computed Axial Tomography, CAT scan) A diagnostic method using ionizing radiation for imaging. The imaging of tissues is based on a densitometric principle; detectors scan the amount of radiation, which after emission from the source of X-ray go through the scanned area of the human body. Absorption of radiation after transition through body structures is measured. CT enables imaging of a particular locality in the transverse plane. The computer converts the values of radiation absorption from digital form into a particular degree of grey and thereby forms the final image of organs and tissues. Based on this data, modern CT scans can also produce subsequent two- and three-dimensional reconstructions. Administration of contrasts (orally, intravenously, intracavity, intrathecally) is used to improve imaging (emphasising density differences) of human tissues.

CT is not used in the diagnosis of rheumatic inflammatory diseases as a basic evaluation method of the extent and distribution of bone change, and is not helpful in evaluating early changes. Compared to conventional radiography, CT, by tomographic visualisation, enables better imaging of articular lesions, erosions, destructions and positional changes, which are only partially visible on plain X-ray.

CT plays an important role in the imaging of acetabular protrusion, precise visualisation of a reduction in acetabular cavity and the extent of proximal femur displacement, which is essential for orthopaedic interventions. It is also useful for imaging areas with difficult accessibility by conventional radiography – sacroiliac joints, sternoclavicular, sternocostal, costotransverse joints and temporomandibular joints. CT supplements the diagnostic rel-

evance of cervical spine changes in rheumatoid arthritis – spondylodiscitis, atlanto-axial subluxation, erosion of the dens; enables distinction between inflammatory and degenerative processes of the spine, disc protrusion and herniation. CT is helpful in the diagnosis of joint complications, e.g. osteomyelitis, septic arthritis, complications after intra-articular aspiration and injection or after surgical intervention.

Arthro-CT

A CT scan is performed after intra-articular administration of contrast. Compared to conventional arthrography, CT is better in the evaluation of joint cartilage and subchondral bone. Arthro-CT enables high quality two-dimensional reconstructions in different planes, which provides more transparent imaging.

As CT is based on ionizing radiation with a low sensitivity to soft tissue imaging, ultrasound and MRI are currently preferred in certain rheumatological diagnostic tests.

Conglutinin A lectin that can be found in the serum and on the surface of various human and other mammalian cells. It specifically recognises and binds to the monosaccharides N-acetyl glucosamine, L-fructose, L-glucose or mannose. Lectin interaction with saccharides induces cell aggregation or activation of the lectin complement pathway (complement).

Conventional antibodies These are produced in individual organisms after accidental, targeted or experimental immunisation by complete antigen (immunogen). They are characterised by heterogeneity. Conventional antibodies do not consist of one population of immunoglobulin molecules whose polypeptide chains have an identical sequence of amino acids, but consist of a mixture of a number of molecule types whose binding sites (immunoglobulin binding site) have a different affinity, and thereby also different specificity to particular epitopes of the complete antigen that induced their production. Each epitope in an antigen molecule stimulates one particular clone of B lymphocytes to produce antibodies. As complete antigens have a number of epitopes, they activate several clones of B lymphocytes and therefore produce polyclonal antibodies. Conventional antibodies are basically a mixture of monoclonal antibodies against a complex antigen containing several epitopes.

Convertases Proteolytic enzymes developing during activation of components and factors of the complement to cleave the C3 or C5 components to C3a and C3b, or C5a and C5b fragments, respectively. Thus, there are two convertases, C3-convertases and C5-convertases. These differ in whether they form during the classical or alternative complement activation pathways. The C3-convertase of the classical pathway consists of C4b2b fragments and the C3-convertase of the alternative pathway consists of C3bBb fragments. The C5-convertase of the classical pathway consists of C4b2b3b fragments and the C5-convertase of the alternative pathway consists of C3bBb3b fragments.

Corticosteroid-induced Osteoporosis
The pathogenesis of osteoporosis in patients with endogenously or exogenously mediated excess of glucocorticoids is complex. The direct influence of glucocorticoids on bone remodelling may be regarded as the most important. Glucocorticoids act via specific glucocorticoid receptors on osteoblasts. Activation of these receptors leads to an inhibition of replication and differentiation of osteoblasts. Glucocorticoids reduce the duodenal absorption and the renal tubular resorption of calcium causing the development of secondary hyperparathyroidism. The other effect of glucocorticoids is their negative influence on the skeletal muscles (protein catabolism), which causes decreased stimulation of new bone formation through relative inactivity. Glucocorticoids also exert a negative influence on the hypothalamic-pituitary axis with a consequent deficiency of sex hormones. The adrenal production of oestrone, dihydroepiandrosterone (DHEA) and androstenedione decreases due to ACTH suppression (in primary hypercorticism and during long-term corticosteroid treatment), and deficiency of these anabolic hormones may contribute to the development of osteoporosis.

Costochondritis → see Tietze's syndrome and costochondritis

COX-1 inhibitors → see Non-steroidal antiinflammatory drugs (NSAIDs)

COX-2 inhibitors → see Non-steroidal antiinflammatory drugs (NSAIDs)

Coxa saltans (snapping hip syndrome)
A voluntary or involuntary movement of the iliotibial tract over the greater trochanter causing an audible click. It can be caused by an uneven length of the lower limbs or some other anatomic anomaly. The irritation of the greater trochanteric bursa can be manifested by tenderness or pain.

C-reactive protein (CRP)
An acute phase reactant produced by the liver and acting mainly as an opsonin for bacteria, fungi, parasites and immune complexes. In the presence of calcium it binds to phosphorylcholine which is a regularly occurring component of phospholipids and complex polysaccharides richly present in the cellular wall of a number of bacteria and in the membranes of eukaryotic cells. It activates the classical pathway of the complement system and is regarded as a primitive antibody protecting the organism until specific antibodies develop. It also binds to certain components of the nucleus of the cell – chromatin, histones and small nuclear nucleoproteins – with reports also of binding to adhesive molecules of fibronectin and laminin types, and certain biological polycations. CRP is the most evaluated acute phase reactant in rheumatology. It has a very low basal serum concentration with rapid and prominent increase within a few hours after inflammatory or infective stimulation and short half-life of less than 24 hours.

Crepitus An audible phenomenon created during movement of joints or tendons. A coarse crepitus is present in degenerative disease involving a major joint, a fine crepitus is present in patello-femoral arthritis; a subcutaneous crepitus is present on the chest and neck, for example, in a superficial emphysema following a traumatic pneumothorax.

CREST (Calcinosis, Raynaud Esophagus, Sclerodactyly, Telangiectasiae) syndrome → see Systemic sclerosis (SSc)

Creutzfeldt-Jakob disease (CJD) A disorder elicited by prions, belonging to the prionoses. In the past, there was an erroneous assumption that it was caused by unconventional ("slow") viruses. The disease occurs in three forms: hereditary, spontaneous (sporadic) and the new variant CJD. The hereditary form is transmitted from the parent to their child and represents approximately 15% of all CJD cases. It is caused by point mutation in the gene for the prion protein. The sporadic form of CJD occurs in mid and late life (50 to 70 years), and has a rapid progression. Dementia and myoclonus (brief muscle spasms) are typical symptoms and signs. The new variant CJD has only recently been recognised. It has been demonstrated that it is caused by the same prion that had caused the epidemic of bovine spongiform encephalopathy (BSE) in Great Britain (first recognized in November 1986). The disease affects younger age categories (18 to 38 years) and ends in death usually within one year. It has developed by the breakthrough of the interspecies barrier most probably by consuming food prepared from inoculated cows. In the years 1996 up to 2004, some 120 young people died from the new variant CJD in Great Britain alone.

Crosslinked telopeptides of type I collagen The C-terminal (CTX) fragment of type I collagen stems from cross-linked C-terminal telopeptides of two α1 chains of type I collagen with the helical area of either the α1 or α2 chain from another collagen molecule and is released during bone resorption. This fragment is probably bone-specific because it contains transverse bonds of a mature collagen that cannot be found in type I collagen from other sources.

One C-terminal propeptide is released from each collagen molecule built into the collagen fibril. It is released as an intact subunit with a molecular weight of 100 kDa.

The N-terminal (NTX) connection of the N-terminal telopeptide with the helical area of another collagen molecule is another site of deoxypyridinoline and pyridinoline production in the bone collagen. These N-telopeptides contain more deoxypyridinoline compared to the C-telopeptides. A substantial advantage of methods assessing the pyridinoline crosslinks is that these fragments carry information of the collagen from which they are cleaved. Using this method to measure urinary pyridinolines, the peptides derived from the type II collagen (for example in the rheumatoid arthritis and osteoarthrosis) should not cross-react. Currently, measurement of serum NTX is preferred in order to eliminate the biovariability of urinary assays. Furthermore, other factors including an incomplete urine collection is excluded.

The degradation products of collagen – NTX and CTX – significantly increase in conditions with accelerated bone turnover, especially in prevailing osteoresorption. They are utilised mainly in the follow-up of efficacy of the antiresorptive treatment.

Crow-Fukase-Takatsuki syndrome → see POEMS syndrome

Cryoglobulins They can be classified into three groups:

Type I – consists of cryoglobulins formed by a single cryoprecipitable immunoglobulin of IgG, IgA or IgM class without known antibody-mediated immunity; rarely this can involve monoclonal light chains (Bence-Jones protein),

Type II – mixed cryoglobulins consisting of a monoclonal immunoglobulin, most frequently IgM (but sometimes IgG or IgA), with antiglobulin activity against the polyclonal IgG,

Type III – mixed cryoglobulins consisting of polyclonal immunoglobulins of one class or sometimes with non-immunoglobulin molecules, for example C3 or lipoproteins.

The mixed cryoglobulins form the circulating immune complexes and often induce symptoms of systemic vasculitis. They occur in systemic lupus erythematosus, Sjögren's syndrome, polyarteritis nodosa and other autoimmune, infectious and lymphoproliferative disorders. Mixed cryoglobulinaemia was usually linked with the hepatitis B virus infection. More recent studies have demonstrated a strong association with chronic hepatitis C virus infection (30–98%) (Della Rossa et al. 2008). The absolute IgG concentration in the cryoglobulin may be a useful indicator in the diagnosing and monitoring of the disease, unlike the qualitative cryocrit test, which only gives limited information.

Crystalline-induced arthropathy A group of inflammatory arthritides caused by intra-articular crystals, such as urate (gout), calcium pyrophosphate (chondrocalcinosis or pseudo-gout), and sometimes other crystals such as calcium hydroxyapatite and calcium oxalate. Diagnosis may be suspected clinically by the history and distribution of joint involvement, but can only be confirmed by joint aspiration and a combination of light and polarised microscopy of the synovial fluid.

CTX → see Crosslinked telopeptides of type I collagen, Markers of osteoresorption, Peptide fragments of collagen type I (NTX, CTX)

Cyclooxygenase The cyclooxygenase enzyme consists of two related isoforms that are about 60% homologous (Figure 1). Both isoforms convert arachidonic acid to endoperoxides (PGH), thereby creating prostaglandins (PG), thromboxanes and prostacyclin. The first isoenzyme (COX-1) was identified a long time ago, when it was found to be the target site of the effect of non-steroidal anti-inflammatory drugs (NSAIDs). The second isoenzyme COX-2 is also sensitive to NSAIDs. Recently a third isoform COX-3 has been detected that is derived from a gene for COX-1. The COX-3 differs from COX-1 and COX-2 in that it is more sensitive to the inhibitory action of paracetamol.

The constitutive isoform of cyclooxygenase (COX-1) is found in almost all cells and fulfils the role of an enzyme responsible for maintenance of homeostasis at the cellular level. It facilitates the mechanisms for protection of gastrointestinal mucosa, perfusion of renal parenchyma, homeostasis on the level of vascular endothelium and platelet function. The inducible isoform COX-2 is present exclusively at the site of inflammation or

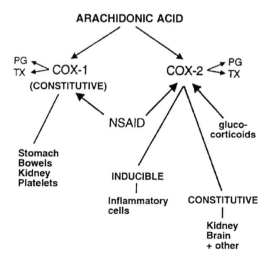

Figure 1. Cyclooxygenase isoenzymes

damaged tissue. It is released after stimulation of the cell by different factors, cytokines and other mediators of the inflammation. The COX-2-dependent prostaglandins can also have physiological roles in certain tissues, especially in the brain, in renal perfusion and glomerular hemodynamics, functions of the uterus, responses to stressful stimuli and in the physiology of embryonic membranes. NSAIDs have been shown to suppress both COX isoforms, i.e. COX-2 and COX-1. They differ, however, in terms of their COX-2/COX-1 inhibition ratio, and so have been labelled as COX-1-specific inhibitors, non-specific COX-2/COX-1 inhibitors, selective COX-2 inhibitors and specific COX-2 inhibitors, the so-called coxibs. COX-1 does not participate in the pathogenesis of inflammation and the onset of pain.

Cyclophosphamide N,N-bis(2-chloroethyl)-tetrahydro-2H-1,3,2-oxazaphosphorin-2-amino-2-oxide, an alkylating agent that after binding to DNA changes its structure, and consequently its properties. In addition to anti-neoplastic action, it possesses significant immunosuppressive effects, predominantly against B-lymphocytes and antibody production.

Dosage and clinical efficacy: It is an alkylating agent that has the ability to interfere with the nucleic acid molecules. Due to its rather high toxicity, it is not a first line treatment, and the risk-to-benefit ratio should be very carefully assessed before proposing it for treatment. It is used most frequently in the treatment of severe forms of systemic vasculitis such as microscopic polyarteritis, Wegener's granulomatosis, and severe systemic lupus erythematosus and now less frequently in rheumatoid vasculitis. The usual initial oral daily low dose regime lies between 1–2.5 mg/kg/day. Once a clinical effect has been achieved (usually after 6 months) the dose is reduced to a maintenance dose of 0.5 mg/kg/day or changed to an alternative less toxic immunosuppressive agent, such as Azothiaprine. Intermittent pulse intravenous treatment is given at doses of 500–1500 mg/m^2/month. The treatment often takes effect between three and six months after oral administration; earlier with parenteral administration. The disadvantage of pulse treatment is a higher number of infectious complications and increased incidence of malignant diseases. A full blood count should be assessed continuously – every 14 days for the first two months, and then every 6 to 8 weeks. When thrombocytopenia or leukopenia occurs, the dose should be reduced, and treatment discontinued if no improvement. It is advisable to monitor the hepatic transaminases every eight weeks and perform regular urinalysis, especially looking for haematuria (a sign of haemorrhagic cystitis).

The most frequent adverse events of cyclophosphamide treatment are nausea and vomiting. Their incidence rises in proportion to the dose, but can be effectively suppressed by ondansetron – a serotonin antagonist. A mild elevation of hepatic transaminases and leukopenia often occur due to bone marrow suppression. In long-term daily use of cyclophosphamide, hemorrhagic cystitis can develop. The acrolein toxicity can be decreased by a high fluid intake and concomitant administration of compounds containing sulfhydryl groups such as sodium 2-mercaptoethansulfonate (MESNA).

Cyclosporin (Ciclosporin) (CyA) A fungal cyclic peptide consisting of 11 amino acid units. The first cyclosporins were derived from the fungal strain *Tolypocladium inflatum* isolated at the turn of 1969 and 1970. Nowadays, however, cyclosporins represent relatively common secondary metabolites of the soil fibrous fungi *Acremonium, Aphanocladium, Beauveria, Fusarium, Verticillium, Tolypocladium* and *Trichoderma*. It has been the most important immunosuppressive agent used as a treatment in clinical medicine, especially transplantology, but also in the treatment of various autoimmune disorders. Its primary mode of action is to bind to cyclophilin causing blockade of IL-2 production and IL-2R expression by T-lymphocytes.

Clinical efficacy: Cyclosporin (A) is used in the treatment of rheumatoid arthritis (RA), either as monotherapy or as part of combination treatment. It is not considered a first-line treatment of RA. Its efficacy in monotherapy is comparable to the other disease modifying anti-rheumatic drugs (DMARDs) such as oral and parenteral gold compounds, antimalarials and sulfasalazine, though it is limited by a narrow therapeutic versus toxicity ratio. The slowing down of the radiological progression of bone erosions has so far not been conclusively confirmed, though there are several studies showing positive evidence of this effect (Zeidler et al. 1998, Forre et al. 1994, Ferraccioli et al. 1997).

Dosage: In the treatment of RA the dosage of CyA is in the range of 2.5–4.0 mg/kg/day, with initiation at the lower dose. CyA is administered in divided dose twice a day, usually with a meal. When necessary, the dose is gradually increased by 0.5 mg/kg/day up to a maximum dose of 4 mg/kg/day. If there is no benefit after using the maximum dose for six months, treatment should be discontinued.

In the course of treatment blood pressure and the serum creatinine level are monitored. If blood pressure rises or the serum creatinine level becomes increased by 30% compared with the pre-treatment value, the dose should be decreased or treatment discontinued.

Adverse effects of CyA treatment:

renal complications: increase in serum creatinine, tubular atrophy, interstitial fibrosis, arterial hypertension,

consequences of immunosuppression: recurrent infection, risk of malignancy,

other: hepatotoxicity, gastrointestinal disturbances, hypertrichosis, gingival hyperplasia, hyperkalaemia.

Cyriax method An exercise of applied and functional anatomy in which assessment of body movements indicates where lesions lie. First described by James Cyriax (1905–1985, Orthopaedic Surgeon in England) as "the method of systematic examination of the moving parts by selective tension".

Cytokines An extremely large group of glycoproteins or proteins that are used in the body as signalling compounds. They affect the direction, intensity and duration of immune and inflammatory reactions, as well as other physiological and pathophysiological manifestations of the cells in a paracrine, autocrine or endocrine way. When they act preferentially within the immune system, they are referred to as immunokines; if their primary target is the central nervous system, they are referred to as neurokines. Cytokines are interconnected in the network responsible for intercellular communication within the nervous system, as well as for information exchange between the immune system and other systems in the body. Cytokines include lymphokines, interleukins, interferons, tumour necrosis factors, colony stimulating factors, transforming growth factors, polypeptide growth factors, chemokines (interkines), stress proteins and others.

Cytophilic antibodies Antibodies that bind to the surface of cells through Fc-receptors and not through their own binding sites. Similarly IgE can bind IgE antibodies to the surface of mast cells and basophils through high affinity receptors for the Fc fragment. After such binding, they still have a free binding site available for the specific antigen epitope.

Cytotaxins Chemotactic factors (chemotaxins) are compounds inducing the chemotactic movement of cells (chemotaxy). This movement can be positive (cells moving towards the source of cytotaxins, i.e. in the direction of rising cytotaxin concentrations), or negative (cells moving in the direction of falling cytotaxin concentrations).

Cytotoxic antibodies Antibodies that specifically react to superficial epitopes of target cells and thereby activate complement. Subsequently, the activated complement damages or even lyses the cell marked in this manner. Cytotoxic antibodies (particularly IgG) may be involved in cell impairment by the ADCC (Antibody dependent cell-mediated cytotoxicity) mechanism.

Dactylitis → see Psoriatic arthritis (PsA)

DAS 28 (**disease activity score** based on a 28 joint assessment)

The disease activity of rheumatoid arthritis can be quantified by official criteria of the European League Against Rheumatism (EULAR), being referred to as DAS (disease activity score). After assessment of 28 tender joints (0–28), 28 swollen joints (0–28), the erythrocyte sedimentation rate, and a patient global assessment (GA) by a Visual Analogue Scale (0–100), the DAS 28 is calculated is as follows: DAS 28 = $0.56\sqrt{t28} + 0.28\sqrt{sw28} + 0.7\ln(ESR) + 0.014GA$ (t – tender joints, sw – swollen joints). The DAS 28 activity evaluation: remission DAS $28<2.6$, low activity DAS $>2.6<3.2$, medium activity DAS$>3.2<5.1$, high activity DAS $28\geq5.1$.

DAS calculation:

Automatic at *http://www.das-score.nl/www.das-score-nl/DAS28calc.htm*

In Excel format at *http://www.das-score.nl/www.das-score-nl/DAS28ne.xls*

de Quervain's stenosing tenosynovitis Roughening of the tendon sheaths of the extensor pollicis longus and brevis muscles and abductor pollicis longus muscle, which evoke pain radiating to the thumb and forearm. The pain worsens when grasping or squeezing the hand. Operative solution – removal of the roughened tendon sheath.

Defect of vitamin D metabolism Hypocalcaemia is not frequent in vitamin D deficiency as a secondary increase in parathormone (PTH) usually retains the serum calcium level within the normal range. However, it is possible in long-term vitamin deficiency and can lead to clinical rickets in children. Failure to supplement vitamin D in a breast-fed child along with other risk factors (insufficient calcium intake in food) may lead to

such a situation. Apart from the typical skeletal X-ray changes, other findings include a high serum PTH level, hypophosphataemia and increased serum alkaline phosphatase. The 25-OH vitamin D level is very low. Deficiency of the active metabolite of vitamin D may also occur in severe chronic liver disease, chronic renal impairment or with certain anticonvulsant drugs. Hereditary defects of vitamin D metabolism include vitamin D-dependent rickets type I with 25-OH vitamin D-1 alpha hydroxylase deficiency or hereditary resistance to calcitriol (previously referred to as vitamin D-dependent rickets type II), which represents the group of rare diseases with a functional defect of vitamin D receptors.

Deficiency of C1-inhibitor This is expressed as hereditary angioedema. This deficiency is inherited as an autosomal dominant trait and there are three mechanisms inducing it: decreased level of C1-INH (partial deficiency), malfunction of its molecule (a mutation in the relevant gene) or the presence of autoantibodies against C1-INH.

Deficiency of complement The deficiency can involve individual components, factors or regulatory glycoproteins of the complement system (C). The vast majority of primary deficiencies are inherited as an autosomal recessive trait. The absence of the first components participating in the classical activation pathway (C1q, C1r, C4 and C2) is expressed as a systemic lupus erythematosus-like syndrome. The deficiency of C3, leading to chronic pyogenic infections, belongs to the most severe deficiencies. The deficiency of the terminal components (C5 to C9) is manifested by increased susceptibility to infections induced predominantly by *Neisseria gonorrhoeae* and *Neisseria meningitidis*. The most severe deficiency of regulatory glycoproteins is the deficiency of C1-inhibitor with angioedema as a consequence, and also DAF or MACIF deficiencies, which cause the development of paroxysmal nocturnal haemoglobinuria.

Deficiency of IgA, selective This is one of the most frequent selective immunoglobulin deficiencies (involving individual immunoglobulin classes or subclasses). Approximately 0.2% of clinically healthy blood donors have a significantly decreased level of IgA in the serum and mucosal secretion. The situation becomes critical when the concentration of serum IgA drops below 1 mg/L. These patients suffer from recurrent respiratory, gastrointestinal and genitourinary tract infections. In addition they are prone to early-type allergic reactions, such as food allergies or atopic bronchial asthma. Treatment with an intravenous immunoglobulin preparation containing IgA is contraindicated due to the possibility of developing an anaphylactic shock. In some patients with IgA deficiency, it is possible to choose a cautious treatment approach by influencing mucosal immunity, where IgA plays an important role (autovaccination, or the administration of bacterial lysates).

Deficiency of phagocytosis Inefficient function of professional phagocytes expressed predominantly as an increased susceptibility to infectious diseases. It is divided into a primary deficiency that is caused by abnormal or missing relevant genes, and secondary deficiency that can be induced physiologically (infants and elderly) through poor nutrition, harmful factors of the external environment, various disorders or the toxic effect of xenobiotics, including drugs. The most important of the primary defects of phagocytosis include: chronic granulomatous disease, leukocyte adhesion deficiency (LAD syndrome), Job's syndrome, Chédiak-Higashi syndrome, the deficiency of specific granules, myeloperoxidase deficiency, glucose-6-phosphate dehydrogenase deficiency and tuftsin deficiency.

Deformities These are often the result of rheumatic inflammatory and degenerative disorders. In rheumatoid arthritis there may be deformities of the hand and fingers (swan-neck deformity, boutonniere deformity, mallet-finger deformity, Z deformation of the thumb, flexion and subluxation deformities or ulnar deviation in the metacarpophalangeal (MCP) joints, bayonet position in the wrist, volar subluxation or luxation of the radiocarpal joint (drop hand).

A flexion and supination position of the forearm with limited movement in the proximal radio-ulnar joint.

An adduction deformity of the shoulder together with a cranial shift of the scapula.

An adduction, flexion and internal rotation deformity in the hip, Knee deformities such as genu varum or valgum, longitudinal and transverse flat-foot, hallux valgus, hammer toes, crossing toes.

Dendrites Thin branched projections arising from the body of the nerve cell. They serve as an input region for stimuli and transmission of electrical impulses to the cell body

Depo-medrone (Methylprednisolone) → see Glucocorticoids, Intraarticular glucocorticoid treatment

Dermatomyositis → see Idiopathic inflammatory myopathies (IIM), Non-inflammatory myopathies, Juvenile dermatomyositis (JDM)

DEXA → see DXA

Diabetes mellitus A metabolic disorder of glucose, lipids and proteins that occurs as a consequence of a relative or absolute lack of insulin, or its insufficient effect. In 1990 the WHO accepted a new classification, according to which diabetes has two basic types. Type I has two subtypes either immunologically conditioned or idiopathic. Insulin resistance or deficit prevails in type II. The other specific types of diabetes are genetic disturbance of β-cell function, genetic disturbances of the effect of insulin, disorders of the endocrine pancreas, endocrinopathies, diabetes induced by drugs and chemical agents and rare forms of immunologically conditioned diabetes.

Immunopathological mechanisms play an important role especially in type I diabetes. The immunogenetic predisposition is provided by an association with major histocompatibility leucocyte antigens HLA-DR3, HLA-DR4, HLA-DQ2 and HLA-DQ8.

Bone and joint manifestations of diabetes mellitus include specific arthropathy of the hands and feet, shoulder joints, spine, and osteopenia.

Arthropathy in the hands is characterised by:
- limitation of joint movement (LJM) – cheiroarthropathy,
- Dupuytren's contracture,
- tenosynovitis of the peritendons of I, III and IV fingers,
- diabetic sclerodactyly or scleroderma diabeticorum,
- carpal tunnel syndrome.

Affection of the foot:
- Charcot's osteoarthropathy,
- limited movement of the joint,

Affection of the shoulder:
- adhesive capsulitis, frozen shoulder syndrome,
- calcified periarthropathy,
- limited movement of the joint,
- generally, the joints are affected by limited movement, osteoarthrosis and chondrocalcinosis.

Changes to the spine:
- Increased susceptibility to DISH (diffuse idiopathic skeletal hyperostosis).
- neuropathic osteoarthropathy of Charcot's joint type.

Changes in bone mass:
- diabetic osteopathy.

Diacerein An acetylated (4,5-diacetyloxy-9, 10-dioxo-anthracene-2-carboxylic acid) form of rhein, an extract of rhubarb, is a drug used in osteoarthritis. Inhibition of the effect of interleukin-1 and other proinflammatory cytokines is its most important action. The preparation is encapsulated in a gelatinous capsule of 50 mg each. It is administered twice a day after food for at least 6 months.

Diadynamic currents (Bernard) Single- or double-phase, one-way connection, modified low-frequency (50–100 Hz) sinus currents applied in various modalities. They have analgesic and hyperaemic effects. A simple impulse current (MF-monophase) has analgesic and vasodilatatory effects. Currents shifting in short periods (CP) have a spasmolytic effect. Currents shifting in long periods (LP) have mainly an analgesic effect. Diadynamic currents are used for acute rather than chronic pain.

Dialysis associated osteoarthropathy A group of musculoskeletal diseases developing in relation to chronic renal failure and chronic dialysis treatment.

Diathermy A treatment with high-frequency currents where the electrical energy is converted in the body to heat (CAVE: pacemaker and metallic implants).

Types of diathermy:
1. *short-wave:* a wavelength of 22.1 metres (deep heating in the condenser or induced field),
2. *microwave:* a wavelength of 12.5 centimetres (relatively better heating of the muscles; not used in children due to the possibility of damage to the growth cartilage and the lens),
3. *ultra short-wave:* a wavelength of 69 centimetres (focusable electromagnetic wave). It has the same indication as for short-wave diathermy, in terms of effects it belongs to thermotherapy.

The shorter the wavelength, the more uniform the heating of the tissue. The application of diathermy induces deep production of heat in a circumscribed region that is expressed by deep hyperaemia leading to increased tissue metabolism and relaxation of striated and smooth muscle spasm. In patients with rheumatoid arthritis, caution needs to be taken due to the possibility of inflammation outbreak (overheating). The main fields of indication for diathermy are osteoarthrosis

D

(except for activated osteoarthrosis), fibrositis, enthesiopathy and chronic periarthritis.

Diffuse cutaneous SSc (dcSSc) → see
Systemic sclerosis (SSc)

Diffuse Idiopathic Skeletal Hyperostosis (DISH; ankylosing hyperostosis; Forestier's disease)
A chronic skeletal disorder of unknown aetiology occurring in middle and later years. The characteristic feature is massive new bone formation in the shape of calcification and ossification of the spinal ligaments, predominantly in the region of the anterior longitudinal ligament causing bony ankylosis of the anterolateral horns of the spine, more frequently on the right and anterior aspects, with significant ossification. Involvement of the peripheral skeleton is generally expressed by extensive enthesopathies. Its aetiology is unknown; several authors classify it amongst the degenerative disorders of the skeleton, whilst others assign it to a metabolic or endocrine disorder. The American College of Rheumatology put it amongst the disorders of bone and cartilage. As a distinct disease, it has only appeared in literature in recent years; previously it was usually mentioned in relation to the differential diagnosis of ankylosing spondylitis and osteoarthrosis.

Clinical symptoms and signs:
- onset of clinical symptoms usually after the 40th birthday,
- centripetal type of obesity,
- insidious, often asymptomatic limitation of spinal movements,
- enthesopathic pain in the periphery (heels, knees, elbows and shoulders),
- neurological signs of compression,
- radiographic evidence of extensive hyperostotic ossifications.

Digitus rigidus → see Toe swelling/deformity and associated diseases

DIL → see Drug-induced Lupus

Disability
A condition or function judged to be significantly physically or mentally impaired relative to the usual standard of an individual of their group. It may be reversible. Refer to "ICF classification" for newer information.

Disease-Modifying Anti Rheumatic Drugs (DMARDs)
Disease-modifying antirheumatic drugs (DMARDs) or slow-acting antirheumatic drugs (SAARDs) are a group of drugs with the potential to suppress disease activity and thus reduce or prevent joint damage and preserve joint function. They were first used in rheumatoid arthritis, but are now indicated in most immunologically-mediated chronic joint inflammatory diseases (psoriatic arthritis, juvenile idiopathic arthritis, etc.). They were initially only used in well established disease, but modern practice is to introduce them very early (3–6 months) to gain the most benefit. DMARDs include methotrexate, sulphasalazine, leflunomide, azathioprine, myocrisin and hydroxychloroquine (see in relevant sections of the text). They require careful monitoring under the supervision of a rheumatology unit to ensure that the effective dosage regime is reached and proper monitoring for toxicity.

Diseases causing diffuse oedema
Diffuse lower extremity oedema may be due to arthritis such as traumatic arthritis, infectious arthritis, gout, seronegative spondyloarthritis and rheumatoid arthritis. Other causes include Sudeck's syndrome, diabetic arthropathy – occurs in poorly controlled diabetics in which leg or foot ulcerations and osteolytic changes on the bones can be observed. Oedema can be caused by lymphoedema or cardiac, renal, hypoalbuminaemia or other aetiology. Among endocrinological disorders, it may be present in myxoedema.

Diseases causing foot oedema: conditions with foot deformity – pes equinus, pes equinovarus, congenital pes varus, pes valgus, pes calcaneovalgus, pes excavatus, pes paralyticus, pes planovalgus.

Also tarsal tunnel syndrome may be involved (see below) in conditions mentioned above.

DISH → see Diffuse Idiopathic Skeletal Hyperostosis (DISH; ankylosing hyperostosis; Forestier's disease)

DMARDs → see Disease-Modifying Anti Rheumatic Drugs (DMARDs)

DNA antibodies Antibodies directed against DNA form a heterogeneous group of antibodies directed against various antigenic determinants on the DNA molecule. Antibodies against double-stranded DNA (dsDNA) are diagnostically specific (97%) for systemic lupus erythematosus (SLE), while antibodies against single-stranded DNA (ssDNA) are present in the course of various diseases, such as rheumatoid arthritis, Sjögren's syndrome, progressive systemic sclerosis, drug induced lupus, chronic active hepatitis or infection. Anti-dsDNA was first described by a number of authors in 1957. A positive correlation between these antibodies and the presence of nephritis in the course of SLE was observed. Circulating anti-dsDNA belongs to IgM, IgG and rarely IgA classes; IgG antibodies are more significant than IgM as their presence correlates with the activity of the disease and with the severity of nephritis. Such a correlation can be found also among antibodies which fix and activate the complement, particularly IgG anti-dsDNA. The pathogenicity of anti-dsDNA depends on their various physical properties. Although single assessment of anti-dsDNA is highly diagnostic, long-term monitoring of these antibody levels is recommended for prognostic purposes, as increasing titres of anti-dsDNA indicate increasing disease activity and may predict disease flare.

DNA (Deoxyribonucleic Acid) The genetic material of all cells and many viruses. The DNA molecule is a dextrorotatory double-helix polymere consisting of two polynucleotide chains interconnected between the purine and pyrimidine bases by a hydrogen bond. DNA contains the two purine bases adenine (A) and guanine (G) and the two pyrimidine bases cytosine (C) and thymine (T); furthermore, 2-deoxyribose and phosphoric acid. In addition to these main bases, it can also contain the so-called minority bases as base modifications with low or no gene expression. The adenine is always linked by the hydrogen bond to the thymine, cytosine to guanine. The presence of complementary pairs of bases in the DNA double-helix enables the existence of a regular structure, because all pairs of bases have the same size. The DNA molecule does not contain all four bases in the same molar proportions. Their contents can be expressed by the following relation $A/T = G/C \approx 1$. The sequence of the bases in the chain is not random, as it is defined and creates the genetic information whose carrier is the DNA. More than 90% of DNA is located in the nucleus of the cell, as a component of chromosomes, while part of it lies in the structure of the cell and mitochondria. The mutation of individual genes (sections) of DNA can lead to the development of genetically determined diseases. In 1953 James Watson, Francis Crick and Maurice Wilkins received the Nobel Prize for the discovery of DNA. An understanding of its structure enabled other discoveries, leading to the development of genetic engineering, reliable identification of an individual on the basis of DNA, but also to the successful mapping the whole human DNA (genome).

Dougados functional index A functional index completed by the patient of 20 questions using activities of daily living (e.g. put on your shoes, breathe deeply), most commonly in patients with spondyloarthropathy. Each question is answered by either yes, yes but with difficulty, or no. It has largely been superseded by the Bath AS functional index (BASFI).

Dougados' system of assessment of SpondyloArthritis (SpA) The system consists of two parts:
1. *articular index* Examined by a physician (pressure on the thorax from the front and from the side, maximum flexion in the hip joint, a pressure on the middle part of gluteus maximus muscles, spine rotation while sitting with the upper limbs crossed

– pressure pain is evaluated in four degrees).

2. *functional index* Evaluation of the ability to perform certain daily activities (Dougados functional index, DFI).

Down's syndrome

Caused by duplication of part of the entire 21st chromosome (trisomy), which manifests in mental retardation, disturbances of immunity and congenital heart disease. The genes for certain proteins important for the immune and nervous systems (CuZn-superoxide dismutase, β-chain of the leukoadhesive integrins, interferon receptors, etc.) are located in the chromosomal region 21q22. The increased expression of these proteins participate in the underdevelopment of the thymus and abnormal maturation of T-lymphocytes that results in their defective function leading to an increased risk of infections, an increased incidence of malignancies and autoimmune disorders (especially hypothyroidism). Patients can also suffer from hypermobility of the joints and atlanto-axial instability with spinal cord compression.

D-penicillamine

A chelating agent which binds copper and other metals. This ability is utilised in the treatment of Wilson's disease, where copper accumulates in tissues. Based on the assumption that it could dissociate immune complexes by disrupting the disulphide bonds between the chains of the immunoglobulin molecule, it was introduced in the treatment of rheumatoid arthritis (RA) many years ago, but is now rarely used. It has also been used in the treatment of systemic sclerosis, though clinical efficacy now appears poor.

Pharmacokinetics: After oral administration, it is detected in the plasma as early as 20 minutes. The maximum plasma concentration is reached in 1.5 to 4 hours. After oral administration 40–70% of the drug is absorbed. Its bioavailability can be significantly decreased by concomitant food intake, antacids and iron preparations. It binds to albumin in the circulation and is largely excreted in the urine within 12 hours.

Efficacy: D-Penicillamine is used in the treatment of RA, juvenile idiopathic arthritis and systemic sclerosis, but is now recognised as only a very mild disease modifying anti-rheumatic drug, and has a high incidence of side effects. Its onset of action takes many months as the dosage regime is start low and increase slowly. It is initiated at 125–250 mg daily in the morning on a empty stomach with increases of 125 mg daily every 4 to 6 weeks to a dose of 500–750mg daily. In systemic sclerosis, it has mild effects in retarding the progress of skin thickening and survival, but usually at a dose of 750–1,500 mg daily. Full blood count and urinalysis are necessary every 1–2 weeks for the first 2 months, then every 4–6 weeks thereafter.

Adverse events:

Mucocutaneous:
- mouth ulcers, stomatitis,
- pruritus, rashes,
- hair loss, dermatitis, pemphigus,
- cutis laxa (elastolysis),*
- elastosis perforans serpiginosa.*

Pulmonary:
- acute pneumonitis,
- acute alveolar haemorrhage,
- bronchiolitis obliterans.

Autoimmune disorders:
- myasthenia gravis,
- polymyositis/dermatomyositis,
- drug-induced lupus erythematosus,
- pemphigoid, pemphigus,
- Goodpasture's syndrome.

Renal:
- proteinuria, haematuria,
- glomerulonephritis.

Haematological:
- thrombocytopenia, leukopenia,
- aplastic anaemia.

Gastrointestinal:
- nausea, loss of taste,
- hepatitis,
- cholestasis.

Gynaecomastia

* detected in patients with Wilson's disease and cystinuria treated with high doses of D-Penicillamine

Drug-induced Lupus

Many drugs, particularly those from the groups of cardiac antiarrhythmics, antihypertensive agents and anticonvulsive drugs may evoke a clinical condition similar to lupus in some patients. More recently, it has been caused by the administration of biologic therapy. Such a clinical condition is called drug-induced lupus (DIL, sometimes also drug-related lupus) and usually recovers after discontinuation of the inducing drug. DIL constitutes less than 10% of diagnosed lupus. Compared to systemic lupus erythematosus, DIL is more frequent in males than in females.

Clinical symptoms:
- most frequent: arthralgia, myalgia, weakness, fever, pleuropericarditis
- less frequent: skin and mucosal symptoms, haematological abnormalities (anaemia, leukopenia, thrombocytopenia),
- rare: central nervous system impairment, nephritis.

Drug induced muscular diseases → see
Non-inflammatory myopathies

Drug-induced Osteoporosis
Several drugs may influence adversely bone turnover and bone mineral density thereby increasing the risk of fracture, when taken in the long term. Most frequently, they are glucocorticoids, heparin, anticonvulsants, high doses of medrooxyprogesterone acetate, and high doses of thyroid hormones.

DXA – Morphometric lateral scans
The newer DEXA devices can perform rapid lateral scans of the thoracic and lumbar spines. This allows evaluation of changes in height and shape of individual vertebrae. These scans are evaluated by special software for measurement of vertebral body height. The differences in the measured height of vertebra in the dorsal, medial and anterior part of its body can indicate wedging, and thus a fracture. Thus the scan enables an evaluation of vertebral fractures at the same time as BMD measurement without the conventional lateral X-ray. Reduction of

the height of the vertebral body without a history of major trauma belongs to the most important risk factors of development of another fracture and independently of the measured BMD. With the combination of BMD and assessment of vertebral morphometry, we may achieve better selection of the patients with a higher risk of fracture. The relatively short duration of the scan and low radiation dose and BMD measurement at the same time are the advantages of this method. The capital cost of the newer densitometers with the necessary software, the not infrequently worse projection of the vertebrae, especially in the upper thoracic part of the spine compared to a classical X-ray, are its disadvantages.

Dynamic aerobic exercise
Greatly increases muscle strength and stamina, as well aerobic capacity compared with a static exercise. In rheumatoid arthritis, muscle strength and stamina are affected by age, concomitant diseases and functional disability.

Dysesthesia
Unpleasant, abnormal sensations occurring spontaneously or after a stimulus.

Dystrophia musculorum progressiva
One form of hereditary non-inflammatory disease of the muscles. Onset can occur in childhood or adulthood. It predominantly affects proximal muscles (shoulder and hip girdles) in a symmetrical fashion which as they weaken, lead to a "duck" gait and climbing the thighs on straightening from a kneesbend. There is a detectable myogenic lesion on EMG (electromyography). The serum creatine kinase and aldolase levels are increased and creatinuria is present. Biopsy confirms a non-inflammatory myogenic atrophy of the muscles with fibre degeneration.

Treatment: There is no effective treatment, but careful physiotherapy. Anabolic hormones and vitamin E are sometimes given.

E

Early T lymphocyte activator 1 → see Osteopontin (OPN)

Ehlers-Danlos' Syndrome (EDS) A group of hereditary connective tissue disorders, characterised by hyperelasticity and fragility of the skin and hypermobility of the joints. Various forms differ by their clinical picture and genetic background. In individual patients, EDS has a very diverse and variable disease severity leading to a highly variable clinical picture. The frequency of EDS is 1:5000 live-born in both genders and all ethnic groups.

Clinical symptoms and signs: The hyperelasticity skin can be folded and distended up to several centimetres. After release, it returns to its original state. Even mild trauma of the skin usually leads to superficial lacerations. Metacarpophalangeal joints and other parts of the body where the bones protrude clearly under the skin are often covered by scars. There is a tendency towards the development of haematomas and pigmentation of the scars. Grape-like swellings, referred to as molluscoid pseudotumors, may occur in these regions. On the calves and forearms small, hard mobile subcutaneous nodules may be detected on palpation. To a varying degree there is joint laxity, excessive movements of the joints and orthopaedic complications are common especially in people with extreme hypermobility. Dermatological, cardiovascular, gastrointestinal, neurological, ophthalmological, urological, respiratory and dental abnormalities may also occur. Dissection of the aorta, rupturing of major arteries, gastrointestinal bleeding and perforations (see below) have all been documented as complications of vascular EDS.

The fragility of tissues and the tendency towards bleeding can complicate surgical procedures and labour. These problems can be minimised by accurate diagnosis of EDS forms.

Eiselsberg's phenomenon → see Acute shoulder pain

Electromyography (EMG) A recording of the electric potentials from striated muscles. The potentials are recorded with surface electrodes, or more accurately by direct needling. The potentials are amplified by the EMG device and displayed on a screen. EMG is used in the diagnosis of peripheral motor neurone lesions. In rheumatology, it is used in the diagnosis of tunnel syndromes and myopathies, such as myositis, where the potentials are narrower, have smaller amplitude and are polyphasic. In myopathic syndromes, the potentials are narrower and smaller, but the velocity is normal. In myasthenia gravis, the amplitude and frequency of the potentials decrease with repeated voluntary contractions.

Electrotherapy The use of various forms of electrical energy in the treatment of diseases, mainly by physiotherapists. A direct current, variously shaped alternating current impulses of low and middle frequencies, high-frequency field and high-frequency ultrasound, laser and transcutaneous nerve stimulation can all be used. Electrotherapy has analgesic, myorelaxing and vasodilatatory effects, as well as stimulating local and general metabolism. Electrical energy is also used in electrodiagnostics.

ELISA (Enzyme-Linked ImmunoSorbent Assay) ELISA is a two step biochemical technique used mainly in immunology to quantify the level of an antibody or an antigen in a sample. The antigen is immobilized on a solid support (usually a polystyrene microtitre plate) either non-specifically (via adsorption to the surface) or specifically (via capture by another antibody specific to the same antigen, in a "sandwich" ELISA). The sample (usually serum) is added and incubated allowing the formation of antibody-antigen immune complexes. A secondary antibody, which is linked to an enzyme through bioconjugation, is then added to link onto the primary antibody or to the antigen-antibody complex (sandwich principle) to determine its level. Between each step the plate is typically washed with a mild detergent solution to remove any proteins or antibodies that are not specifically bound. After the final wash step the plate is developed by adding an enzymatic substrate to produce a visible signal, which indicates the quantity of bound secondary antibody and indirectly the amount of antigen in the sample. Older ELISAs utilize chromogenic substrates, though newer assays employ fluorogenic substrates with much higher sensitivity. This is now a universal, efficient and automated technique employed in modern laboratories for detecting serum antibody levels.

Enteropathic arthritis (EA) Defined as arthritis induced by an intestinal disorder (ulcerative colitis, Crohn's disease), or as arthritis occurring concomitantly with the intestinal disorder. These are acute, recurrent oligo- or polyarthritis often following the inflammatory activity of the enteric disorder.
   Clinical symptoms and signs:
- peripheral arthritis, usually oligoarticular, asymmetric, with predilection the lower limb joints,
- frequent involvement of the axial skeleton in terms of sacroileitis and/or spondylitis,
- dactylitis (in post-enteric reactive arthritis),
- enthesitis,
- involvement of the skin and mucous membranes: iritis, erythema nodosum, pyoderma gangrenosum and other ocular involvement.

Eosinophilic fasciitis (Shulman's Syndrome) A disorder characterised by the sudden onset of painful swelling replaced later by a stiffness of the skin and dermis of the trunk and limbs. This condition is caused by inflammatory, fibrotic and sclerotic changes in the fascia of the adjacent muscle, fibrous sep-

ta of the subcutaneous adipose tissue lobules, or the deep dermis. The clinical picture is expressed by an orange peel appearance and rough surface to the affected skin. The uneven surface is caused by retraction of the adipose tissue septa. There may also be subcutaneous induration fixed to the deep tissues. In addition, there may be arthralgias, arthritis, joint contractures, tunnel compression syndromes, involvement of striated muscles, and occasionally interstitial pulmonary fibrosis and dysmotility of the oesophagus.

In laboratory tests, there is eosinophilia (more than 10% of the whole leukocyte count), especially at the onset of the disease. Generally, there is hypergammaglobulinaemia and increased erythrocyte sedimentation rate. Histological examination shows a picture of inflammatory changes in the cutaneous fascia. The disease generally has a benign course. Treatment usually only requires small doses of glucocorticosteroids and antimalarials, but with a severe disease, pulse corticosteroid treatment with cyclophosphamide may be necessary.

Epicondylitis humeri Painful insertions on the lateral (tennis elbow), or less frequently the medial (golfer's elbow), epicondyle of the humerus. Causes include posttraumatic and degenerative changes or splitting of the tendon; more rarely there are painful tendon insertions as part of a generalised rheumatic condition (fibrositis syndrome).

Epitheses Prostheses that cosmetically help to cover up a physical imperfection. They are mainly dental and ocular prostheses and breast implants. Their importance is to help eliminate any secondary mental consequences arising from aesthetically prominent damage.

Ergometry (bicycle, winch, treadmill) Exercise functional diagnostics dealing with the examination and assessment of the fitness and adaptation of the cardiorespiratory, metabolic and other physiological or pathophysiological function to various forms of exertion. The exercise treadmill test is used in the diagnosis of the severity of heart disease and allows modification of the treatment and rehabilitation regime. The most frequently used measure is cycle ergometry which allows graduated increase in the load, ECG recording and the measuring of blood pressure. In patients with rheumatic disorders, a regime of gradual and fixed aerobic training is utilised.

Ergotherapy Utilised with different specific activities for improving the functional condition of the patient. Working therapy is included.

Erosive osteoarthritis This primarily affects middle aged and older females and particularly affects the small joints of the hand. Initially, it manifests itself by DIP (distal interphalangeal) and PIP (proximal interphalangeal) joints inflammation and inflammation of the wrist; with subsequent deformities of these joints. The ESR or CRP may be slightly raised, and the latex fixation test may be weakly positive. The radiological picture shows arthritic changes of affected joints and the development of marginal erosions.

Treatment: Non-steroidal anti-inflammatory drugs; physiotherapy to help maintain the joint function and provide an analgesic effect.

Erythema nodosum (EN) → see Arthritis associated with erythema nodosum in the course of infection

Erythrocyte Sedimentation Rate (ESR) The simplest and commonest parameter of inflammation. It is best at assessing disease activity in certain diseases (polymyalgia rheumatica) and in systemic diseases of the connective tissue (systemic lupus erythematosus, systemic sclerosis, Sjögren's syndrome) in which C-reactive protein (CRP) is often not significantly increased. The combination of ESR and CRP is often very useful in assessing the disease activity of rheumatoid arthritis, ankylosing spondylitis and other diseases.

Erythromelalgia A disorder characterised by reddening of the skin on the limbs associated with burning pain and swelling. It can occur at any age, but most frequently in middle age; men are more often affected than women. The disease is either primary or secondary to disorders such as hypertension, polycythaemia vera, essential thrombocythaemia, angiitis obliterans or other vascular, haematological or neurological diseases. Certain drugs (nifedipine or bromocryptine) can also induce this disease. The aetiology of skin involvement is acute arterial hyperaemia.

Clinical symptoms and signs: A reddening in the region of the limbs dominates the clinical picture, with lower limbs being more frequently affected than upper limbs. The reddening is associated with a burning pain and swelling, and worsens when the limbs are exposed to heat or hang below the level of the body. On the other hand, exposing the limb to cold air or immersion into cold water, or limb elevation brings relief. The skin is sensitive to touch and hyperhidrosis is present.

Erythromelalgia should be distinguished from ischaemia in occlusive arterial disorders and from peripheral neuropathy. In contrast to these conditions, the peripheral pulses are easily felt, and neurological examination is normal.

ESR → see Erythrocyte Sedimentation Rate (ESR)

Essential mixed cryoglobulinemia (EMC) This is characterised by the presence of immunoglobulins that precipitate reversibly in the cold. These are cryoglobulins of types II and III (a mixture of at least two types of antibodies against a polyclonal IgG). The onset of the disease is in the 4th and 5th decade, more frequently in women.

Clinical symptoms and signs: Characteristic signs include purpura and ulcerations on the lower limbs, hepatosplenomegaly, proteinuria, microscopic haematuria, arthralgias or arthritis, and detection of the cryoglobulin on blood tests.

Etanercept A recombinant-DNA drug made by combining two proteins to a fusion protein which combines with the Fc fragment of human IgG on the soluble TNF receptor (sTNF-R) to block the effect of TNF. The majority of cells have two kinds of receptors for TNF, transmitting different signals: TNF-RI (55 kDa) and TNF-RII (75 kDa). The soluble forms of TNF-R are important inhibitors of TNF. In active rheumatoid arthritis (RA), soluble TNF-R is present in an increased concentration in the serum and synovial fluid, however, not even this increased concentration is able to neutralise the overproduction of TNF in high inflammatory activity. Etanercept is licensed for patients with severely active rheumatoid arthritis and psoriatic arthritis who have failed treatment with at least two disease-modifying antirheumatic drugs, including methotrexate. More recently, it has received a license for severe ankylosing spondylitis. Studies have demonstrated the increased efficacy when combined with methotrexate (MTX) (Weinblatt et al. 1999, Klareskog et al. 2004). The preparation is given subcutaneously at a dose of 25 mg twice or 50 mg once a week. It has a rapid onset of action with some patients reporting an improvement within two weeks of treatment. Recent studies have shown very good responses when etanercept is administered in early RA with severe disease activity inducing remission and preventing progression of radiological changes (Bathon et al. 2000, Emery et al. 2008).

Adverse events: Local skin reaction in the region of administration, increased susceptibility to infection of the upper respiratory tract, pneumonia, pyelonephritis, generalised sepsis, and reactivation of tuberculosis, leukocytoclastic vasculitis, positive anti ds-DNA antibodies, discoid lupus, hypertension, heart failure and demyelinating diseases.

Euro Quol questionnaire → see Instruments of assessing (health status measurements, outcome measurement)

Eutony method → see Exercise techniques

Exercising Classification according to target and effect

- *training strength* This constitutes short-term exercise with maximum exertion on the muscles, where mostly tonic fibres are being stretched. Includes resistance exercises – movements with a short trajectory, but a lot of strength.
- *training speed* Mainly phasic muscle fibres are activated here. A lot of output is achieved through a relatively small amount of work. With this exercise, the connective tissue accumulates and fat is not deposited in the muscle.
- *training endurance* This incorporates long-term exercises (work therapy) that do not require maximum muscle strength. They are frequently repeated and long-term.
- *training dexterity* This is also referred to as training neuromuscular coordination and is based on the principle that repetition leads to stabilisation of the dynamic stereotype. This includes the training of balance, as well as the training of all new and sophisticated movements.

Exercise techniques *Alexander technique* A technique that endeavours to produce normal body posture and movement habits in our everyday life and activities. It is a method of posture control that releases the increased tone of postural muscles and leads to easy natural body-control. It is targeted at people with bad body posture, back pain, migraine and living in stressful situations.

Feldenkrais technique An exercise technique that tries to uncover and prevent faulty movement patterns and substitute them gradually with a targeted mental activity, which is also accompanied by improvement of the psyche, positive thinking and mental health. The essence of the Feldenkrais method is to relearn the movements that we were able to perform in childhood (exercises in prone and supine position, crawling, walking on all fours). Regained mobility of the body also manifests in greater mental flexibility.

Rolf technique – rolfing By returning to a normal body posture and anatomically normal movement habits, this decreases or eliminates pain in the locomotor organs. It uses certain elements of yoga as well as techniques of deep massage of the connective tissues.

Eutony method It places the main emphasis on balanced muscle and mental tone (eutony), which stabilises itself by perception of the whole environment (smell, sound, touch, gravitation) and also by conscious perception of the movement of one's own body.

Pilates technique – The Pilates techniques place emphasis on proper performance of movement patterns together with quality breathing and principles of biofeedback. It is the training of deep-seated muscles creating a stabilisation system, the so called powerhouse – central muscle girdle. The aim is to acquire a synergy of transversus abdominis, multifidi, longissimus, iliocostalis and pelvic girdle muscles, posterior fibres of the obliquus internus muscle and diaphragm. Pilates called his system "The art of control". The system has six basic pillars: breathing, concentration, control, powerhouse, accuracy and fluency.

Extra-articular rheumatism (extra-articular rheumatism; rheumatism of soft tissues) Diseases affecting extra-articular soft tissues of the musculoskeletal system such as muscles, tendons, peritendons, tendinous insertions, fascia and bursae. The causes vary, but most frequently are due to local overuse, acute or repeated trauma and microtrauma during sporting activity or work, impaired movement coordination, incorrect gait, inflammation etc.

Extra-articular rheumatism has three forms:

generalised – fibromyalgia, chronic fatigue syndrome, myofascial syndrome,

regional – complex shoulder pain syndrome (humeroscapular periarthropathy) and hip (hip periarthropathy),

localised – bursitis, tendinitis etc.

F

Fab fragment A fragment (part) of the immunoglobulin molecule (usually IgG) able to bind to an antigen. It is formed by its proteolytic degradation and contains one binding site between the variable domains of the light and heavy chains.

F(ab)₂ fragment A double Fab fragment. It contains both binding sites of the original molecule. It is practically an immunoglobulin molecule without the C-terminal halves of the heavy chains that form the Fc-fragment.

Fabry's disease Belongs to the group of sphingolipidoses. It is an inherited X-linked recessive inborn error of the glycosphingolipid metabolism. It occurs due to a deficiency of the enzyme α-galactosidase A which is coded by a gene localised on the long arm of the X-chromosome (Xq22). As a consequence of this enzyme defect, a glycolipid known as globotriaosylceramide accumulates in blood vessels, other tissues and organs.
   Clinical symptoms and signs:
- episodes of painful acroparaesthesia,
- a significant reduction or absence of perspiration (anhidrosis),
- characteristic skin lesions (angiokeratomas),
- ocular changes,
- decreased activity of α-galactosidase A.

FACS (Fluorescence Activated Cell Sorter) A separator of fluorescence activated cells (flow cytometer). This device allows the analyses and division of a mixture of cells based on their diverse ability to bind a certain antibody labelled by a fluorescence dye. It is a technique referred to as flow cytometry (cytofluorography). The device has two detectors, one of which separates the cells according to the intensity of their fluorescence, and the other one according to their size. Newer cell analysers make it possible to use three differ-

ent fluorescence labelling of cells simultaneously, thereby giving the whole device a higher sorting ability. Using fluorescence labelled monoclonal antibodies against the differentiation antigen CD4, it is possible to determine, for example, the T-lymphocyte count in the peripheral blood; using the antibody against CD8, the cytotoxic T-lymphocyte count; using the antibody against CD3, the total T-lymphocyte count, etc.

Factor P → see Properdin

Familial hypocalciuric hypercalcaemia A condition characterised by mild hypercalcaemia with relative hypocalciuria (i.e. normal value of calcium excretion in the urine with serum hypercalcaemia). It is inherited as an autosomal dominant trait and is caused by mutation of the gene for CaSR (calcium-sensing receptor). Patients are usually asymptomatic, only rarely do they feel mild tiredness, weakness, lack of concentration or polydipsia. Recurrent pancreatitis, cholelithiasis, diabetes mellitus and myocardial infarction occur more frequently in the families. Bone turnover assessed by biochemical parameters can be slightly increased but bone mineral density is normal and patients are not more susceptible to fractures. The serum calcium level (total and ionised) is elevated throughout life with a tendency to fall with age. The serum magnesium can also be slightly elevated; conversely serum phosphate is slightly decreased. Renal function remains normal. Parathormone and calcitriol levels are within the physiological range, except in a minority of patients when it can be mildly elevated.

Familial Mediterranean fever (FMF) A genetically determined autosomal recessive disorder occurring only in certain ethnic groups such as Sephardi Jews, Anatolia Turks and Arabs. The gene, called MEFV, has been localised on chromosome 16. Typically the onset is in adolescence, usually before the age of 20.

Clinical symptoms and signs:
- recurrent attacks of fever, peritonitis, unilateral pleuritis and arthritis,
- periods of remission are usually asymptomatic,
- in untreated patients type AA amyloidosis may develop,
- regular treatment with colchicine prevents attacks and prevents the development of amyloidosis.

Farber's disease A disease belonging to the sphingolipidoses, with musculoskeletal manifestation, characterised by an accumulation of lipids in tissues due to an enzyme deficiency. Farber's lipogranulomatosis is an autosomal recessive defect caused by a deficiency of ceramidase, an enzyme which cleaves fatty acids from ceramide producing sphingosine. It appears in the neonatal period.

Clinical symptoms and signs: Red painful xanthomas form around joints and the peritendons, which lead to the development of joint and tendon contractures. Motor development retardation, macular degeneration and mental retardation are present. Patients die early. The primary cause of death is oedema in the laryngeal region and epiglottis leading to recurrent pulmonary infections. A mild form of this disease allows longer survival, and these children may present to a rheumatologist with their joint problems and mental retardation. There is no curative treatment.

Farnesyl diphosphate synthetase (FPPS) → see Bisphosphonates

Fc fragment A crystallisable fragment of the immunoglobulin molecule formed by its proteolytic fragmentation. It represents the C-terminal end of both heavy chains connected by a disulphide bond. It is unable to bind antigen, but has other important biological effects, the most important of which is its ability to bind to Fc-receptors.

Fc-receptors The binding sites for the Fc domains of the immunoglobulin molecules localised on surface of leukocytes and other cells. Every class of immunoglobulins has its own type of FcR. There are specific Fc-receptors for IgG, IgE, IgM and IgA. The FcR for IgG and IgE can be found in multiple isoforms, usually as high-affinity and low-affinity receptors. They are important in the processes of phagocytosis and antibody-dependent cellular cytotoxicity (ADCC).

Feldenkrais technique → see Exercise techniques

Felty's syndrome The combination of rheumatoid arthritis with splenomegaly and leukopenia. The syndrome mainly affects patients with long-term seropositive, nodular and deforming rheumatoid arthritis. Some patients have low articular activity at the time of Felty's syndrome manifestation. Many of these patients test positive for antinuclear antibodies, have leg ulcers and hyperpigmentation.

Fever Fever or pyrexia is a transient increase in body temperature above the normal value of 37.5°C, when taken orally. It can be graded as low (<39°C), moderate (39–40°C) or high (>40°C). It is one of the systemic changes accompanying a protective or impairing inflammation. It is part of the physiological protective reaction of the organism. It occurs due to an upregulation of the thermoregulation centre in the hypothalamus by endogenous pyrogens (especially IL-1, IL-6 and TNF-α) from a normal value to a higher one. This stimulation is indirect, mediated by PGE as the second messenger. The cellular metabolism and many immune processes are activated in fever leading to more rapid elimination of the infectious agent or other factors inducing the inflammatory reaction. The pattern of fever can help to clinically diagnose diseases (e.g. malaria, Still's disease).

Fibroblast growth factors (FGF) Belong to a family of 23 members in humans, which are structurally-related signalling molecules.

Initially, two isoforms were recognised – an acidic aFGF (FGF-1) and basic bFGF (FGF-2) factor. Both of these are members of the cytokine family and belong to the oldest known growth factors. They act on mesenchymal and endothelial cells, provide important signals during the body's development and have angiogenic activity (angiogenesis). Moreover, FGF directly stimulates the migration and proliferation of cultured endothelial cells and induces the production of differentiated blood capillaries, so are important in wound healing.

Fibrodysplasia ossificans progressiva

A very rare but interesting connective tissue disorder sometimes referred to as myositis ossificans progressiva. Patients are born with short big toes and usually develop recurrent episodes of painful swelling of the soft tissue leading to heterotropic ossifications in childhood. The disease affects all ethnic groups with a frequency of approximately 1:1,000,000 births. It is inherited as an autosomal dominant allele on chromosome 2q23-24 with variable expressivity, but most cases are sporadic due to a new mutation. Gonadal mosaicism is possible. A very similar disorder in cats has become the animal model for studying this disease.

Pathogenesis and histological picture: Initially, there is an accumulation of B- and T-lymphocytes in the perivascular spaces of muscle that otherwise appear normal. Among the oedematous muscle fibres there is a visible T-lymphocytic infiltrate followed by angiogenic proliferation of the fibres. The lymphocytes present in the muscle synthesise excess bone morphogenetic protein-4 BMP4, a product that contributes to the development of the skeleton in the normal embryo. Enchondral ossification takes place with the subsequent formation of healthy bone tissue with a normal haverian system. The trabecular bone contains haematopoietic bone marrow. The diagnostic difficulty and concerns over aggressive juvenile fibromatosis or sarcoma often result in a biopsy of the acute lesion if the clinician doesn't recognise the clinical picture.

Clinical picture: Suspicion of this disorder should be considered in the newborn, before the occurrence of calcifications, due to the characteristic finding of shortening and malformation of the big toes. Some patients have shortened and malformed thumbs. Synostosis and phalangeal hypoplasia is common. Other malformations of the fingers, however, are not typical for this disease. Later, swelling of the soft tissues with subsequent extra-skeletal calcification confirms the diagnosis. Some patients are wheelchair-dependent in adulthood. The painful swelling of the soft tissues occurs more frequently in the first decade of life, either spontaneously or after a minor trauma (for example an intramuscular injection). These lesions swell over several days, become indurated and their formation is accompanied by fever. Some of them resemble an infectious process. Typical localisation is in the paravertebral and limb girdle muscles. After varying periods (weeks to months), some regress spontaneously, but most pass through enchondral ossification with subsequent development of bone tissue. Once ossification occurs, it is permanent. The bone matrix gradually ankyloses certain joints and contractures or deformities occur, initially around the neck and shoulders. When the muscles of mastication are affected following local anaesthetic injection for dental surgery, the limitation of movement of jaw can significantly limit food intake and chewing. Ankylosis of the spine and thorax consequently reduces lung and cardiovascular function, leading to frequent chest infections. The disease does not affect the vocal cords, diaphragm, oculomotor muscles and smooth muscle. Hearing impairment and alopecia is observed more frequently than in the healthy population.

Fibromyalgia (FM) A chronic, non-inflammatory myofascial (musculoskeletal) syndrome characterised by widespread pain and points of increased tenderness to pressure and typically accompanied by profound fatigue. It may be primary and secondary; the latter is usually associated with a rheumatic disorder. Some patients fulfil the diagnostic

F

criteria of chronic fatigue syndrome (CFS). Although the long term course of the disease causes much hardship, it does not reduce life expectancy, nor lead to deformities, cosmetic changes or locomotor disability.

Clinical symptoms and signs:
- widespread musculoskeletal pain,
- multiple tender points,
- painful spasms,
- fatigue, sleep and mood disturbance, post-exercise pain,
- headache, paraesthesia and functional organic syndromes.

Fibromyalgia impact questionnaire

(FIQ) → see Instruments of assessing (health status measurements, outcome measurement)

Fibrous dysplasia A skeletal disorder with sporadic incidence.

Pathogenesis: All types of the disease originate in the activating mutation of the gene coding for the Gs-alfa subunit of the G-protein that stimulates the production of cyclic adenosine monophosphate. Insufficient differentiation of mesenchymal cells to osteoblasts leads to the skeletal lesions. The nascent cells form imperfect bone tissue. The overproduction of interleukin 6 seems to be an important pathogenic factor.

Clinical symptoms and signs: The onset of the disease occurs in the first decade of life affecting both genders equally. Foci of expanding fibrous tissue appear in one or more bones. They are most frequently visible on the long bones and the skull. Patients suffer from pain in the bones; deformities and fractures may occur. However, in many cases the foci are asymptomatic and found incidentally on radiographs performed for some other indication.

Flat foot (pes planus) The commonest static defect of the civilized population. It is characterised by gradual retrogression of the physiological longitudinal arch of the foot. In a typical case, the longitudinal arch flattens or disappears, the posterior part of foot is in the valgus position, and fibularis (peroneal) muscles are shortened, which causes abduction and supination of the anterior part of the foot. In such a case of impaired mechanics, the transverse arch of the foot extends and the heads of the medial metatarsal bones descend in a plantar direction. This leads to callosities under the feet. Medial incurvation and typical three-point load are missing on the plantogram.

Treatment is based on prevention with foot exercises, arch supports or orthotics.

Fluorides Belong to the stimulators of osteoformation with a consequent increase of bone density in the region of trabecular bone (spine). Their influence on the density of cortical bone and decrease of incidence of fractures has not been unambiguously documented with some studies showing an increased risk of non vertebral fractures. They are therefore no longer advocated in treatment of osteoporosis. (Lane and Leboff 2005).

FMF → see Familial Mediterranean fever (FMF)

Foreign-body induced arthritis This arthritis develops post-traumatically by the penetration of a foreign body into the articular cavity and after intra-articular implants. Chronic inflammatory monoarthritis of non-infectious origin can develop. Sometimes an infection is spread along with the foreign body. The foreign body can be of plant origin (thorns, hawthorn, rose, cactus and others), mixed kind (splinters of wood, fish bone, stone debris, rubble, glass, rubber, plastic) or could be fragments of joint prostheses (cement, silicone, metal, methyl metacrylate).

Clinical picture: Pain, swelling and oedema of the joint immediately after trauma, or sometimes after a delayed period of time. Suspicion of this diagnosis relies on a good history (contiguous trauma) and the exclusion of other causes of monoarthritis. Sometimes it is difficult to confirm the diagnosis, especially in children and the elderly, who often do not remember, e.g. a thorn prick. To demonstrate the foreign body we use an ultrasound arthroscopy, but mainly joint sonography or magnetic resonance imaging.

Therapy lies in the surgical removal of the foreign body.

Forestier's Disease → see Diffuse Idiopathic Skeletal Hyperostosis (DISH; ankylosing hyperostosis; Forestier's disease)

Frozen shoulder → see Adhesive capsulitis

Functional muscle chains This refers to a sequence of integrated muscle groups necessary for performing a certain activity (creeping, crawling, bipedal gait, and breathing). They are programmed in the central nervous system.

F

Galvanisation A treatment which uses low-frequency direct current. Included are:
- downstream galvanic current (anode proximally, cathode distally) – having analgesic and spasmolytic effects,
- upstream galvanic current (anode distally, cathode proximally) – stimulating the nerves and muscles,
- Kowarschik's galvanic current (two electrodes placed lengthwise, the direction of the current is transversal) – having an analgesic effect,
- four-chamber hydro galvanic bath – the limbs are put into special baths with water (the direction in the current is from top to bottom or vice versa); it has an analgesic effect and causes hyperaemia. It is used with benefit in patients with involvement of the peripheral joints (rheumatoid arthritis, ankylosing spondylitis, Sjögren's syndrome).

Gamma/delta T-lymphocytes These are T-lymphocytes which have a T-cell receptor consisting of gamma and delta polypeptide chains on their surface. They make up about 5% of the T-lymphocyte population

Gammaglobulins These are fractions of blood serum glycoproteins that have the lowest mobility in alkaline pH during electrophoresis and migrate in the direction of the anode. The majority of immunoglobulins and antibodies belong to this fraction.

Gammopathy A disorder characterised by the overproduction of undesirable immunoglobulins (Ig). Unlike normal Ig, these molecules represent a structurally and functionally homogeneous population. The term is derived from a serum protein fraction in which Ig's are found (gammaglobulins). Gammopathies (G) develop when a clone of plasma cells or lymphocytes uncontrollably secrete a homogeneous immunoglobulin or its components. Gammopathies may be monoclonal or polyclonal.

In monoclonal G, only one clone of cells (plasma cells or their precursors belonging to B cells) reproduces beyond control and releases identical immunoglobulin molecules of a certain class or parts of the immunoglobulin molecule (light or heavy chains). With polyclonal G, two or rarely more cell clones reproduce, each of which produces an antibody with different specificity. The undesirable Ig (s) are released into the blood in great abundance and can be determined in the serum by protein electrophoresis or immunofixation technique. Monoclonal gammopathy of undetermined significance (MGUS) is asymptomatic and can have a benign course with a low rate of conversion to malignancy. However, most monoclonal gammopathies are a malignant growth of antibody-producing cells including multiple myeloma, Waldenström's macroglobulinaemia and heavy chain disease. In multiple myeloma, malignantly growing plasma cells can be found in the bone marrow and produce monoclonal myeloma IgG, IgA, IgD, or IgE often together with Bence-Jones proteins, whose molecule consists of one of the two light chains. In Waldenström's macroglobulinaemia, there is a malignant growth of atypical lymphocytes secreting an excessive amount of monoclonal IgM. In heavy chain disease, there are incomplete heavy chains of γ (characteristically of the IgG class), α (IgA) or μ (IgM) found in the serum of patients.

Gate control theory of pain Pain is not simply perceived but is modulated by interacting neurons, according to Melzack and Wall. Based on this theory, the nociceptive signal is conducted by thin nerve fibres to the spine where the existence of neurons (in the dorsal horn of the spinal canal) with gate function is suggested. These neurons transmit less or more signals to the brain depending on how wide the 'gate' is open. The 'gate' is opened by afferentation from thin fibres and closed by afferentation from coarse nerve fibres. The existence of an 'interpretation centre' in the subcortical region is suggested. The centre modulates when and under what circumstances these signals are conducted into consciousness as pain. It has been found that nociceptive afferentation can be blocked by 'closure' of synapses conducting nociceptive afferentation by the use of substances similar to morphine. These are referred to as endorphins, which are synthesised by the brain (psychological modulation of pain).

Gaucher's disease A disorder inherited by autosomal recessive trait. Due to a deficiency of the lysosomal enzyme glucocerebrosidase (also known as β-glucosidase) the membrane glycolipid glucocerebroside accumulates in body organs and tissues forming the so-called Gaucher cells.

Clinical symptoms and signs: Often hepatosplenomegaly, bone pain and osteopenia, disturbances of the bone marrow (anaemia, thrombocytopenia) are present caused by an infiltration by Gaucher cells. Aside from clinical signs, the disorder can be suspected by high activity of alkaline phosphatase in the serum.

Gene The basic unit of inheritance localised on a certain position of the chromosome (locus). The gene can be defined functionally (its product underlying a certain trait in the phenotype) or structurally (a particular section of the DNA molecule or RNA molecule when RNA viruses are implicated). The gene can manifest phenotypically (phenotype) in three cardinal functional forms:
1. as a section of the DNA chain coding for the primary structure of a polypeptide (structural gene),
2. as a section of the DNA chain transcribing itself into the primary structure of tRNA, rRNA or other types of RNA that are not subject to translation,

3. as a section of the DNA (or RNA in the case of RNA viruses) with a regulatory function (regulatory gene).

Generalised nodal osteoarthritis (GNOA) → see Osteoarthritis – primary generalised nodal osteoarthritis (GNOA)

Genome All of the genes in a cell (cell genome) or a virus (viral genome) containing the whole hereditary information. Not all these genes must be functionally expressed in the given environment and stage of development. The genome of a prokaryotic cell consists of genes situated in the nuclear DNA and plasmids; the genome of a eukaryotic cell comprises a gene situated in the nucleus and mitochondria, and chloroplasts in herbal cells.

Genu recurvatum (backward curvature of the knee)
1. unilateral – hyperextension of the knee associated with instability; most frequently post-traumatically (meniscus, cruciate ligaments),
2. bilateral – as the manifestation of local joint laxity or generalised hypermobility (hypermobility syndrome).

Genu valgum (knock kneed) A knee with an increased internal angle. It occurs as a consequence of tibial overload after rickets, in renal osteodystrophy in children and certain metabolic disorders. Women may have a physiological valgosity of 8°. In adults, it can occur in rheumatoid arthritis and osteoarthritis as a consequence of the compensatory mechanism of the adduction contracture in the hip, advanced destruction of the knee joint and damaged medial collateral ligament.

Genu varum (bowleggedness) A knee with a reduced internal angle. It occurs in the proximal part of the tibia or distal part of the femur in metabolic or systemic disorders. A mild physiological varosity is seen in 2 to 3 year old children, but it is necessary to exclude rickets, or osteochondritis of the medial

G

part of the proximal tibia (Blount's disease). More severe forms occur in adults secondary to osteomalacia and Paget's disease. In middle-age, it causes rapid development of gonarthrosis (more frequently in women). It is accompanied by instability of the knee.

Gestagens Their androgenic activities have a beneficial influence on bone production and mineralisation. They also compete with cortisol for the binding site on osteocyte receptors.

Giant Cell Arteritis → see Temporal Arteritis (TA)

Glandular fever → see Infectious mononucleosis

Glomerulonephritis (GN) A group of disorders characterised by inflammation and lesions of the renal glomeruli. Immune mechanisms participate in the pathogenesis of the majority of primary and secondary glomerulonephritis. More than 70% of patients with GN have deposits of immunoglobulins in the glomeruli, frequently in association with complement deposition. Damage to the glomeruli is induced by an inflammatory reaction initiated by either deposits of circulating immune complexes (as for example in systemic lupus erythematosus) or by cytotoxic antibodies against glomerular antigens. Goodpasture's syndrome is one example of a cytotoxic antibody reacting with the basal membrane of the glomerulus. The so formed immune complexes (similar to deposits of circulating immune complexes) activate complement which leads to damage of the basement membrane either directly or its chemotactic fragments attract neutrophils which cause damaging inflammation.

Glucocorticoids A group of steroid hormones with the ability to bind to the glucocorticoid receptor and secreted by the suprarenal (adrenal) cortex. They have been used for many years as antiinflammatory drugs, immunosuppressants and replacement treatment in endocrinology. Even though gluco-

corticoids do not cure, and likely do not change the prognosis of rheumatoid arthritis (RA), they are amongst the most effective symptomatic anti-inflammatory drugs. There is increasing evidence that they slow the progression of erosive changes in early RA. Their use in rheumatology is frequent, and indispensable in many cases. The effect of glucocorticoids is determined by the concentration and density of their peripheral cellular receptors. Due to the extensive physiological influence (anti-inflammatory, immunological, metabolic, mineralocorticoid effects, and the feedback inhibition of the function of hypothalamic-pituitary-adrenal axis), it is advisable in the interest of the patient to follow the guideline of giving the minimally effective dose for the shortest period to minimize adverse toxicity and minimise suppression of the hypothalamic-pituitary-adrenal axis on withdrawal. It is one of the major disadvantages of glucocorticoids that withdrawal after long-term systemic (mainly oral) administration is possible only in a limited number of RA patients.

Adverse effects:

Preventive measures against suppression of the hypothalamic-pituitary-adrenal axis function during long-term treatment:
- do not use corticosteroids with extended biological activity – corticosteroids with a medium biological half-life are recommended (prednisolone, methylprednisolone),
- always give the lowest possible, effective dose,
- consider administering the dose on an alternate day regime, though may not be possible as it may be ineffective in controlling the disease
- when decreasing the dose:
  - if the period of administration is two weeks or less, it is usually possible to decrease the dose by 1 tablet daily (5 mg of prednisone/prednisolone) every week,
  - if the administration is longer than two weeks and especially longer than six months, then decrease very slowly by 1 tablet daily every 15–30 days.

Indications for the systemic administration of glucocorticoids:

- persisting synovitis in several joints in spite of regular administration of non-steroidal anti-inflammatory drugs (NSAIDs) and a DMARD (disease-modifying antirheumatic drug),
- severe systemic signs (for example fever and loss of weight) or extraarticular involvement (vasculitis, episcleritis or pleuritis),
- occasionally glucocorticoids are prescribed early in disease for a limited period to suppress the signs of inflammation, until the expected effect of DMARDs occurs.

Systemic administration of glucocorticoids: glucocorticoids are given usually in a daily dose below or up to 7.5 mg of prednisone.

The following are treatment regimens in RA:
- *continuous:* administration of the daily dose several times a day – in the morning, at noon and in the evening, where the evening dose is the lowest,
- *daily:* administration of a single daily dose, usually in the morning,
- *alternating:* twofold dose every other day,
- *intermittent:* administration over 2 to 3 days, then 2 to 3 days drug free,
- *intramuscularly:* administration of 120 mg methylprednisolone (Depo-medrone),
- *pulse:* intravenous administration of high doses of methylprednisolone (250–1000 mg) daily for 3 to 5 days.

The therapeutic plan should take into account the length of the overall activity of glucocorticoids: hydrocortisone, prednisone, prednisolone and methylprednisolone act for a short term (24 to 36 hours), triamcinolone for a middle term (up to 48 hours) and dexamethasone and betamethasone for a long term (more than 48 hours).

Glucosamine sulphate (GS) The basic substrate for glycosaminoglycan synthesis. It is used in the treatment of osteoarthritis (Rovati 1997, Reginster et al. 2001, Pavelka et al. 2002). Glucosamine sulphate is well absorbed from the gastrointestinal tract. Stimulating effects on the biological function of chondrocytes are attributed to glucosamine in vitro. Dosage: tablets and capsules containing 250 mg of GS; 3 tablets are given twice a day or 1 sachet (1500 mg) of GS once daily. The treatment lasts usually 2 to 3 months. The treatment course is repeated twice a year. GS is also given intramuscularly twice a week. A possible structure-modifying effect of glucosamine sulphate is hypothesised, though the results of good evidence based studies are awaited

Glucose-6-phosphate dehydrogenase This enzyme participates in the metabolism of glucose (its oxidation in the hexose monophosphate shunt). In professional phagocytes, it ensures the production of nucleotide reductase (NADPH), which is essential for the respiratory burst and the formation of necessary antimicrobial substances. In glucose-6-phosphate dehydrogenase deficiency, there is a decrease of its activity in neutrophils to less than 1% of the average normal value.

Glycoproteins Biomolecules composed of both amino acid units and saccharides.

Glycosylation The process whereby glycoproteins are formed. The addition of sugar chains (saccharides) to these compound proteins occurs in a posttranslational modification by virtue of glycosyl transferase enzymes.

Gm allotypes An allotypic determinant localised to the constant region of the heavy chains of human IgG1, IgG2 and IgG3. The allotypes are products of individual alleles of the same structural gene. To date there are 25 different known Gm allotypes in the human population.

Gold salts They started to be used in the treatment of tuberculosis and other infectious diseases at the end of the last century. It was accidentally discovered that during treatment of tuberculosis with gold salts, patients with co-existent rheumatoid arthritis noticed an improvement in their arthritis.

Myocrisin

Gold has a number of oxidative forms. The gold agents used in the treatment of RA consist exclusively of monovalent Au^+, which binds to the organic molecule through a sulphur atom. From three gold compounds, which contain sulphur (sodium aurothiomalate, sodium salt of aurothiomalic acid, aurothioglucose and aurothiosulphate), sodium aurothiomalate is now used by intra-muscular injection.

Auranofin

This triethylphosphine compound of gold differs from other compounds by its better solubility in lipids. Compared to other gold agents, auranofin is well absorbed after oral administration. The reactivity of auranofin with sulphydryl groups is less than in other gold compounds. As such reactivity determines the biological activity of gold agents, compared to sodium aurothiomalate and aurothioglucose, the efficacy of auranofin is lower.

Pharmacokinetics: Sodium aurothiomalate (25 to 50 mg every 1 to 4 weeks) and auranofin (6 to 9 mg daily) bind to plasma proteins, especially albumin. The maximum plasma concentration of gold (4 to 7 mg/L) is achieved within 2 to 3 hours of intramuscular administration. Initially, it is excreted from the blood with a plasma half life of approximately 6 days, but an equilibrium between absorption and excretion is achieved after 5 to 7 weeks and deposits of gold form in the body. The gold bound to albumin is transported into synovial fluid where it reaches 50% of its plasma concentration. Gold has an affinity towards inflamed synovial tissue.

Mechanism of action

Properties of salts of gold:

- Inhibitory effect on expression of the endothelial adhesion molecule for leukocytes (ELAM 1) on synovial blood vessel cells and therefore they reduce the transfer of inflammatory cells into synovial tissue,
- In vitro inhibition of proliferation of synovial fibroblasts, synovial cells and collagen,
- Gold influences polymorphonuclear leukocytes (PMN): gold inhibits phagocytosis, chemiluminescence, chemotaxis of PMN and the release of reactive oxygen forms; in vitro it stabilises the cellular membranes

and inhibits the release of lysosomal enzymes from phagocytosing cells,

- Influence on monocytes: salts of gold inhibit the production of IL-1, chemotaxis, chemiluminescence and the production of reactive oxygen forms,
- Influence on lymphocytes: gold binds to HLA-DR antigens of lymphocytes, modifies their structure and therefore inhibits antigen presentation with subsequent activation of specific T-cells; in vivo particular subpopulations of T-cells do not change; in vitro salts of gold inhibit mitogen induced proliferation of lymphocytes.
- Cytokines: gold inhibits the production of IFN-γ, IL-1, IL-2 and IL-2 receptor, IL-6, IL-8,
- Influence on B lymphocytes: in vivo the salts of gold reduce the increased number of circulating $CD5^+$ B-lymphocytes, decrease the level of immunoglobulins, rheumatoid factor and immune complexes.

Adverse effects:

- *Skin and mucosa* – dermatitis, mouth ulceration, pruritus, erythema, eczema, urticaria, erythroderma, morbilliform or scarlatiniform exanthema, nail changes, chrysiasis greyish pigmentation, gingivitis, vesicular, bullous and ulcerative stomatitis, hypersalivation, alopecia, photosensitivity, metallic taste,
- *Vasomotoric (nitroid) reactions* – facial rash, hot flushes, nausea, hypotension, fatigue,
- *Renal* – proteinuria, haematuria, membranous glomerulonephritis, nephrotic syndrome, renal impairment – associated with HLA-DR3 and HLA-B8,
- *Haematopoietic system* – eosinophilia, thrombocytopenia, neutropenia, aplastic anaemia,
- *Pulmonary system* – hypersensitivity pneumonitis with pulmonary infiltrations, obliterating bronchiolitis,
- *Liver* – cholestatic jaundice, hepatocellular damage, occasionally acute liver dystrophy,
- *Pancreas* – pancreatitis,
- *Gastrointestinal system* – enterocolitis, nausea, vomiting, diarrhoea,

- *Nervous system* – peripheral and cranial neuropathy, encephalopathy, Guillain-Barre syndrome,
- *Eyes* – chrysiasis (pigmentation) of cornea or lens, conjunctivitis, corneal ulceration
- *Miscellaneous* – metallic taste, headache.

Goniometry A method used for measuring the range of movement within individual joints. In physiotherapy it is important to determine the range of motion of the joints and spine. Passive movements are measured (arthrotest). It is universally accepted that the method "neutral-0" depending on the planes, referred to as SFTR (sagittal, frontal, transverse, and rotatory), be measured. Every movement is recorded using three values: outer limit value (e.g. extension), zero position and outer limit value (e.g. flexion). For example, the limitation of flexion in the knee is expressed as 0–0–45°.

Goodpasture's syndrome An autoimmune disorder induced by antibodies against the basement membrane of the glomeruli and/or alveoli, or against the non-collagen domain type IV collagen molecule. As a result, a highly progressive vasculitis develops, especially of small vessels in the lungs and kidney, leading to pulmonary haemorrhage and acute membranous-proliferative glomerulonephritis with the potential to rapid death of the patient if not treated.

Gottron's sign → see Idiopathic inflammatory myopathies (IIM), Juvenile dermatomyositis (JDM)

Gout (gouty arthritis) A clinical disease developing in people with hyperuricaemia due to an inflammatory reaction of the body to the presence of sodium urate crystals. It can be classified as primary or secondary.

Clinical symptoms and signs: It most frequently affects middle-aged men. Acute episodic severe arthritis is typical. In its chronic form, tophi often occur. The most frequently affected joints include the first MTP (metatarsophalangeal) joint, the ankles and knees. Gout may be associated with an increased alcohol intake, obesity, hypertension, hyperlipidaemia, glucose intolerance and kidney disease.

Granulocytopenia Abnormally low granulocyte count in the peripheral blood.

Granulocytes Leukocytes with a nucleus usually lobed into three segments and a cytoplasma containing characteristic granules (mostly typically lysosomes). According to the pigment type where the granules can be histologically stained, they are divided into neutrophilic (neutrophils), eosinophilic (eosinophils) and basophilic (basophils) granulocytes depending on the pigment type determined by histological staining. An alternative term for granulocytes is polymorphonuclear leukocytes (PMN), but this is not exactly true as the term polymorphonuclear leukocyte is synonymous with neutrophils. Granulocytes represent 40–70% of all leukocytes in the peripheral blood.

Granuloma An organised structure of mononuclear cells that is a typical feature of cell-mediated immunity. The immunological granuloma is characterised by a central core consisting of epithelioid cells and macrophages, occasionally with multinucleated giant cells (hypothesised to be the final developmental stage of the monocyte-macrophage cell-line). Sometimes (for example in tuberculosis) this central part contains a necrotic zone of destroyed cells. The macrophage-epithelioid part of the granuloma is surrounded with lymphocytes.

Granzymes The serine proteases found in the granules of cytotoxic T-lymphocytes and NK-cells. They participate in cytotoxic reactions performed by these cells. They are also referred to as fragmentins.

Growth factors These belong to cytokines. They regulate the growth and metabolic activity of various cell populations and are termed accordingly. When they influence the proliferation of colony-forming haematopoietic cells, they are referred to as colony-

G

stimulating factors; when they influence leukocytes, they are called interleukins; and when they influence other cells, they have different terms such as nerve growth factor (NGF), epidermal growth factor (EGF), fibroblast growth factor (FGF), platelet-derived growth factor (PDGF), etc.

Growth hormone Affects bone by several mechanisms. It increases metabolic turnover with a presumed influence on osteoformation and influences calcium resorption. It plays an important role in achieving peak bone mineral density. It stimulates proliferation and differentiation of osteoblasts. Its effects are mediated directly (interaction with specific growth hormone receptor) or indirectly (via growth factors – insulin like growth factors – IGF-1 and IGF-2). Growth hormone and growth factors also possess other important effects influencing bone metabolism. Stimulation of 1-alpha-hydroxylase increases the concentration of 1,25-dihydroxy vitamin D, thereby increasing absorption of calcium and phosphate in the small intestine. Other effects include influencing gonadal steroids, modulation of the immune system as well as an anabolic effect on skeletal muscle.

G

Haemochromatosis (HMCH) A hereditary (autosomal recessive) disorder in which mutations of the HFE gene (a MHC class 1-type gene) causes increased intestinal iron absorption. This diagnosis should be considered in patients with early onset osteoarthritis (especially involving the metacarpophalangeal joints) in association with liver or other endocrine diseases. The diagnosis can now be made by genotyping for the HFE mutation in patients with very high serum iron studies (Olsson 2008). Involvement of joints is characterised by the accumulation of iron pigment causing the degeneration of articular cartilages. The disorder can be associated with the occurrence of chondrocalcinosis (CCA). The radiographic appearance can be divided into two categories:

1. Articular calcification develops in approximately 30% of patients. The hyaline cartilage in HMCH heavily protrudes into the joint. The fibrous cartilage in the symphysis is affected in HMCH more frequently than in CCA.
2. Structural damage of the joints develops in almost 50% of cases. These are similar to those seen in CCA except on the radial side of the metacarpophalangeal joints where hooky osteophytes are formed in patients with HMCH. In CCA, the 2nd and 3rd MCP joint are affected, in HMCH the 4th MCP joints is also involved.

Treatment of the underlying disease involves regular venesection to normalise the serum iron studies, though this has little effect on the joint symptoms. Consideration should be given to screening 1st degree relatives of the patient for the disease (Olsson 2008).

Haemoglobinopathies and involvement of the locomotor organs Haemoglobinopathies are inherited disturbances of the production and function of haemoglobin. As a consequence of the gene mutation, two kinds of disturbance have been identified: deficient production of the globin chains (so-called thalassaemias), or a mismatch of the sequence of amino acid (so-called true haemoglobinopathies).

Clinical symptoms and signs:
- painful crises in the juxta-articular regions of the long bones, spine and ribs
- dactylitis
- osteonecrosis
- osteomyelitis
- gout.

Haemophilia → see Musculoskeletal complication in rare inherited haemorrhagic diatheses

Haemophilic arthropathy This can occur following repeated bleeding into the joint after microtrauma or spontaneously in patients with haemophilia, a group of related inherited bleeding disorders. Recurrent protracted bleeding can result in synovitis, haemosiderosis and functional disturbance of the joint, eventually leading to joint destruction. Bleeding into muscles can also occur and can create a so-called haemophilic pseudotumour. The radiographic findings are characterised initially by the formation of cysts and erosions, but later the articular surfaces flatten and sclerosis occurs at the edges, eventually leading to severe osteoarthritis. Prophylactic use of Factor VIII or intensive on-demand Factor VIII replacement therapy to reduce the frequency or severity of joint bleeds delays the progress of joint disease.

Hallux rigidus (Stiff big toe) The big toe is stiff with marked limitation in the movement of the first metatarsophalangeal joint making the normal push off of the foot when walking difficult. There may be a pain in the big toe.

Hallux valgus → see Toe swelling/deformity and associated diseases

Hammer toe → see Toe swelling/deformity and associated diseases

Hand silhouette Similar to a palmogram, the contour of the hand with all fingers adducted and then with all fingers maximally abducted is traced; the lateral shape of the hand is also traced (the 5th finger lies on the paper). The method can be utilised for monitoring treatment targeted at the hand. For example, it is used in systemic sclerosis, but also in other disorders of hand function.

Handicap A category expressing an irreversible loss of a certain physical or mental function that decreases the ability of the individual to assert oneself in occupation, family or other sphere of his/her social life. The IDH (impairment–disability–handicap) classification is now expanded and modified in the new "ICF classification".

Hauffe's bath A branch of hydrotherapy characterised by a gradual increase in the temperature of a bath, for example, for the feet of patients with a disturbance of macro- or microcirculation (in diabetes or systemic sclerosis), in which the sudden immersion in a hyperthermic bath would produce an undesirable initial vasoconstriction.

HBeAg Hepatitis B virus nucleocapsid antigen. Its presence in the serum is a feature of the contagious stage of the disease.

HBsAg Hepatitis B virus surface antigen.

Head's zones In diseases of certain internal organs, regions of altered sensation appear on the skin at relevant spinal cord segments, named Head's zones after their discoverer (Sir Henry Head, neurologist in England, 1861–1940). They can be used diagnostically and therapeutically to influence the affected organs.

Health assessment questionnaire (HAQ) → see Instruments of assessing (health status measurements, outcome measurement)

Health status measurements → see Instruments of assessing (health status measurements, outcome measurement)

Heat shock proteins (HSP) They are synthesised in two ways:
1. after induction by increased temperature or by other stress factors. These are inducable HSPs,
2. constantly synthesised without the effect of any stress factor called constitutive or cognitive HSPs, which are more commonly referred to as HSCs.

The production of HSPs can also be induced by pathophysiological conditions (infections, inflammation, malignancies etc.), immunological factors (e.g. phagocytosis, certain cytokines, free radicals, organ transplants) as well as normal physiological conditions (cell cycle, embryonic development, cell differentiation etc.). HSPs have a similar amino acid structure in the cells of different organisms, from single celled organisms to humans. They act as chaperone proteins (attendant proteins) to protect the structure (biologically active form) of other proteins, play an important role in the protection of cells against proteotoxic agents and are involved in various immune mechanisms.

Heberden's nodes → see Osteoarthritis – hands (Heberden and Bouchard type)

Henoch-Schönlein purpura A leukocytoclastic vasculitis involving small vessels with deposits of immune complexes containing predominantly IgA. The disorder typically affects the skin, bowels, and kidneys (glomeruli) and is associated with arthritis. It occurs predominantly in childhood, more frequently in boys. The inciting agent can be an infection, allergic reactions to medications, food, insect bite or exposition to cold. A purpuric rash on the lower extremities and/or buttocks together with swelling of the large joints is a typical presentation. Some patients suffer from abdominal pain and may have blood in the stools and micro- or macroscopic haematuria. More severe manifestations in the gastrointestinal tract (changes to the mesenteric vessels, diarrhoea) and the involvement of the central nervous system (CNS) or testicles are indications for treatment with glucocorticoids.

In tests, rheumatoid factors of IgA class are often present. A recurrent purpuric rash appears in 1/3 to 1/2 of patients, mostly within 6 weeks, rarely after several years. Antibiotics are usually given when concomitant infection is suspected. The prognosis depends on the extent of renal and CNS involvement. In severe forms the administration of glucocorticoids in various forms is necessary combined with immunosuppressant treatment or plasmapheresis.

Hepatitis An inflammation of the liver that can present as jaundice. It appears in multiple forms that can be infectious or chronic. Infectious hepatitis is induced by viruses and can be of several types – A, B, C (formerly nonA, nonB), D or E. The type A hepatitis (infectious jaundice) is caused by type A virus from the *Picornaviridae* family. It is manifested by tiredness, malaise, anorexia, disturbance of liver functions, and eventually jaundice. The disease is transmitted through food and water though the source of the infection is always a human. The virus causing type B hepatitis belongs to a group of "hepdna" viruses (hepatitis-DNA virus). It contains the following diagnostically significant antigens: surface HBsAg, the nuclear HBcAg and HBeAg. Infection is transmitted exclusively parenterally (via blood). The incubation period is 2 to 7 weeks. HBsAg is positive as early as two weeks before the onset of clinical symptoms and signs that are similar to those seen in hepatitis A. It vanishes within 6 weeks after the infection unless the disease becomes chronic. The occurrence of antibodies against HBeAg is a sign of immunity and the beginning of subsidence of the infection. Increased levels of antiHBc antibodies of the IgM class indicates a new acute infection. AntiHBs antibodies appear in the course of several

months after the fadeout of HBsAg and are a sign of acquired immunity. The most at-risk groups for contracting hepatitis B are health professionals, haemodialysis patients, haemophiliacs, drug addicts and homosexuals. Hepatitis C is caused by an RNA virus that is often transmitted parenterally mainly by blood transfusions, less frequently via infected needles in drug addicts or via sexual intercourse. The disease has a milder course than hepatitis A or hepatitis B.

Chronic hepatitis

The inflammation of the liver lasts longer than six months and includes a heterogeneous group of liver diseases with typical inflammatory infiltrations, necrosis of hepatocytes and signs of regeneration processes as well as fibrosis, but without the signs of a cirrhotic transformation. They include viral hepatitides such us hepatitis B, C and D, autoimmune hepatitis, primary biliary cirrhosis, primary sclerosing cholangitis and some overlapping syndromes whose diagnostic, histological, or clinical signs are typical for different nosological diseases classified under chronic hepatitis.

Heterobispecific antibodies These are monoclonal antibodies that are not produced during normal immune responses. They can be prepared by hybridoma technology or by gene engineering methods. They possess two binding sites with different specificity (each binds a different epitope).

Heterocytotropic antibodies These are antibodies of a particular animal species, which also have a high affinity for the Fc-receptors of cells of another animal species.

Hippotherapy A complex physiotherapeutic method based on neurophysiological principles that uses a living instrument – a horse – for treatment purposes. Hippotherapy is classified as a proprioceptive neuromuscular facilitatory method. It is closest to the Bobath and Kabat methods.

HIV (human immunodeficiency virus)
The abbreviation for the human immunode-

ficiency virus that causes the acquired immunodeficiency syndrome (AIDS). It is a retrovirus (a virus family whose genome is composed of RNA that after penetration into a susceptible cell transcribes its information into the cellular DNA), which has a typical envelope glycoprotein gp120 on its surface. This glycoprotein can specifically bind to the CD4 molecule, which allows it to enter and infect cells having this feature on their surface (T-helper lymphocytes, macrophages, follicular dendritic cells, microglia). After the HIV particle has penetrated T-helper lymphocytes, it can start reproducing, thereby causing cell death with a serious disturbance of immune homeostasis leading to clinical signs related to AIDS. To date, two types of these viruses are well-characterised – HIV-1 and HIV-2. In the diagnosis and prognosis of AIDS, an essential role is played by the demonstration of viral antigens p24 and gp120, as well as the antibodies against them in the serum of the infected individual.

HLA The commonly used abbreviation for human leukocyte antigens which belong to the histocompatibility antigens. They are products of the human major histocompatibility complex (HLA complex) and according to their structure and function are divided into HLA antigens of class I and class II. The molecules of HLA class I consist of two polypeptide chains (α- and β_2-microglobulins, while only the α-chain is coded from the HLA complex) and are localised on the surface of all nucleated cells. The molecules of HLA class II also consist of two polypeptide chains (α and β), forming a heterodimer and are routinely found on the surface of immune system cells, as well as on other activated cells.

HLA complex A complex of genes located on the short arm of the 6th chromosome and codes the human major histocompatibility system. These genes comprise several regions and sub-regions and their products represent the HLA antigens of class I (HLA-A, HLA-B, HLA-C, HLA-E, HLA-F and HLA-G) or class II (HLA-D, HLA-DP, HLA-DQ and HLA-DR). Among the loci coding for HLA classes I and II, we can also find genes for certain components of complement, cytokines and other proteins (more than 40 in total) that are usually termed HLA antigens of class III, even though they do not participate directly in the major histocompatibility system.

Homocystinuria Homocystinuria is an autosomal recessive inherited enzymatic defect of methionine metabolism that is characterised by cystathionine β-synthetase deficiency.

Clinical symptoms and signs: The disease manifests in mental retardation, often accompanied by ectopy of the lens, glaucoma, arachnodactyly and other signs of Marfan syndrome, such as osteoporosis, muscle weakness, connective tissue dysplasia and kyphoscoliosis. Also coxa valgum, genu valgum, deformities of the feet (pes cavus), laxity of joints and signs of hypermobility can be present. Hepatomegaly often occurs in homocystinuria; epileptic seizures can occur. There is often hyperreflexia and mild spasticity of the limb muscles. In tests, hypermethioninemia, hypergammaglobulinaemia and hyperhomocysteinemia can be found. Examination of the urine shows homocystinuria.

Homocytotropic antibodies These are antibodies which have a higher affinity to Fc-receptors of the cells of the animal species in which they are produced than to Fc-receptors of the cells of other animal species. In humans, IgE antibodies belong to this group.

Hormonal effects The sexual hormones, growth hormone, calciotropic hormones, cortisol, insulin, local factors and thyroid hormones all have important effects on the regulation of bone remodelling.

Hormonal Replacement Therapy (HRT) From a pathophysiological point of view, it was the treatment of choice in patients with the postmenopausal osteoporosis. Oestrogens prevent osteoresorption (a vicarious effect on the osteoclasts and reduction of osteoblast apoptosis). Oestrogens with or without progesterone significantly reduce the risk of osteoporotic fractures (femoral neck, spine, forearm). The optimal duration of administration is more than 5 years. After termination of treatment, osteoresorption dominates again over osteoformation. Due to an increased risk of invasive breast cancer, thromboembolic events, cardiovascular and cerebrovascular complications, HRT is no longer the treatment of choice in postmenopausal osteoporosis. However, some postmenopausal ladies, after counselling on the risks and benefits of HRT, still decide that HRT is their treatment of choice to improve their quality of life.

Hormones of the thymus The hormones produced by the thymus. There are more than 40 peptides and polypeptides whose main function is the regulation of T-lymphocyte development and maintenance of the delicate balance between various subgroups. Thymopoetins, thymosins and thymulin belong to the most studied hormones.

5-HPETE 5-hydroperoxyeicosatetraenoic acid is an intermediate product formed in the metabolic cascade of arachidonic acid. By virtue of the lipooxygenase enzymes, it is converted to leukotrienes and lipoxins. Similar to LTB$_4$, it is an effective chemotactic factor for the neutrophils, monocytes and macrophages. It also causes the release of histamine and other mediators by degranulation of mast cells.

HSP Abbreviation for heat shock proteins, which belong to stress proteins. Their production within the cell is increased by a elevated temperature, ionised radiation, heavy metals, anoxia, glucose deficiency and other stressful conditions. The HSP form a superfamily of several tens of molecules differing in their molecular weight and cellular function. Their best known function includes the chaperone function (i.e. the ability to protect the molecules of other proteins against denaturation and diverse proteotoxic agents that could induce the loss of their biological activity). They regulate the production of immunoglobulins, expression of HLA antigens and other molecules participating in the immune responses.

Hubbard's tank A special bath shaped like a butterfly which allows the physiotherapist to access the patient from either side. There are different jets in the basin and an underwater massage is also possible using a water hose. A suspension mechanism enables the immersion of a patient with polyarticular impairment in the water for the subsequent application of physiotherapeutic procedures.

Hughes syndrome → see Antiphospholipid syndrome (APS)

Human leukocyte antigens → see HLA

Humanised antibodies Monoclonal antibodies prepared by recombinant DNA technology. Their molecules possess binding sites or whole variable domains originating from mice or rats, while the rest of the molecule (constant domains) is encoded by human genes. The humanised molecule, after administration to humans for diagnostic or therapeutic purposes, significantly decreases the immune response to foreign antigen which would have occurred if the entire molecule had been encoded by mouse or rat genome alone.

Hungry bone syndrome Occurs in the presence of rapid termination of resorption and/or increased activity of osteoblasts. The causes include the early phase of treatment of vitamin D deficiency with rapid mineralisation of excessive amounts of osteoid without adequate calcium supplementation, after surgery for hyperparathyroidism or hyperthyroidism; or rarely in children due to the activity of osteoblastic metastasis. Biochemical results include hypocalcaemia, and possibly hypophosphataemia and hypomagnesaemia with corresponding clinical manifestations, such as tetany.

Hunter's disease → see Mucopolysaccharidosis (MPS)

Hurler's disease → see Mucopolysaccharidosis (MPS)

Hyaline cartilage A non-vascular, non-neural and non-lymphatic type of dense connective tissue. It is a hard translucent smooth tissue covering the ends of bones to form a smooth articular surface to joints. In a young body it has a blue-white colour and is slightly transparent, in an older body it becomes yellow-white and opaque. It is composed of chondrocytes (derived from mesochymal cells) which secrete a matrix composed mainly of type II collagen fibres and proteoglycans, though also has a high water content (65–80%). Nutrition of chondrocytes is provided by the diffusion of compounds through the synovial membrane. The intensity of nutrition of the tissue is low, but the metabolic turnover of chondrocytes is high. As chondrocytes are bound in lacunae and cartilage has no blood supply, cartilage has a poor repair mechanism.

During embryonic development, mesenchymal cells condense in regions where cartilage normally develops, and differentiate into chondroblasts which then produce the macromolecular components of the cartilaginous matrix. In the circumference of these cells a fibrous envelope called perichondrium begins to form. Chondroblasts stem from the cells of the inner perichondrium layer. This layer is referred to as the chondrogenic layer of the perichondrium. The chondroblasts deposit new cartilaginous matrix on the surface of previously formed cartilage, leading to apposition growth of the cartilage. The cells of the outer perichondrium layer differentiate into fibroblasts producing collagen and creating the fibrous layer of the perichondrium that persists on certain cartilages up to adulthood (e.g. the cartilaginous rings of the trachea and the cartilages attaching the anterior ends of the ribs to the sternum). Both layers of the perichondrium vanish from the articular cartilage leaving the articular cartilage in the synovial joint no longer covered by the perichondrium.

After the intercellular matrix of the cartilage covers the chondroblasts they are referred to as chondrocytes. The components of the cartilaginous matrix are self-synthesised and self-produced. Chondrocytes can be found in the tiny spaces of the matrix called lacunae. The primary lacuna is one containing a chondrocyte that stopped secretion of the intercellular substance into its surrounding environment. However, such a chondrocyte is able to reproduce, which is demonstrated by mitosis and is called the interstitial growth of the cartilage. The daughter cell is located in the same lacuna and a tiny barrier of intercellular matrix is formed between the cells. Sometimes the daughter cells undergo further mitotic reproduction so that up to four cells are located in one lacuna. Such an aggregate is called a chondrocyte nest. The chondrocytes situated in one nest represent a clone (that is descent from the original cell of the primary lacuna). The size and shape of chondrocytes are very variable; the young ones are usually flattened; the adult ones are big and oval. The chondrocytes of articular cartilage retain their ability to produce components of the intercellular cartilaginous matrix during their life, however, under normal conditions they do not reproduce. The production of new matrix is the only mechanism by which articular cartilage can compensate for the loss caused by everyday use. This limitation has been recognised by estimations of chondrocyte proportions in the matrix showing that the relative cell count in articular cartilage decreases with age. Chondrocytes in adult cartilage are longliving cells that rarely reproduce. However, their reproductive ability remains preserved and can be regenerated when the matrix collagen network in their proximity is impaired, such as in osteoarthritis.

Hyaluronic acid The sodium salt of hyaluronic acid is the main component of synovial fluid and the intercellular matrix of hyaline cartilage and can be administered in the treatment of osteoarthrosis. The preparation Hyalgan (500–730 kDa) is administered intraarticularly at weekly intervals up to a total of five times. The treatment cycle can be repeated twice yearly. The preparation Synvisc (Hylan G-F 20) is a high molecular polysaccharide (6000 kDa) that has a viscosupplemental effect and regulates synovial fluid homeostasis. Synvisc is administered intra-articularly in three weekly doses. Both preparations are administered strictly intra-articularly, especially in osteoarthrosis.

Hydrocortisone → see Glucocorticoids

Hydrops articulorum intermittens (intermittent hydrops of the joint) A recurrent joint effusion occurring without demonstrable cause, mainly affecting the knee joint. There is no synovitis, with the joint usually being cool and non-tender. The swelling usually lasts 2 to 6 days and recurs at various time intervals (for example over 7, 14 or 21 days).

    Treatment: Joint aspiration, intraarticular injection of glucocorticoids, or rarely synovectomy may be necessary. Nonsteroidal antiinflammatory drugs or mild disease modifying antirheumatic drugs may be administered. The disease is often referred to as prerheumatoid as approximately half of cases go onto develop rheumatoid arthritis.

Hydrotherapy The use of water of various temperatures for therapeutic and prophylactic purposes. The procedure can involve simple methods such as applying thermal stimuli (hot and/or cold), or mechanical stimuli such as bead bath, whirlpool bath, various showers, and chemical stimuli applied through baths with ingredients. Hydrotherapy can be combined with kinesiotherapy, so-called hydrokinesiotherapy.

Hydroxychloroquine → see Antimalarial drugs

Hydroxyproline It represents approximately 13% of the total aminoacid composition of collagen. It is formed by posttranslational hydroxylation of proline in the collagen chain. Approximately 10% of the total hydroxyproline produced during degradation of collagen is excreted in the urine. Even though hydroxyproline is regarded mainly as a marker of bone resorption, it also produced from degradation of the C1q component of complement and in the rheumatoid arthritis and other inflammatory disorders can be responsible for up to 40% of hydroxyproline in the urine. Moreover, this method demands a diet lasting at least 24 hours because the collagen content in food may influence its concentration in the urine. Therefore, more specific markers of bone breakdown of the pyridinoline type are now used.

Hyperaesthesia Increased sensitivity to various stimuli (increased sensation).

Hyperalgesia An increased response to stimulus that normally elicits pain:
• primary – in the area of damage,
• secondary – a pain felt in the undamaged area surrounding the damaged area.

Hyperalgesic zones (HAZ) Areas in the skin, subcutaneous tissues, muscles, fascias or periosteum with altered sensitivity that develop as a manifestation of reflex events in a segment elicited by nociceptive irritation. By eliminating HAZ (using reflex massage or by injecting the site with Bupivacaine (Marcaine, etc.) it is possible to interrupt the reflex events in, for example, vertebrogenic pain syndromes.

Hypergammaglobulinemia An increased concentration of serum immunoglobulins.

Hyperkinesis A pathological involuntary movement caused by a disturbance of the central motor neuron. Hyperkinesis includes tics, tremors, spasms, manifestations of spinal cord automatisms, choreaform and athetoid movements.

Hyperlipidaemias → see Musculoskeletal symptoms in primary hyperlipidaemias

Hypermobility syndrome (HMS) It is characterised by the occurrence of musculoskeletal symptoms in individuals with joint hypermobility who do not suffer from any

H

other rheumatic disease. When the syndrome was first described in 1967, many rheumatologists were very sceptical – such a syndrome was considered more as a clinical curiosity than a rheumatic disease. The set of five manoeuvres referred to as Beighton criteria with nine grades are characteristic for the diagnosis of HMS:

1. Dorsal flexion in the 5th MCP (metacarpophalangeal joint) by 90°,
2. Apposition of the thumb to the volar aspect of forearm,
3. Hyperextension of the elbow by 10°,
4. Hyperextension of the knee by 10°,
5. Place the palms on the floor without bending the knees.

One point is awarded to each manoeuvre, with two points for bilateral involvement, giving a maximum score of nine. A score >3 is considered indicative of generalised hypermobility.

Clinical symptoms: Are characterised by a wide range of easily detectable traumatic lesions and lesions due to overloading, e.g. traction traumas of tendons and ligaments, synovitis of joints and bursae, chondromalacia patellae, rotator cuff lesions of the shoulder, or back pain. Some patients suffer from joint instability and recurrent dislocations. In others, chronic arthritis develops either low grade synovitis of traumatic origin or osteoarthrosis, which many authors consider to be a complication of HMS. Inflammation markers are negative in laboratory tests. Therapeutic techniques consist of establishing the correct diagnosis, proper therapeutic rehabilitation and elimination of provoking factors.

Hypermobility test 2 (according to Janda)

- Head rotation – greater than 80°,
- Scarf test – elbow is placed behind the vertical axis of the body; fingers are placed behind spinous processes of the cervical vertebrae,
- Arms swinging downward/backward test – fingers and palms are interlocked to a certain extent,
- Arms swinging behind head test – fingers from one arm are crossed behind the head

overlapping contralateral acromion, even reaching the scapula,
- Extended elbows test – elbows can touch during gradual extension, even above the angle of 110°,
- clasped hands test – palms remain in contact during elevation of elbows, even in a wrist angle of 90°,
- Forward bend test – the whole palms can touch the floor in the fingers-floor test,
- Bend to side test – vertical line arising from axilla reaches the contralateral side during lateral flexion of the lumbar segment of the spine,
- Behind the heel sit down test – gluteal muscles reach the floor between the heels when the patient is sitting between the heels,
- Forward bend in sitting position test – trunk rests completely on the thighs,
- Bend to side in kneeling position test (informative) – the extent of the side bend is increased.

Hyperostosis A common term for multiple disorders having an increased bone density. These disorders may be detected radiographically as an increase in bone density. However, without a histomorphological examination, it is impossible to differentiate an increase of new bone formation from a decrease of its destruction. The aetiology of these disorders is currently unknown. It is a complex of factors decreasing the resorptive activity of the osteoclasts. A disturbance in the lysosomes, viral inclusions, abnormal PTH synthesis and disturbance of interleukin-2 production have all been implicated. Carboanhydrase II deficiency in erythrocytes causes a specific form of hyperostosis (osteopetrosis, renal tubular acidosis and cerebral calcification). Usually, the disorders are not accompanied by an excess of minerals when compared to bone matrix substance, but osteopetrosis is an exception. Hyperostosis may also be encountered in hyperparathyroidism. If successfully treated, the degree of bone resorption reduces very rapidly and sites with increased new bone formation followed by increased density, mainly in areas of healing brown tumours may occur. In hypothyroidism and acromegaly, an increase in bone density with preserved architecture may occur. Skeletal hyperostosis can be found after a long-term treatment with synthetic retinoids.

Hyperpathy Exaggerated response to painful stimulus.

Hyperphosphatasia This syndrome is characterised by high serum activity of alkaline phosphatase. At present there is no consensus regarding the use of these terms (hyperphosphatasaemia and hyperphosphatasia). Hyperphosphatasaemia represents a heterogeneous group of conditions characterised predominantly by high alkaline phosphatase levels in serum (S-ALP). The hyperphosphatasaemia (hyperphosphatasia) group includes completely benign conditions that are biochemical abnormalities accompanied by a significant increase in S-ALP, but also clinical conditions associated with severe bone deformities that are a form of bone dysplasias.

Hyperphosphataemia Occurring when the ability of the kidneys to eliminate phosphate in the urine is decreased (renal insufficiency, hypo- and pseudohypoparathyroidism) or in excessive delivery of phosphate to extracellular fluid during enhanced catabolism or tissue destruction (long-lasting excessive intake of beverages with a high phosphoric acid content or recurrent rectal enemas of phosphates, acute leukaemias, haemolytic anaemias, cytotoxic treatment, injuries or non-traumatic rhabdomyolysis). Clinical manifestations include tetany and other manifestations of hypocalcaemia, eventually leading to hyperparathyroidism and soft tissue calcifications.

Hypersensitive reactions → see Immunopathology

Hyperuricaemia The presence of an elevated serum uric acid level. Levels of serum uric acid depend on gender and age. In the pre-pubertal period, the concentration of serum uric acid is low in both genders. At puberty, they rise sharply in boys to an average value of 0.36 mmols/l and remain around this level throughout life. In girls, the levels of serum uric acid rise very little at puberty but rise to levels similar to men after the menopause (pre-menopausal average value of 0.24 mmols/l). Using the oxidation-reduction method with phosphotungstic acid for determining the level of serum uric acid, levels greater than 0.42 mmols/l and 0.36 mmols/l are regarded as hyperuricaemia in men and women, respectively. Using the uricase method, serum urate levels are 0.04 mmols/l lower. The occurrence of hyperuricaemia in the population varies in different studies between 4 to 40% (Pavelka 2000). It seems that the worldwide incidence of hyperuricaemia is rising. In the Central-European region, the estimated incidence of hyperuricaemia is 10 to 20% (Pavelka 2000).

Hypoalgesia Decreased or impaired sensation of painful stimulus.

Hypochondroplasia → see Achondroplasia and hypochondroplasia

Hypoesthesia A decreased sense of touch or sensation.

Hypogonadism This is characterised by sex hormone deficiency. This may be primary due to testicular and ovarian failure, or secondary due to hypothalamus – pituitary dysfunction. Hypogonadism can lead to osteoporosis.

Hypomagnesaemia Magnesium (Mg) depletion is substantially more frequent than its accumulation. Hypomagnesaemia occurs with the serum concentration of magnesium below 0.7 mmol/L.
  Pathogenesis: Magnesium deficiency can occur due to a lack of intake, malabsorption in the gastrointestinal tract or increased renal loss.
  Causes of magnesium deficiency (according to Rude 1993, Whang 1994):
  • *decreased intake of Mg in food:* malnutrition,

- *gastrointestinal causes:* vomiting, malabsorption syndrome, resection of the bowel, acute and chronic diarrhoea, intestinal fistula, acute pancreatitis (saponification of Mg in the fat necrosis), primary infantile hypomagnesaemia,
- *renal losses:* long-term parenteral nutrition, osmotic diuresis (glucose, mannitol, urea), metabolic acidosis, hypercalciuria, hyperaldosteronism, Bartter's syndrome, chronic pyelonephritis, interstitial nephritis, chronic glomerulonephritis, polyuric phase of the acute tubular necrosis, renal tubular acidosis, renal transplantation, isolated familial hypomagnesaemia,
- *treatments:* diuretics (furosemide, bumetanide), aminoglycosides, cisplatin, cyclosporin, amphotericin B, glycosides,
- *other mechanisms:* hungry bone syndrome, burn injuries, excessive perspiration, exchange transfusion.

Long term (>3-weeks) magnesium deficiency leads to depletion of the intracellular Mg resulting in a decrease in parathormone (PTH) secretion along with resistance of end organs (bone and kidneys) to the biological effects of PTH and disturbed production of cAMP (cyclic adenosine monophosphate). As a consequence, hypocalcaemia develops with all its associated symptoms.

Hypoparathyroidism This disorder is characterised by parathormone deficiency or its insufficient action on target tissues. There is an increased neuromuscular irritability, psychosis and trophic changes in the lens, nails and teeth. Blood tests reveal hypocalcaemia and hyperphosphataemia. The treatment of choice involves the administration of calcium and active forms of vitamin D.

Hypophosphatasia Characterised by low serum activity of alkaline phosphatase.

Pathogenesis: There are approximately 50 described mutations of the gene that codes tissue non-specific alkaline phosphatase which is localised on chromosome 1, with further mutations being recognised. Osteoblasts lack alkaline phosphatase activity. The accumulation of inorganic pyrophosphate suppresses the growth of hydroxyapatite crystals and impairs mineralisation of the skeleton. The zones of insufficient mineralisation are expanded and osteoid accumulates.

Clinical symptoms and signs: The bone has a primitive structure and remodelling does not occur, leading to a picture resembling rickets. Ossification of the flat bones is substantially limited.

The congenital form is inherited by an autosomal recessive trait. The skeleton of affected individuals is demineralised and involvement of the skull is called "caput membranaceum" (soft calvarium). Intracranial bleeding can occur. The extremities are deformed by multiple fractures. The condition is usually fatal. The infantile form manifests itself within the first six months of life. The child fails to thrive, is hypotonic and has wide opened fontanelles and the skull is hypomineralised. The condition resembles severe rickets, though the hypocalcaemia is associated with hypercalciuria leading to vomiting and renal impairment. Functional craniostenosis and skull deformation may occur. Respiratory difficulties, due to a demineralisation of the thorax, leads to death in up to a half of patients. A juvenile form leads to premature loss of milk teeth before the 5th year. Afflicted persons have weak growth and dolichocephalia (a long narrow head). Besides retarded growth, there is also bone pain and deformities develop (coxa vara, genu varum, kyphoscoliosis, etc.), which are the most frequent symptoms and signs of hypophosphatasia. Individual limbs are strikingly short, while the head, neck and trunk are normally developed. The gait is often waddling due to marked muscle weakness. In adults the disease manifests in middle age by fractures and pseudofractures.

The signs of hypophosphatasia first manifest after reaching the first year of life. Children lag behind in growth and do not thrive in weight. The fontanelles close prematurely and development of craniostenosis with subsequent changes to the shape of the skull. During growth, the clinical signs may improve in early childhood. In addition to the above mentioned symptoms, tetany and spontaneous fractures rarely occur in familial hypo-phosphatasia. X-rays show changes similar to those seen in rickets or osteomalacia.

Hypoxaemic reperfusion (hypoxic reperfusion oxidative injury) inducing joint damage

This is the method by which hypoxaemic reperfusion of reactive oxygen species complexes in the joint cause joint damage. The intra-articular pressure in a healthy joint is lower than atmospheric pressure and after activity does not increase. An inflamed joint has increased intra-articular pressure at rest which increases following activity causing compression of the capillary vasculature of the synovial membrane with subsequent hypoxia. This induces the production of hypoxanthine or xanthine, which in a healthy synovial membrane in the presence of xanthine dehydrogenase can be degraded, in an inflamed synovial membrane the hypoxanthine is converted to xanthine by the enzyme xanthine oxidase, thereby enabling the production of reactive oxygen species. Once joint activity ceases, the complex of reactive oxygen species penetrates the joint cavity where it participates in the degradation processes of proteins, lipids and proteoglycans, and so perpetuates inflammation and joint destruction.

H

I

Ibandronate A bisphosphonate licensed for the treatment of postmenopausal osteoporosis. The drug can be administered orally or by slow intravenous injection. Orally, it is given before meals and washed down with a cup of water; afterwards, the patient must sit and not lie down for 30 minutes. The oral dose of 150 mg is given once a month, a regimen thought to improve compliance. It can also be administered by slow intravenous injection at a dose of 3mg in 3mls every 3 months. This is particularly useful in patients with gastrointestinal intolerance of bisphosphonates.

ICAM → see Intercellular adhesion molecule (ICAM)

ICF → see International classification of functioning (ICF)

Idiopathic infantile hypercalcaemia
Patients resemble children with Williams-Beuren-syndrome; some of them can have heart disease, facial dysmorphism, hypertension and radio-ulnar synostosis. Further there can be strabismus (squint), inguinal hernia and hyperacusis, which are persistent. Polyuria and polydipsia are frequent. In some patients, an elevated PTHrP (parathyroid hormone-related protein) level can be detected. The hypercalcaemia persists much longer than in Williams-Beuren-syndrome and sometimes requires limitation of the calcium intake, exclusion of vitamin D and administration of glucocorticoids.

Idiopathic inflammatory myopathies
(IIM) Acquired inflammatory disorders of the striated muscles of unknown aetiology. They can be sub-divided into primary idiopathic polymyositis (PM), primary idiopathic dermatomyositis (DM), PM–DM in childhood, myositis associated with malignancy, and myositis combined with other systemic rheumatic disorders (such as scleroderma, systemic lupus erythematosus, Sjögren's syndrome or rheumatoid arthritis). Certain other disorders are included such as inclusion-body myositis (IBM), granulomatous myositis, and eosinophilic myositis or focal and nodular myositis.

Clinical symptoms and signs: Idiopathic inflammatory myopathies are characterised by the presence of symmetrical, predominantly proximal muscle weakness, biopsy evidence of muscle fibre impairment, elevated serum levels of muscle enzymes or myoglobin and the presence of multifocal myopathic signs on electromyography. In DM characteristic changes of the skin appear. Impairment of other systems such as joints, lungs, heart and gastrointestinal tract occur with variable frequency. There may be an association with malignancy, especially in the older population.

Criteria of classification Minimally modified criteria of Bohan and Peter are used and include the following manifestations:
- predominant or strictly proximal, usually symmetrical muscle weakness, progressive over weeks or months, with or without myalgias,
- biopsy evidence of muscle fibre necrosis and regeneration with a mononuclear inflammatory infiltrate (perivascular or intravascular) with or without perifascicular atrophy,
- elevated serum creatine kinase (MM-isoenzyme), aldolase and myoglobin levels,
- multifocal myopathic changes on electromyography (small, short and polyphasic potentials) with increased insertion activity, with or without spontaneous potentials,
- a rash typical for DM, especially heliotropic exanthema and Gottron's signs.

A diagnosis of IIM is definite when 4 or more criteria are present, it is probable when three criteria are present.

A diagnosis of DM is definite in the presence of a rash and three other criteria; it is probable in the presence of a rash and two other criteria.

Laboratory tests: Serum levels of creatine kinase (CK), lactate dehydrogenase, serum glutamic oxaloacetic (SGOT) or aspartate transaminase (AST), aldolase and myoglobin are raised. The rise occurs in the course of active disease and often normalises during remission. The level of MM-CK isoenzyme is especially elevated but also the MB-CK fraction which comes from a repeatedly damaged regenerating muscle. Occasionally the level of CK is normal due to the presence of inhibitors or in association with malignancy. Autoantibodies are present in the serum of 70–80% of patients. The erythrocyte sedimentation rate (ESR) and acute phase proteins are often normal. Mild anaemia can be present. The autoantibodies probably play a role in

the pathogenic process, and often associate with other clinical signs (table 3).

Idiotope An idiotope is a unique set of antigen determinants found in variable domains of immunoglobulin polypeptide chains.

Idiotype It is a shared characteristic between a group of immunoglobulin or T cell receptor (TCR) molecules based upon the antigen binding specificity and therefore structure of their variable region. Also it is a set of idiotopes at the binding site for a certain antibody. Antiidiotypic antibodies that are one's own anti-antibodies can develop against the idiotypes. Their binding site is complementary to the binding site of the first antibodies and so it has a spatial structure identical to the antigen determinant that is specific for this first antibody. These antiidiotypic antibodies are therefore referred to as

Table 3. Associations for myositis-specific autoantibodies (modified according to: Miller, F.W., JAMA, 270, 1993) (Miller 1993)

Myositis-specific autoantibody	Clinical picture	Onset of myositis			Response to treatment	Prognosis	HLA association*	Frequency of incidence in myositis
		rate	severity	season				
Antisynthetases (anti-Jo-1)	Arthritis, interstitial pulmonary fibrosis, fever, "hand mechanics", Raynaud phenomenon	Acute	Severe	Spring	Moderate, outbreak at dose decrement	Poor, 5-year survival in 70% of cases	DR3 DRw52 DQA1*0501	20–40%
Anti-SRP	Cardiac involvement, myalgia	Very acute	Very severe	Autumn	Poor, aggressive chemotherapy needed	Very poor, 5-year survival in 25% of cases	DR5 DRw52 DQA1*0301	5%
Anti-Mi-2	DM classification with a distribution of rash in the V and shawl shape type	Acute	Mild	Anytime	Good, but the rash persists long	Good, 5-year survival in almost 100% of cases	DR7 DRw53 DQA1*0201	15–20%

DM – dermatomyositis, SRP – signal recognition particle

the inner antigen picture of homoantibodies. It is assumed that the idiotypes and antiidiotypes form a regulatory network in the body.

IgA A class of immunoglobulins whose molecules can exist in two forms, either serum IgA (a monomer) or secretory IgA (a dimer whose molecule also contains a J-chain and a secretory component SC). Secretory IgA (S-IgA) can be found in mucosal secretions where it participates in local immune reactions. Penetration of epithelial cells onto the surface of the mucous membrane is facilitated by the secretory component. There are two known isotypes of heavy chains $\alpha - \alpha_1$ and α_2 – which produce antibodies of IgA1 and IgA2 subclasses.

IgD Immunoglobulins with a less well understood biological function. IgD molecules are, together with IgM monomers, most frequently incorporated in the cytoplasmic membrane of B-lymphocytes, having a discriminative function of the antigen receptor component.

IgE In physiological circumstances, their serum concentration is the lowest of all immunoglobulins. These antibodies participate in the protection of the body against parasitic infections and, just like reagins, are responsible for early hypersensitive reactions (allergies, anaphylaxis). Serum IgE levels are raised in parasitic infections and are especially high in allergic reactions.

IGF → see Insulin-like growth factor (IGF)

IgG This class of immunoglobulins is the most widespread in extracellular fluids. Their molecules consist of two identical light and two identical heavy chains that are spatially organised into domains. There are four known heavy chains γ distinct in antigen structure, which form the four subclasses IgG1, IgG2, IgG3, and IgG4. The antibodies of IgG class are formed mainly during the response to the repeated administration of soluble antigens. They are the only antibodies to cross the human foetal-maternal barrier in

the placenta. They activate complement after binding with the antigen (immune complexes) or in the form of self aggregates (clusters of one's own molecules).

IgM They have the biggest relative molecular weight (900,000 Da) and sedimentation coefficient (19S). Their molecule consists of five identical subunits (each with 180 kDa and 8S), thus forming a pentamere that aside from 10 light chains and 10 heavy chains contains also one J-chain. A small amount of circulating IgM (up to 5%) forms a hexamere. The basic subunit 8S of IgM is not circulating, but remains in membrane form as a component of the antigen receptor on the surface of B-lymphocytes. Antibodies belonging to the IgM class are produced mainly upon first contact of the organism with a corpuscular antigen. They have the greatest additive effect of multivalency, which makes them particularly effective in the agglutination of bacteria and in activating complement via the classical pathway (after formation of immune complexes or aggregates).

IL-1 to 18 → see Interleukin 1 to 18

IL-1R The IL-1 receptor occurs in two isotypes – I and II. The type II has a shorter cytoplasmic part compared to the type I which consequently causes insufficient intracellular transmission of the signal after binding IL-1.

IL-1RA An antagonist of the IL-1 receptor. IL-1 is a cytokine participating in normal physiological processes as well as regulation of the inflammatory responses. IL-1RA occurs in three isoforms: one secretory (sIL-1-RA) and two intracellular (icIL-1RAI and icIL-1RAII). The function of secretory IL-1RA consists in local inhibition of IL-1 and blockade of acute phase proteins, while the function of the intracellular IL-1RA is unknown.

Immune complexes Complexes arising from the reaction between an antigen and an antibody. They can occur either *in vitro* (where they are the essence of immunochemical assays and diagnostic methods) or *in vivo* (in which case they facilitate phagocytosis of bacteria or other particles opsonised by the antibodies, or can induce immune complex disorders if the immune complexes are soluble, or autoimmune disorders when the reaction between an autoantibody and autoantigen occurs in an organ). With *in vivo* conditions or in the presence of blood serum, the immune complexes can also bind to certain components of complement.

Immune system (IS) This is a diffuse (not strictly delineated) organ that weighs around 1,000 grams in an adult and consists of multiple tissues, cells and molecules. It is a component of the neuro-endocrine-immune supersystem, ensuring the input and processing of all information necessary for the survival of humans and other superior organisms. The fundament component of the IS is lymphatic tissue either condensed in lymphoid organs or existing in the form of free cells (lymphocytes, leukocytes). The lymphoid organs are divided into central (primary) or peripheral (secondary). As well as lymphocytes, the other important cells include antigen presenting cells and phagocytes (especially macrophages and neutrophils). Essential molecules involved in the reactions of the IS include antibodies (immunoglobulins), components and factors of the complement system (complement), various immunohormones, cytokines and other immunoregulatory substances, and numerous receptors on the surface of immunologically active cells, such as antigen and immunoadherence receptors, Fc-receptors etc. The basic function of the IS is to obtain information from the internal and external environment, their logical processing and response (immune response), the result of which is usually a defence-adaptation reaction (induction of immunity), but can also sometimes cause damage to one's own tissues, cells and their structure in the autoimmune or other immunopathological responses (immunopathology). In this respect the immune system is similar to the neuroendocrine system, with which it is closely linked, thus forming a single superinformation system that is a prerequisite for the existence of all superior animals. The most important property of the IS is its ability to differentiate its own molecular structures from foreign ones (antigen). Proper and fully-functioning antigens are normally tolerated; heterogeneous (on the surface of microorganisms or transplanted cells) or proper but functionally altered (estranged as for example on tumour-transformed or virus infected cells) are inactivated and destroyed in the course of an immune response.

Immunity The capability of an organism to withstand infectious germs (viruses, bacteria, fungi, cytozoon), foreign and estranged cells (cells transplanted from a genetically different individual and one's own altered cells (cancerous) or cells invaded by viruses) and their products, producing the ability to react against the antigen by the immune response to the benefit of the body. This immunity can be either non-specific (natural, innate) or specific (acquired, adaptive). Both are determined by an individual's genetic makeup (genome).

Numerous anatomical structures (for example the skin and mucous membranes) and physiological systems (for example haemocoagulation) that are not directly part of the immune system (they represent a natural resistance), as well as specialised molecules (the complement system, many cytokines) and cellular mechanisms (phagocytosis) participate in non-specific immunity. The activity of innate immune mechanisms is not conditioned to prior sensitisation with a certain antigen, and so they are effective against various antigens and do not possess an immunological memory.

Contrary to these, the mechanisms of specific immunity are activated only after contact with a certain antigen and referred to as acquired or adaptive immunity. They are specific in acting only against the antigen that has activated it, possess immunological memory and are evolutionary younger than components of the natural immunity. Cells and molecules can participate in both non-specific and specific immunity. Phagocytosis and NK-cells are basic mechanisms of non-specific cellular immunity, while the executive (cytotoxic) and regulatory (helper and suppressive) T-lymphocytes are responsible for specific cellular immunity. The complement system (complement) is the most important component of non-specific humoral (molecular) immunity, while acquired humoral immunity is executed by antibodies (immunoglobulins).

Immunity – cellular immunity Immunity executed by cells belonging to the immune system (lymphocytes and professional phagocytes for specific and natural or non-specific cellular immunity, respectively)

Immunity – humoral immunity The immunity mediated by executive molecules belonging to the immune system and often found in body fluids (= humors). These molecules are mostly antibodies. This type of immunity is also called antibody-mediated immunity.

Immunity – non-specific immunity This is a set of reactions at the tissue, cellular and molecular level that are congenitally present in the body and whose activity is independent of prior contact with the antigen. This allows them to respond immediately after contact of the body with an infectious agent. Non-specific immunity is activated predominantly in the elimination of heterogeneous substances from tissues and in anti-infectious and anti-neoplastic defence.

Immunity – specific immunity It is also referred to as acquired immunity. It is the ability of the body to react against a heterogeneous antigen with a specific immunological response. Specific antibodies, effector lymphocytes and lymphocytes with an immunological memory able to react solely with the antigen that has induced their production occur in specific immunity. They do not exert action immediately after contact of the immune system with a specific antigen, but instead require a latent period of several days during which the relevant clones of cells pro-

liferate and differentiate and the production of antibodies is induced.

Immunity – transplantation immunity An acquired immunity against the cells, tissues and their antigens (major histocompatibility antigens) induced following their transfer from a genetically non-identical donor. There can be two responses to heterogeneous histocompatibility antigens: host versus graft rejection (HvG) or graft versus host reaction (GvHR). The host versus graft rejection can be hyperacute (executed by the antibodies, for example, in blood group differences or xenotransplantations), acute (reaction of cytotoxic T-lymphocytes against heterogeneous HLA antigens) or chronic (participation of antibodies against weak histocompatibility antigens).

Immunoadherence This is the ability of professional phagocytes to adhere to their immunoadherent receptors (FcR or CR) of bacteria or other particles opsonised by antibodies or the C3b fragment of complement.

Immunoadherent receptors These are present particularly on the surface of professional phagocytes where they are involved in phagocytosis with the binding and ingestion of bacteria, immune complexes and other particles covered by antibodies or C3b, iC3b, or possibly C4b fragments of complement. The particles covered by antibodies are recognised by Fc-receptors while particles opsonised by C3b or C4b fragments are bound to CR1 and CR3. In primates, CR1 is present on erythrocytes and is involved in the clearance of immune complexes from the circulation.

Immunoadsorbent An insoluble substance (carrier) with a bound antigen or antibody used as a functional ligand. If the antibody is bound to the carrier, a simple separation of a specific antigen is possible or vice versa (immunoadsorbent chromatography).

Immunoassay, chemiluminescence An immunochemical method used to measure the concentration of antigen (hapten) or antibody, in which one of these reactants is labelled by a chemiluminophore (chemiluminescence).

Immunoassay, enzymatic An immunochemical method used for determining the concentration of a certain antigen (hapten) or antibody in which one of these reacting components is labelled with an enzyme. After interaction, the resultant immune complex is also labelled with this enzyme and the precise level of immune complexes can be quantified by an enzymatic reaction with a suitable, usually coloured substrate.

Immunoassay, fluorescence Fluoroimmunoanalysis is an immunochemical method for determining the concentration of antigen (hapten) or antibody in a compound mixture of different substances in which the antigen or antibody is labelled by a fluorescent agent (a fluorophore). The level of analysed substance is then measured by fluorimetry or photon absorptiometry.

Immunoassay, particle-enhanced An immunochemical method for determining the concentration of antigen (hapten) or antibody in which one of these reactants is adsorbed or chemically linked to the surface or a particle (erythrocyte, latex particles, colloid gold, etc.). Following interaction with the other reactant, agglutination or particle lysis occurs, which can be measured by various techniques.

Immunoassay, radioisotope An immunochemical method used to determine the concentration of an antigen or hapten, in which added external antigen is labelled by a radioactive isotope giving rise to the term, radioimmunoassay (RIA). Conversely, if the antibody is labelled with the radioactive isotope, the method is called an immunoradiometric assay (IRMA).

Immunoblotting A method used to detect a specific protein in a given sample of tissue homogenate or extract.

Immunocompetence A genetically determined ability of certain lymphocytes to react against an antigen with a specific immune response in a quantitative and qualitative sense. This is the ability of the body to produce a normal immune response following exposure to an antigen. When applied to lymphocytes, it means that a B or T lymphocyte is mature and can recognise antigens and is capable of mounting an immune response.

Immunodeficiency A deficiency of immunity caused by disturbances in the mechanisms of specific and/or non-specific immunity in which T-cells, B-cells or both types of lymphocytes, antigen-presenting cells, professional phagocytes, other accessory cells, antibodies, cytokines, complement system, or other components of the immune system participate. The aetiology can be due to reduced numbers or abnormal activity of these cells, the absence, malfunction or decreased synthesis of executive and regulatory molecules of the immune system. These disturbances can involve immune system cells at different stages of development. This produces a broad range of clinical symptoms and signs, the most common of which are disturbances of anti-infectious and anti-neoplastic immunity. Depending on their origin, the immunodeficiency can be divided into primary (hereditary, innate), whose aetiology is a missing or defective gene or even a group of genes, or secondary (acquired during development of the individual). Secondary immunodeficiency can be induced by various unfavourable physical, chemical, biological and psychosocial factors, or by insufficient or improper nutrition. If the activity of the unfavourable factor wears off, secondary immunodeficiency usually normalises, in contrast to primary immunodeficiencies. A list of the most important primary immunodeficiencies is given in table 4.

Immunodiffusion A diffuse movement of the antigen and antibody molecule, usually in agar or agarose gel. The movement velocity depends on the concentration of both components and diffusion constants. A gel pre-

Table 4. Human primary immunodeficiencies

Primary specific immunodeficiencies	
Antibody – mediated immunodeficiency	X-linked agammaglobulinemia selective deficiency of immunoglobulin classes (mostly IgA) selective deficiency of IgG subclass selective deficiency of specific antibodies transient infantile hypogammaglobulinaemia common variable immunodeficiency (CVID)
Specific cell-mediated immunodeficiencies	
• severe combined immunodeficiency (SCID)	adenosine deaminase deficiency (ADA) SCID T⁻–B⁻ (absence of T- and B-lymphocytes) SCID T⁻–B⁺ (absence of T-lymphocytes and NK-cells) Protein kinase Jak-3 deficiency Protein kinase ZAP-70 deficiency
• disturbance of phagocytosis function of T-lymphocytes	DiGeorge's syndrome Nude lymphocyte syndrome (absence of HLA class II molecules) Failure of HLA class I molecules expression hyper-IgM syndrome Chédiak-Higashi syndrome (CHS) Omenn's syndrome familial haemophagocytosing lymphohistiocytosis lymphoproliferative X-linked syndrome familial lymphoproliferative hyper-IgE autoimmunity syndrome (Job syndrome)
• other antibody- and cell-mediated immunodeficiencies	hyper-IgD syndrome mucocutaneous candidiasis ataxia-telangiectasia
Primary non-specific immunodeficiencies	
Phagocytosis deficiency	
• disturbance of neutrophil count	Kostmann syndrome cyclic neutropenia reticular dysgenesis glycogenosis of IIb type
• disturbances of phagocyte function	chronic granulomatous disease (CGD) LAD-syndrome I LAD-syndrome II Deficiency of certain lysosomal enzymes (thesaurismosis, storage diseases) α-chain of IFN-α receptor deficiency deficiency of specific granules
Complement deficiency	defects in individual components C1-inhibitor deficiency Disturbance of iC3b receptors (LAD-syndrome I) Mannose binding protein (MBP) deficiency

cipitate can be seen in the presence of the sought antigen or antibody at the point where they meet and their concentration is approximately equal. Under the correct conditions, it is also possible from the surface of the precipitate to determine the concentration of the evaluated component, in a similar fashion to simple radial immunodiffusion. Immunodiffusion methods are used for confirmation of diagnostically significant antigens (where a specific antibody is available) or antibodies (where a specific antigen is available).

Immunoelectrophoresis This laboratory technique is a combination of electrophoresis and immunodiffusion in agar or agarose gel. Using immunoelectrophoresis techniques, it is possible to determine the presence and amount (concentration) of antigens substantially faster than by a simple immunodiffusion method. Depending on technique, immunoelectrophoresis can be subdivided into 5 groups: classical immunoelectrophoresis according to Grabar and Williams (used especially for confirming multiple myeloma immunoglobulins), rocket immunoelectrophoresis, counterimmunoelectrophoresis, two-dimensional immunoelectrophoresis and immunofixation.

Immunofixation An immunoelectrophoresis method in which the separated antigens are detected directly in the gel on the basis of their precipitation with a specific antibody.

Immunofluorescence A property of certain molecules to absorb light or other form of energy and show it in the form of a photon (light with longer wave-length than that of absorbed light). It is used in immunohistochemistry and immunoassay techniques. Using the antibodies labelled by an immunofluorescent stain it is possible to localise the applicable antigens in histological slides, or study the fluorescent immune complexes through a fluorescent microscope. The same principle is also applied in sensitive fluorescent immunoassays (immunoassay, fluorescent).

Immunogenetics A branch of science representing the boundary between immunology and genetics and dealing with the genetic analysis of executive and regulatory molecules of the immune system (especially antigens of the major histocompatibility complex, immunoglobulins, cytokines and components and factors of complement), as well as the genetic regulation of immune responses.

Immunoglobulin deficiency This can be induced by abnormal function of B-lymphocytes or both B- and T-lymphocytes. Affected individuals manifest with a low level of immunoglobulins (hypogammaglobulinemia), abnormal function of immunoglobulins (gammopathy), hypercatabolism (excessively rapid degradation of the immunoglobulin molecules), excessive loss (upon heavy haemorrhage) or damage to lymphocytes (for example by drugs or lymphocytotrophic viruses). These can all lead to diseases in which the pathogenesis is a decreased immunity against most infectious agents. Subsequent severe recurrent infections are usually resistant to conventional antibiotic treatment. Primary immunoglobulin deficiencies include agammaglobulinaemia and selective deficiency of IgA, or also other immunoglobulin classes and subclasses, severe combined immunodeficiency and hereditary ataxia-telangiectasia.

Immunoglobulin, normal human Intravenously applicable immunoglobulin preparation made from the blood plasma of at least 1,000 healthy donors. It contains predominantly IgG and is used for substitution treatment (in deficiencies of antibody production), for prophylaxis and the treatment of certain infectious and auto-immune disorders (immunoglobulins, therapeutic preparations).

Immunoglobulin superfamily A complex of glycoprotein molecules coded for by genes with an evolutional homology, i.e. a common predecessor. The members of the immunoglobulin superfamily have several common sections of polypeptide chains in their molecules, with the same stereometric structure as the immunoglobulin chains (immunoglobulin domains). There are three types of stereometrically homologous domains identified among the members of the Ig superfamily: the variable (V), the constant (C) and the H domain. Currently, there are more than 40 known members of this superfamily whose basic functions are discriminative (immunoglobulins, antigenic receptors on T-cells, antigens of class I and II of the major histocompatibility complex, differentiation antigens CD2, CD3, CD4, CD8 and receptors for Fc domain of immunoglobulins – FcR), adhesive (connecting) or regulatory interactions between cells. The group of adhesive molecules include for example ICAM-1 (CD54 – intercellular adhesion molecule-1), ICAM-2 (CD102), VCAM-1 (CD106 – vascular cell adhesion molecule) and PECAM-1 (CD31 – platelet-endothelial cell adhesion molecule). Besides the discriminative molecules, the receptor for polymeric immunoglobulins (p-IgR) and platelet-derived growth factor receptor also possess a regulatory function.

Immunoglobulins (Ig) These are glycoproteins of animal origin and include all antibodies. Their molecules consist of two identical light chains and two identical heavy polypeptide chains interconnected by disulphide bonds. The chains are spatially organised into domains (immunoglobulin domains) and modules. The first domains of the light and heavy chains are variable, while the others are constant. In the variable domains, the sequence of amino acids of the polypeptide chains changes amongst the antibody molecules with diverse specificity, while in the constant domains remains unchanged. The sections of variable domains with particularly intensive changes of amino acids in individual positions are called hypervariable sections. The hypervariable sections of light and heavy chains are positioned in the Ig molecule side by side and form the antibody binding site, accounting for antibody-mediated specificity. There are two types of light chains (Kappa and Lambda). Heavy chain immunoglobulins are classified into five classes (IgA, IgD, IgE, IgG and IgM).

Immunoglobulins – chains Polypeptide chains constituting the immunoglobulin molecule. Each of the molecules contains at least two identical light (L) chains and two identical heavy (H) chains: There are two types of light chain: kappa (κ) or lambda (λ); they determine the type of immunoglobulin molecule (K or L). The heavy chains belong to five different isotypes: gamma (γ), mu (μ), alpha (α), delta (δ) and epsilon (ε); each of them determines membership to a specific immunoglobulin class. In addition to these

two types of chains, the molecule of polymeric immunoglobulins (IgM and secretory IgA) also contains one joining (J) chain and the secretory IgA molecule a secretory component (SC).

Immunoglobulins – classes Isotypic variants that differ from one another by the antigenic structure of constant domains of the heavy chains of their molecules (immunoglobulins, chains). There are five known classes of immunoglobulins: IgG (having the heavy chain (γ), IgM (μ), IgA (α), IgD (δ) and IgE (ε)).

Immunoglobulins – effector functions All functions except those serving at the binding site. These include the ability to activate the complement, bind to the cellular Fc-receptors, pass through the placenta, etc.

Immunoglobulins – genetics → see Genetics of immunoglobulins.

Immunoglobulins – hypervariable regions This is the section of polypeptide chains in the variable domains where individual amino acids are able to a greater extent to change positions, and thus allow immense diversity to generate millions of antigen-specific antibodies. There are six such sections in general – three on the light chain and three on the heavy chain. During the final stereometric arrangement of the immunoglobulin molecule, they become mutually close and form an antibody binding site. The hypervariable sections are also called complementary determining regions (CDR).

Immunoglobulins – idiotypes Immunoglobulin variants determined by a set of antigenic determinants, mainly in the hypervariable sections of both light and heavy chains. Such an idiotype represents the antigenicity of the antibody binding site. Some idiotypes can be found only in the organism of a certain individual (private idiotypes), while other can be confirmed in multiple individuals (common or cross-reacting idiotypes).

Immunoglobulins – isotypes These represent individual classes (sub-classes) and types of immunoglobulins. They identify their antigenic determinants localised in the constant domains of heavy and light chains and are identical in all individuals of the given animal species. They are products of different structural genes and can be identified using xenogenic antisera (for example, rabbit antiserum against human IgG will react with the IgG of all individuals of the human population, but not with the IgG of other biological species).

Immunoglobulins – J chain A additional glycopeptide chain that is a component part of all polymeric immunoglobulin molecules (secretory IgA and IgM). The J (= joining) chain is linked by disulfide bridges to the Fc region of immunoglobulin molecules.

Immunoglobulins – modules The highest form of stereometric arrangement of the immunoglobulin molecule. It is an aggregate arising from the mutual stereometric arrangement of the polypeptide chains of two adjacent variable or constant domains.

Immunoglobulins – molecule fragments They develop as a result of enzymatic or chemical fragmentation (cleavage) of Ig molecules. For example, the papain enzyme splits the molecule into the fragment antigen binding (Fab) and fragment crystallisable (Fc) regions, while pepsin creates the $F(ab')_2$ and pFc' fragments. Fab contains one binding site of the original IgG molecule and $F(ab')_2$ two of them. Chemical degradation causes the cleavage of interchain disulphide or certain peptide bonds.

Immunoglobulins, monoclonal → see Monoclonal antibodies

Immunoglobulins, myeloma Whole immunoglobulin molecules or their parts produced by malignant plasma cells or their precursors. They can be found in the serum of patients with multiple myeloma (monoclonal gammapathy).

Immunoglobulins – secretory component (SC) A polypeptide chain synthesized by epithelial cells to be a component of their receptor for polymeric immunoglobulins. It is a component part of the secretory IgA molecule. In IgA deficiencies, the SC binds to a secretory IgM molecule. The poly-Ig-receptor and from it the resulting SC regulate the transport of these polymeric immunoglobulins to the surface of mucous membranes, where they participate in the mechanisms of local immunity.

Immunoglobulins – subclasses Immunoglobulin variants determined by the characteristic antigenic determinants on the constant domains of heavy chains. There are four known subclasses of human immunoglobulins of the IgG class (IgG1, IgG2, IgG3, and IgG4) and two subclasses of the IgA class (IgA1 and IgA2).

Immunoglobulins – therapeutic preparations These are pure immunoglobulin preparations suitable for clinical use. They are made from plasma collected from at least 1,000 healthy donors. First generation preparations (immune serum gamma globulin) can be administered only subcutaneously or intramuscularly (Subcuvia and Subgam), while second and third generation preparations (normal human immunoglobulin) can also be administered intravenously. However, they have to match safety and efficacy requirements, such as the requirement to contain pure IgG, which must not be in the form of aggregates that could induce adverse anaphylactoid reactions. The presence of IgA in intravenous preparations can induce the production of anti-IgA autoantibodies in IgA-deficient individuals and in the event of subsequent administration, cause the reoccurrence of anaphylactoid, or the occurrence of anaphylactic adverse reactions. Normal human immunoglobulin preparations such as Sandoglobulin, Flebogamma, Gammagard, Octagam and Vigam are used as substitution treatment for primary and secondary antibody-mediated immunodeficiency, or can even be effective in several other disorders

Table 5. Overview of disorders that can be effectively treated using intravenous preparations of normal human immunoglobulin

Very likely effective	
Primary immuno-deficiencies	X-linked agammaglobuli-naemia common variable immunodeficiency selective IgG deficiency severe combined immunodeficiency (SCID)
Secondary immunodeficien-cies	transplant acceptors chronic lymphocytic leukaemia high-risk newborns AIDS in children Kawasaki's disease
Other disorders	idiopathic thrombocy-topenic purpura (acute) haemophilia, autoanti-bodies against the factor VIII
Possibly effective	
Burns Multiple myeloma Autoimmune disorders (SLE, APS) Juvenile rheumatoid arthritis Myasthenia gravis Rheumatoid arthritis AIDS	

(table 5). They can be administered as a prophylaxis to persons whose antibody-mediated immunity has not adequately developed at the time of definite or probable exposure to a certain contagion. These preparations contain an increased volume of antibodies, for example, against the diphtheria toxin, hepatitis B virus or rabies virus. When using immunoglobulin preparations one has to consider not only their substituting effects, but also their regulatory influence, which is why they can influence the immune homeostasis of the individual in both a positive, but also a negative way.

Immunohormones Immunoregulatory active substances possessing the nature of hormones. They are synthesised in certain immunologically active cells and influence the development, differentiation and func-

tional activity of other cells by acting on specific receptors. Some of them have a typical hormonal character (hormones of the thymus – thymosins), whereas others act mainly as local hormones (cytokines). The hormones are secreted in an endocrine manner and their target cells, to which a specific signal is transmitted, can be localised anywhere in the body. The secretion of local hormones is done in a paracrine or autocrine manner and their principal effect is usually limited to the neighbouring cells. Lymphocytes, however, have the ability to move around in the whole body, and so their immunoregulatory products (interleukins, lymphokines) can also have a systemic effect, despite having the character of local hormones.

Immunological tolerance A state of specific unresponsiveness (inhibition) of the immune system to a specific antigen that under normal circumstances would induce an immune response. In these circumstances, the reactivity of the lymphocyte clone capable of responding to this antigen is decreased or completely suppressed, or this clone has been eliminated from the body. The ability to respond to other antigens is preserved in an individual tolerant to a certain antigen (known as a tolerogen). Immunological tolerance has therefore the same specificity as the immunity itself. It can be either natural (spontaneous non-response to one's own antigens emerging during the individual's ontogenetic development also called "autotolerance") or secondary (non-responsiveness to extrinsic antigens). Under experimental conditions, tolerance to a specific antigen can be induced artificially.

Immunomodulation The therapeutic influence on the immune response performed for the purpose of stimulation (immunostimulation), suppression (immunosuppression) or normalisation of the immune response. Drugs normalising the immune response are those modulating a decrease or increase in the immune system activity towards normal function.

Immunomodulation therapy Treatment aimed at modulating the immune system activity of an individual. It is done either to increase the actual activity of the immune system (immunostimulation) or to suppress its activity (immunosuppression). The objective is immune normalisation, when activity of the immune system is restored to normal levels.

Immunopathology This is a sub-specialisation with the application of immunological techniques in the field to the practice of pathology. It studies the pathological changes occurring as a consequence of abnormal, increased (hypersensitive) or defective (immunodeficiencies) immune responses, their aetiology and diagnosis. Immunopathological (hypersensitive) reactions are nowadays classified according to Coombs and Gell into four types:

1. immediate or anaphylactic reactions (anaphylaxis) mediated in humans by the IgE class of antibodies,
2. cytotoxic type mediated by IgG or IgM antibodies against one's own cellular or tissue antigens; the tissue damage is caused primarily by activated complement,
3. immune complex reactions where soluble immune complexes are formed and are deposited in various tissues and organs, such as the vascular system, the kidneys, the connective tissue or skin. Subsequently, reactive oxygen species and lysosomal enzymes are released from neutrophils leading to tissue damage mediated by the immune complex deposition,
4. delayed type hypersensitivity where T-lymphocytes, macrophages and certain cytokines are involved.

Recently, a fifth type of immunopathological response has been proposed with involvement of autoantibodies against the cellular receptors. These autoantibodies can influence organ function via pathological stimulation (as agonists) or inhibition (as antagonists). Thyrotoxicosis is an example of stimulatory hypersensitivity in which the autoantibodies can falsely stimulate the TSH-receptors in the thyroid, whereas in primary myxoede-ma (TSH-receptor blockade) or myasthenia gravis (acetylcholine receptor blockade), the autoantibodies inhibit function. The majority of autoimmune reactions belong to the second type of hypersensitivity according to this manner of classification.

Immunophilins Intracellular proteins with peptidyl-prolyl-cis-trans-isomerase activity specifically bind immunosuppressive drugs such as cyclosporine (CyA), FK506 and rapamycin. There is a specific cytosolic immunophilin for each of them (cyclophilin for CyA), which after binding to the relevant immunosuppressant loses its enzymatic activity and thereby the ability to transmit the activation signal from the T-lymphocyte receptor to the nucleus. This is the principle of their immunosuppressant activity.

Immunopotency The ability of a certain antigen molecule to serve as an antigenic determinant, thereby inducing the production of a specific antibody.

Immunopotentiation An increase in immune system efficacy (stimulation).

Immunoprecipitation This is the production of a precipitate upon the reaction between a soluble antigen and its specific antibody. It can occur in a solution or a semisolid (gel) environment (usually in agarose gel). The technique is carried out in a qualitative or quantitative manner. Using qualitative immunoprecipitation, it is possible to determine the relationship between the amount of precipitate and the antigen-antibody concentration ratio. Huge excess of one of the two reactants can redissolve the immunoprecipitation (according to the precipitation curve or Heidelberger curve)

Immunoprophylaxis Prevention of a disease by either vaccination that induces active immunisation, or by administering an immune serum (containing specific antibodies), or by administering specific active lymphocytes, which induce passive immunity.

Immunoradiometry Immunoradiometric analysis (IRMA) by which the antibody, not the antigen, is labelled by an active radioisotope.

Immunostimulation A non-specific increase in the level of natural (innate) or specific immunity of an individual, manifested by increased rapidity and intensity of the immune response against various antigens, especially bacteria, viruses and neoplastic cells. Various immunostimulatory drugs which act on the immune system can elicit this.

Immunosuppression The suppression of the body's immune responses by external intervention either intentionally during immunosuppressive treatment, or incidentally as an adverse event (for example by the influence of ionizing radiation or certain drugs – especially cytostatic agents, xenobiotics and bacterial toxins). Immunosuppressive treatment is used in organ (especially kidney), tissue and bone marrow transplants to prevent rejection, and in the treatment of certain autoimmune disorders and other diseases with an immunopathogenesis.

Immunotherapy The treatment of abnormal immune responses by an immunostimulating or immunosuppressive agent, or by biological products of either natural or recombinant origin (for example certain cytokines), vaccines and immune sera. It also includes desensitisation in allergic disorders.

Immunotoxicology The investigation of the toxic and adverse effects of various natural and industrial toxins, harmful substances and toxic agrochemicals (xenobiotics) in the living and working environment, as well as the adverse effects of drugs on the immune system. The immunotoxic effects of these agents can manifest itself through suppression of the immune system (immunosuppression), which leads to reduced immunity in the affected individuals against infectious and neoplastic disorders, or on the contrary, through immunopathological stimulation (immunostimulation) when an increase in

the occurrence of allergic and autoimmune disorders is observed.

Immunotoxins Conjugates (complexes) of monoclonal antibodies and cytotoxic compounds can bind through a binding site of the antibody to a specific antigen of the target cell, most frequently a neoplastic cell, and so by the action of the toxic agent can kill the cell without causing injury to other cells in the body. Various vegetable or animal toxins, cytostatic agents and radionuclides can be used as the toxic component of immunotoxins. Currently, immunotoxins have only been experimentally tested in the treatment of certain tumours.

Impairment A term which describes a transient or permanent decrease in the function of an organ or body when compared with the norm in the anatomical, physiological or mental sphere. These are, for example, impairments of speech and sensory organs, joint function, etc. For newer approaches see "ICF classification".

Impingement syndrome of the shoulder Narrowing of the subacromial space leads to painful friction of the affected structures as a consequence of various influences, such as trauma, microtrauma or inflammation. Typical is the so-called painful arc, i.e. pain during abduction of the shoulder from 60° to 120° when the head of the humerus has a pathologically altered subacromial space.

Impulse waves These are pneumatically generated ballistic waves with optional impulse frequency varying from 5 to 10 Hz, adjustable level of energy 1 to 4 bars and a power density on the impulse transmitter of 0.01–0.23 mJ/mm. It is used in the management of painful body areas. The impulse generated in the device is accelerated, thus creating the impulse wave, which penetrates the area of the body exposed to the wave. Indications of impulse waves include area application in the soft tissues, e.g. treatment of enthesopathy and tendinopathy; spatially restricted application used to influence trigger points and tender points; and point application for acupuncture points.

Indications:

- Tendon injury,
- Calcar calcanei (painful heel),
- Dupuytren's contracture,
- Trigger points.

Incisura scapulae syndrome The suprascapular nerve is compressed in the suprascapular notch. Dull pain and tenderness to palpation is present in supraspinatous fossa. The abduction test is positive. The patient places the hand of the affected site on the contralateral shoulder, so that the elbow is in a horizontal line at the level of both shoulders. Then the patient makes a movement of the elbow towards the healthy shoulder. When the suprascapular nerve is compressed, the patient experiences a sharp pain. No changes are visible on X-ray.

Treatment: Injections are administered locally (mesocaine + glucocorticoid) in the proximity of suprascapular notch.

Infectious mononucleosis Also commonly known as glandular fever or Pfeiffer's disease. It is caused by the Epstein-Barr virus (EBV), which infects B lymphocytes. It is most prevalent in adolescents and causes fever, lymphadenopathy, sore throat and fatigue, though can cause arthralgias. The Paul-Bunnell test is positive, though the monospot test looking for heterphile antibodies is now more commonly used.

Inflammation The body's complex biological response of vascular tissues to harmful stimuli, such as pathogens, damaged cells, or irritants. The aim of inflammation is liquidation, dilution or elimination of the injurious stimuli and damaged tissue, or at least its demarcation and reparation. Based on various criteria, the inflammation can be split into protective or harming, acute or chronic, superficial or deep etc. Four phases can be observed during the inflammatory response: vascular response, acute cellular response, chronic cellular response and healing. A number of cells that are a part of the immune system

(particularly neutrophils, macrophages, T lymphocytes, endothelial cells, eosinophils, mast cells, thrombocytes), multi-enzymatic systems of blood plasma (complement, haemocoagulation system, fibrinolytic and kinin system), pro-inflammatory and anti-inflammatory cytokines, acute phase proteins, prostaglandins and other metabolites of arachidonic acid, as well as certain other mediators of inflammation, are involved in an inflammatory reaction.

A fundamental cell of acute inflammation, which reacts to its development, and which as the first cell translocated into the locus of inflammation, is the neutrophil. Macrophages and T lymphocytes are particularly involved in chronic inflammation. At the required time, these cells produce the required amount of mediators, enzymes and cytotoxins, which kill and decompose invading pathogens or damaged tissue in the course of protective inflammation. If the inflammatory stimulus still persists or if the above mentioned products are synthesised in an excessive amount, harming inflammation develops, the result of which is damage to its own cells and tissues, leading to impairment of function of various organs and systems, and possibly death. Inflammatory cells can put their activities into effect only if they translocate from the circulation into the tissue where the inflammatory reaction develops. This transendothelial migration (diapedesis) of leukocytes takes place in postcapillary venules by a number of adhesive interactions between adhesive molecules on the surfaces of leukocytes and endothelium. It is a multi-step process, in which selectins, integrins and immunoglobulin superfamilies, such as ICAM-1, ICAM-2, VCAM-1 and others, are involved.

Inflammatory bowel diseases → see Arthropathy in the course of inflammatory bowel diseases, Enteropathic arthritis (EA)

Infliximab (Remicade) A chimeric monoclonal antibody (consisting of murine and human components) of the IgG1 class, which binds specifically to human TNFα. It is administered by intravenous infusions at regular intervals in doses of 3 mg/kg (rheumatoid arthritis), 5 mg/kg (ankylosing spondylitis, psoriatic arthritis or psoriasis, and Crohn's disease) over 2 hours. After the initial infusion, subsequent infusions are administered after two weeks, six weeks after the first dose, and then all subsequent doses are administered every eight weeks. The serum concentrations of infliximab are more sustained with concomitantly administered methotrexate (MTX; a fixed oral dose of 15–25 mg/week). The co-administration of infliximab and MTX (or an alternative immunosuppressant drug if MTX is not tolerated) not only significantly suppresses the inflammatory activity of rheumatoid arthritis, but also seems to improve the immunological tolerance of infliximab. The onset of action of infliximab is relatively rapid, usually seen soon after the first doses of the drug, and usually persists during the whole treatment period. However, relapse of the disease occurs in the majority of patients on withdrawal of treatment, which can be suppressed by restarting anti-TNF treatment.

Treatment: It should only be indicated in severely active RA with unfavourable prognostic factors, which is refractory to treatment with at least two disease-modifying anti-rheumatic drugs (DMARDs), one of which should be MTX. Infliximab is sometimes administered in early RA with significant activity and progression. Treatment with infliximab has very favourable results in the treatment of severe ankylosing spondylitis unresponsive to conventional high dose NSAIDs, and also in active and resistant forms of psoriatic arthritis.

Adverse effects: Headache, nausea, upper respiratory airways infections, urinary infections, tuberculosis, leukoclastic vasculitis, exanthema, allergies, pruritus, anti-dsDNA antibody positivity, and rarely drug induced systemic lupus erythematosus.

Infrared radiation The invisible part of the optic spectrum, with a wavelength longer than that of visible light. It is divided into three bands according to wavelength:
1. short-wave band IR-A (wave-length of 760–1400 nm), the initial radiation band,
2. middle-wave band IR-B (1400–3000 nm),
3. long-wave band IR-C (over 3000 nm).
IR-A has a superficial thermal effect and penetrates to a depth of up to 1 cm; it is used for diathermy of tissue. IR-B and IR-C are used for warming-up of tissue.

Inherited complete heart block → see Neonatal Lupus

Instruments of assessing (health status measurements, outcome measurement) Questionnaires that are either completed in a controlled patient/physician interview or are self administered by the patient. The questions are directed to obtain relevant answers as to the quality of life of the patient in relation to his/her health status. They contain items (dimensions, domains) that focus on the patient's physical, mental and social status. Individual items or domains are scored separately. Some systems express the result as a score.

There are two main groups of instruments: generic, used in different diseases to assess the overall state of health of the patient, and condition-specific, for the given disease.

Generic instruments

MOS-SF – medical outcome study – short form 36

MOS-SF-36 8-item questionnaire with 36 questions was designed specifically for global assessment of the population health status. The questionnaire investigates the limitations in physical functions, limitations of normal daily activities caused by decreased function, limitations in social activities, body pain, and mental health, limitations in normal role activities because of emotional problems, vitality, and general health perceptions. The questionnaire is filled in by the patient/proband.

Nottingham health profile (Hunt et al. 1985).

There are 38 questions answered simply with yes/no. The patient/proband fills in the questionnaire alone, usually over 5 to 10 minutes. Each question is assigned a weighted value. The best score is 0, the worst is 100.

Sickness impact profile – SIP (Bergner et al. 1985).

It has 6 main items containing 136 questions. It monitors the level of self-attendance, mobility, ambulation, sleep, eating, work, home management, social interactions, recreation, communication, alertness and emotional behaviour. Individual items are scored and the profile is formed by summation of similar items.

Condition-specific

For rheumatoid arthritis:

Health assessment questionnaire (HAQ Fries et al. 1980).

Originally developed for RA it has also proved useful in osteoarthritis. It is also commonly used in many other chronic diseases. There are national versions of the questionnaire. It contains 20 items for the assessment of activities such as dressing, cleaning, rising from a chair, eating, walking, doing body care, arising and reaching for various remote items and activities outside the house. The visual analogue scale (VAS) for pain assessment is also part of it. The score from these items is averaged out and the disability index obtained. The questionnaire takes about 5 minutes to complete.

Arthritis impact measurement scale (AIMS; Meenan et al. 1980). AIMS has 9 items containing a total of 46 questions. Mobility, physical activity, dexterity, social sphere, household activities, activities of daily living (ADL), pain, depression and anxiety are all assessed. Subsequently other questions were added relating to the function of the upper and lower limbs and activities needed for working, leisure time utilisation and the independence of the patient. Similarly to HAQ, it is often used in RA but in contrast to HAQ is time-consuming.

McMaster Toronto arthritis patient preference disability index (MACTAR; Tugwell et al. 1987).

Beside demographic questions are 25 questions related to the possibility of performing certain activities, which are assessed by three possible answers rating between no problem performing the activity, performing the activity with a little difficulty and performing the activity is impossible.

Signals of functional impairment (SOFI; Eberhardt et al. 1988).

Nine simple tasks (for the hand, the whole upper and lower extremity) performed by the patient and assessed by a physician revealing any functional limitations. They can be easily used in daily rheumatological and rehabilitation practice.

Rapid assessment of disease activity in rheumatology (RADAR; Mason et al. 1992 a, b).

The patient self assesses the course of the disease over the last 6 months. Morning stiffness is assessed in 6 time intervals using the VAS. According to the ARA criteria, the patient is classified to the relevant class of functional disability; and assesses pain and tenderness at 10 chosen joints.

Rheumatoid arthritis disease activity index (RADAI; Stucki et al. 1995).

Besides being a model for indicating painful joints, the system contains the Likert's scale for assessing joint stiffness, and also psychometric data.

Overall status in rheumatoid arthritis (OSRA; Symmons et al. 1995).

Using a 3-degree scale (0, 1, 2) it assesses questions in 4 divisions (demographic data, disease activity index, impairment in the functional and social sphere and treatment in the given time). The system is valid and rapid and is undertaken by directed interview.

Rheumatoid arthritis pain scale (RASP; Anderson et al. 1987).

This is a valid and reliable system for assessing pain in patients with RA. It contains 24 items, each of which is evaluated on a scale from 0 to 7.

Piper fatigue scale (PFS; Piper et al. 1990).

It contains 41 questions (the revised version 22 items) divided into 4 sections. All questions are answered using the VAS. Some of them contradict each another. The total score is evaluated.

For ankylosing spondylitis:

Bath ankylosing spondylitis indices (BAS-indices; Calin 1995).

BASG is a global assessment tool to assess the total impact of the disease on the patient over a time interval. The patient's assessments are made using the VAS.

BASDAI (BAS disease activity index) consists of 6 questions, 5 of which are related to 5 main symptoms: tiredness, pain in the spine, pain and swelling of the joints, localised regions of increased sensitivity and morning stiffness; the question assesses both the degree and duration of stiffness. All questions are measured using the VAS.

BASFI (BAS functional index) assesses responses to 10 questions affecting activities of daily living using the VAS.

BASRI (BAS radiological index) has 4 degrees of radiographic assessment of sacroileitis.

BASMI (BAS metrology index) rates measurements of rotation in the cervical spine, the distance between the tragus of the ear and the wall (Forestier fleche), both lateral deviations, Schober's distance in a modified version and intermalleolar distance.

Dougados' functional index (DFI) – (Dougados et al. 1988).

It has 20 items focusing on activities of daily living and evaluated by three possible answers. The testimony of this questionnaire is more valid than metric measurement. The results are similar to those obtained by BASFI.

For systemic lupus erythematosus:
Systemic lupus erythematosus disease activity index (SLEDAI; Bombardier et al. 1992).

The assessment of clinical symptoms by the severity level of the symptoms. 8 symptoms are rated with 8 points, 6 with 3 points, 7 with 2 points and 3 with 1 point.

For fibromyalgia:
Fibromyalgia impact questionnaire (FIG; Burckhardt et al. 1991).

This assessment consists of 4 items. The first item contains 10 questions focusing on daily and social activities; the second one focuses on the overall well-being in the past week; the third one focuses on the possibility of work; and the fourth one focuses on how fibromyalgia problems influence the patient's work capacity. It is evaluated using the VAS and individual items are scored.

Euro Quol questionnaire (Hurst et al. 1994).

This contains 5 items, each of which contains 3 questions. For each question there are 3 possible answers. The best score is 5, the worst is 15. In addition to questions it contains a vertical visual analogue score. It is the most widespread questionnaire for assessment of patient's quality of life.

Oswestry low back pain disability questionnaire (Haas and Nyiendo 1992).

It contains 10 items (pain intensity, personal care, lifting, walking, sitting, standing, sleeping, social life, travelling and changing degree of pain). Each item has a choice of 6 answers.

For osteoarthrosis:
Lequesne's algofunctional test and assessment of the severity of hip joint impairment (Lequesne et al. 1987).

Contains the 3 items pain, walking and daily activities. The assessment of each item uses a severity scale from 1 to 6. The activities are rated with 3 points. One number expresses the function. A score of 1 to 4 indicates normal hip joint function; a score of 4 to 8 indicates moderate impairment; a score of 8 to 10 indicates significant impairment; and a score over 11 represents an indication for total joint replacement.

Western Ontario and McMaster universities osteoarthritis index (WOMAC; Bellamy et al., 1988).

This specific questionnaire is designed for assessing the function in patients with hip- or knee-OA. The patient him/herself answers 24 questions divided into 3 sections. Five questions deal with pain, 2 with stiffness and 17 with the activities of daily living. It is evaluated on a 5-point scale.

Insulin As well as its most important role on glucose metabolism, insulin has effects on the normal development of the skeleton. It stimulates the synthesis of bone matrix and has an influence on its mineralisation. The effect on the osseous bone tissue is direct as well as mediated by IGF-1.

Insulin-like growth factor (IGF) IGF-1 and IGF-2 increase the production of the collagens of bone, the synthesis of matrix and stimulate replication of the osteoblasts. In addition, IGF-1 inhibits the degradation of the bone collagen.

INT Test An analytical method using iodonitrotetrazolium (INT) solution, which changes colour when incubated with leukocytes in the presence of phagocytosable particles, which is evidence of the ability to produce superoxide and other reactive oxygen intermediates (ROI). The intensity of the red colour is measured photometrically (485nm) and is proportional to the ability of the leukocytes to kill bacteria after phagocytosis.

Integrins A family of heterodimeric glycoproteins whose molecules contain two types of polypeptide chain – α and β. They are divided into subfamilies whose members have a common β chain but different α chains. In humans, 19 α and 8 β subunits have been characterised. The subfamily of β_1-integrins is referred to as very late antigens (VLA-1 to VLA-6); the subfamily of β_2-integrins is composed of leukocyte adhesins and has three very well characterised members: LFA-1 (CD11a/CD18), CR3 (CD11b/CD18) and CR4 (CD11c/CD18), while the cytoadhesins of the β_3-integrin subfamily represent the receptors for vitronectin. Integrins are surface adhesion molecules responsible for tissue coherence, cellular interactions during embryonic development and for immune responses, including the binding of cells to molecules of the extracellular matrix, including collagens and fibronectin. They play a major role in the colonisation of lymphoid tissues and organs by lymphocytes and other immune system cells, in the migration of leukocytes from the microcirculation to the tissues during inflammation (diapedesis) and in the interaction of lymphocytes with antigen presenting cells.

The dominant osteoclastic integrin $\alpha v\beta 3$ is a member of αv family of integrins. It is expressed on osteoclasts following activation with RANKL and is an essential part of physiological bone resorption. The competitive ligands for $\alpha v\beta 3$ are able to slow down the osteoresorption and are candidates for antiresorptive treatment of bones

Intercellular adhesion molecule (ICAM)
At present, there are four types known – ICAM-1, ICAM-2, ICAM-3 and ICAM-4 – all belonging structurally to the immunoglobulin superfamily. ICAM-1 (CD54) is a membrane glycoprotein found on various cells, including endothelial and dendritic cells. ICAM-1 binds specifically to the β_2-integrin receptor LFA-1, thereby helping to perform various interactions between T-lymphocytes and antigen-presenting cells (immune response initiation), between neutrophils and cells of the vascular endothelium (initiation of the inflammatory reaction), or between other pairs of cells. IFN-γ, TNF-α and IL-1 stimulate its production. ICAM-2 (CD102) and ICAM-3 (CD50) have similar properties to ICAM-1. Apart from LFA-1, they can also bind to the complement receptors CR3 and CR4.

Intercellular substance of cartilage matrix
Basically an amorphous gel consisting mostly of proteoglycans, but also containing proteins and glycoproteins. This gel is reinforced by a fine, strong network of type II collagen with small amounts of type VI, IX and XI collagens. Among glycoproteins, the matrix contains chondronectin and chondrocalcin.

Approximately half of the organic matter of the matrix consists of viscous hydrophilic proteoglycans. The presence of large macromolecular arrangements of glycoproteins, which provide a molecular substrate for the considerable elasticity (resilience) of the cartilage, is a typical attribute of the matrix. Molecules of proteoglycans form the skeleton in which molecules of interstitial fluid and ions are present. Certain molecules of interstitial fluid even bind through hydrogen bridges to negatively charged units in the glycosaminoglycan chains of proteoglycans. Enormous, for cartilage specific, proteoglycan is denoted as aggrecan. Its molecules are immobilized in the skeleton of collagen fibrils. Approximately 100 chains of chondroitin sulphate and 30 chains of keratan sulphate are bound to the protein nucleus of aggrecan. Aggrecan belongs to the group of hyaluronan binding proteins. The bond between aggrecan and hyaluronan is stabilised by a protein called link protein. Negative charge and high osmotic pressure are formed in the skeleton of

I

proteoglycans as each molecule of aggrecan contains amounts of sulfone groups. It is the reason that the cartilage tends to seal up. The sealing up is controlled by the skeleton of collagen fibrils, which are permanently stretched, even in uncharged cartilage. Charged cartilage reacts by a change of osmotic and hydrostatic pressure and interstitial fluid moves from charged to uncharged areas of the cartilage, while aggrecan remains bound to hyaluronan and immobilised in the collagen skeleton.

Intergrins A family of small cytokines more commonly referred to as chemokines.

Interferential currents (IC) The application of two medium-frequency currents that easily overcome skin resistance. An effective low frequency current develops in the depth of the affected tissue after their interference and its size is determined by the difference between the frequencies of both alternate currents.

Modulations used:
- constant 0–10 Hz: used for muscle gymnastics,
- constant 90–100 Hz: has a sedative and spasmolytic effect,
- constant 100 Hz: spasmolytic effect,
- rhythmic 0–10 Hz: for muscle gymnastics,
- rhythmic 50–100 Hz: has an analgesic and spasmolytic effect and causes hyperaemia,
- rhythmic 90–100 Hz: has an analgesic and spasmolytic effect,
- rhythmic 0–100 Hz: has an alternating suppressive and irritating effect; used in pathologically altered cellular functions (oedema).

Interferon alpha (IFN-α) The main type of interferon produced by leukocytes. It is induced by foreign cells, cells infected by a virus, neoplastic cells and bacteria. It has about 15 isotypes whose genes are localised on chromosome 9 in man. Recombinant IFN-α (Intron A, Roferon A) is used in the treatment of hairy-cell leukaemia, chronic myeloid leukaemia, Kaposi sarcoma, malignant melanoma, multiple myeloma, chronic hepatitis B and C and several other disorders.

Interferon beta (IFN-β) It is produced mainly by fibroblasts with nucleic acids of viral or other origins serving as its inductors. Its gene is also localised on chromosome 9. Recombinant IFN-β (Betaferon) is used in the treatment of relapsing multiple sclerosis. IFN-α and IFN-β have antiviral and antiproliferative effects, and to a lesser extent immunoregulatory effects.

Interferon gamma (IFN-γ) A product of activated T-helper (T_H1) and T-cytotoxic (T_C) lymphocytes or NK-cells synthesized by them in response to a specific antigen or mitogens. It is therefore considered a typical lymphokine whose gene is localised on chromosome 12. Its main function is immunoregulatory, but it does have antiviral and antiproliferative effects as well. It is able to activate many different genes allowing activation of macrophages, giving them the ability to kill intracellular bacteria, to lyse neoplastic cells and exprime HLA class II antigens on their surface. It also stimulates the expression of HLA class I antigens on different cells, thereby making them more sensitive to the activity of cytotoxic T-lymphocytes. It facilitates the differentiation of B- and T-lymphocytes. Recombinant IFN-γ (Actimmun) is used for the prevention and treatment of the chronic granulomatous disease and certain viral disorders. IFN-α and IFN-β exert their activity via the same receptor, while IFN-γ has a unique receptor.

Interferon omega (IFN-ω) Originally referred to as IFN-$α_2$. It has similar properties to IFN-α.

Interferons Classed amongst the cytokines. In mammals, there are five known types of interferons (IFN) which are divided into two classes. IFN-α, IFN-β, IFN-ω and IFN-τ belong to the first class, while the second class is represented by IFN-γ.

Interleukin 1 (IL-1) A glycoprotein with MW 17 kDa. It exists in two forms – IL-1α and IL-1β – which are coded for by separate genes on chromosome 2. They act via a common receptor (IL-1R), which is found on different types of cells. The biological effects of IL-1 are therefore pleiotropic. IL-1α and IL-1β are typical pro-inflammatory cytokines synthesised by macrophages, monocytes and dendritic cells involved in the immune responses, inflammatory processes and haematopoiesis. They stimulate the proliferation of B- and T-lymphocytes, cause the expression of receptors for IL-2, leukoadhesive molecules on neutrophils and endothelial cells, the chemotaxy of neutrophils, macrophages and lymphocytes, and the cytotoxic activity of NK-cells. Further actions include the proliferation and synthesis of collagen by epithelial cells and fibroblasts, the synthesis of prostaglandins in macrophages and the hypothalamus, and the synthesis of acute phase proteins in hepatocytes. It participates in the majority of overreactive and pathological immune reactions. It exerts a damaging effect in rheumatoid arthritis and chronic inflammatory bowel diseases (ulcerative colitis, Crohn's disease). This harmful effect can be therapeutically blocked by monoclonal antibodies against IL-1 or by the natural antagonist of its receptor (IL-1RA).

Interleukin 2 (IL-2) A glycoprotein with MW 15.5 kDa coded for by a gene localised on human chromosome 4. It acts via its receptor IL-2R, which can have low-affinity, medium-affinity or high-affinity forms. It is produced by T_H1-lymphocytes after their activation with an antigen and IL-1. IL-2 is a growth factor for T- and B-lymphocytes and an activating factor of T_C-lymphocytes and NK-cells. In T_H-lymphocytes, it stimulates the production of other cytokines such as IL-4 and IFN-γ, as well as the antineoplastic activity of LAK-cells. Sufficient production of IL-2 and expression of IL-2R is of crucial importance for adequate T-cell immunity. A decreased production of IL-2 is observed in patients with severe combined immunodeficiency, Nezelof's syndrome, AIDS, type I diabetes mellitus and systemic lupus erythematosus. The stimulation of LAK-cells has gained ground in the treatment of certain neoplasms.

Interleukin 3 (IL-3) A glycoprotein with MW 20 kDa secreted mainly by T_H1- and T_H2-lymphocytes, NK-cells and mast cells. Its gene is localised on chromosome 5 in the proximity of the gene for GM-CSF. In the past it was referred to as a multipotent colony-stimulating factor (multi-CSF, colony-stimulating growth factors). It acts via a common receptor for IL-3 and GM-CSF. It is a growth factor of haematopoietic stem cells, megakaryocytes, erythrocytes, granulocytes, mast cells and macrophages.

Interleukin 4 (IL-4) It is produced mainly by T_H2-lymphocytes, but also by mast cells and basophils. It is coded for by a gene localised on human chromosome 5. It stimulates the proliferation of early B-cells inducing their differentiation and production of IgM, IgG1 and IgE. Furthermore, IL-4 stimulates the proliferation of T-lymphocytes, the production of antigen-specific cytotoxic T-cells, the expression of HLA antigens and is an activating factor of macrophages and a growth factor of mast cells. With its capability to switch antibody production from IgM to IgE, it can greatly influence the development of the immediate type of allergic reactions which are mediated by IgE antibodies. It has an antiinflammatory effect.

Interleukin 5 (IL-5) Secreted mainly by T_H2-lymphocytes and activated mast cells. Its gene is localised on chromosome 5. It's most important pleiotropic effects include the activation and stimulation of B-cell and eosinophil proliferation, stimulation of cytotoxic T-lymphocytes and the capability of switching between the production of IgM antibody isotype to IgA antibody isotype, and the ability to increase the expression of receptors for IL-2. During these activities it has a synergic action, especially with IL-2 and IL-4. Together with IL-3 and GM-CSF it controls the development of eosinophils.

Interleukin 6 (IL-6) A glycoprotein whose gene is localised on chromosome 7. Originally it was termed IFN-β_2. It is synthesised by various cells including T_H2- and B-lymphocytes, macrophages, endothelial cells, fibroblasts, mast cells and a number of neoplastic cell lines. It is considered a typical proinflammatory cytokine. Its production is also induced by a number of other cytokines (IL-1, IL-2, TNF-α, IFN-γ, etc.). It acts as an endogenous pyrogen and an activator of synthesis of acute phase proteins in hepatocytes, as well as a final growth factor for the differentiation of the B-cell to plasma cells, and as growth factors of plasmocytomas and myelomas. Increased IL-6 synthesis is observed in a number of disorders, such as rheumatoid arthritis, systemic lupus erythematosus, AIDS, other infections, a number of neoplasms, and in acute transplant rejection.

Interleukin 7 (IL-7) It facilitates the differentiation of lymphoid stem cells into early precursor B- and T-cells, and acts as a growth factor of T-lymphocytes. It is synthesised by stromal cells of the bone marrow and thymus. It activates macrophages and stimulates the proliferation of thymocytes. It acts via high-affinity receptors belonging to the haematopoietin receptor superfamily.

Interleukin 8 (IL-8) It belongs to chemokines and was originally called neutrophil-activating peptide-1 (NAP-1). Its gene is localised on human chromosome 4 and codes for a small protein containing only 79 amino-acid units (MW 8.4 kDa). It is produced mainly by monocytes, macrophages and endothelial cells during a response to various factors inducing an inflammatory reaction. It acts via a specific receptor that can be found only on neutrophils, and so IL-8 is their crucial chemotactic and activating cytokine. In addition, it also induces the expression of β_2-integrins on neutrophils, which is of crucial importance for their transendothelial migration to the focus of inflammation. Its effect is hypothesised in pathological reactions involving the neutrophils, such as in adult respiratory distress syndrome (ARDS), idiopathic pulmonary fibrosis or the late phase of bronchial asthma.

Interleukin 9 (IL-9) It acts predominantly as a helping, co-stimulatory factor of other cytokines during the development of haematopoietic cells. It thus potentiates the proliferation of certain clones of T-helper cells, foetal thymocytes in the presence of IL-2, mast cells after their induction by IL-3 and erythrocytes in co-operation with erythropoietin. It is produced mainly by T_H2-lymphocytes under the influence of IL-1. Its gene is localised on chromosome 5 together with the genes coding for IL-3, IL-4, IL-5 and GM-CSF. The deletion of this chromosomal section is linked to the occurrence of malignancies (myelodysplastic syndrome, acute non-lymphocytic leukaemia).

Interleukin 10 (IL-10) It is produced mainly by T_H2-lymphocytes and to a lesser extent by T_H0-lymphocytes, monocytes, macrophages and activated B-lymphocytes. It is a pure protein (contains no saccharides) with a MW 18KDa. It inhibits the production of other cytokines (IFN-γ, TNF-β, IL-2 and IL-3) by T_H1-lymphocytes, cytotoxic T-lymphocytes and NK-cells. It inhibits the synthesis of pro-inflammatory cytokines IL-1, IL-6, IL-8, GM-CSF and TNF-α in macrophages. It blocks the presentation of proteinous antigens. It acts as a natural immunosuppressive and anti-inflammatory agent. Therefore, it is of possible clinical use in chronic inflammatory conditions and autoimmune disorders.

Interleukin 11 (IL-11) It has multiple biological properties similar to IL-6. Both these cytokines, however, have separate receptors. IL-11 particularly controls the lymphopoietic and haematopoietic systems, hepatic cells and adipogenesis. It is a growth factor of megakaryocytes and, together with IL-3, participates in the development of thrombocytes. It stimulates B-lymphocytes during the antibody-mediated response to T-independent antigens. It is produced by the supporting fibrous tissue in bone marrow and by fibroblasts. Its gene is localised on chromosome 5. It facilitates the development of plasmocytoma, which indicates its role in tumour production.

Interleukin 12 (IL-12) Its molecule consists of a heterodimer of two glycoprotein chains linked together by disulphide bonds. The genes for both chains in a human are localised on different chromosomes. The gene coding for the polypeptide chain p35 is localised on chromosome 3 and a gene coding for p40 is localised on chromosome 5. The principal producers of IL-12 are monocytes and macrophages. It is an activation factor of NK-cells, stimulating their cytotoxicity in the ADCC reaction (antibody-dependent cell cytotoxicity), and increasing the expression of the CD56 molecule which is their typical surface marker. By its activity, NK-cells develop into the more effective LAK-cells. In this activity it resembles IL-2, but with a lower effect (about 50%). In addition, IL-12 facilitates the occurrence of specific human cytotoxic T-lymphocytes against certain neoplasms, stimulates the proliferation of T_H- and T_C-cells and inhibits the secretion of IgE stimulated by IL-4. It is considered to be the principal stimulator of IFN-γ production by T_H1-lymphocytes. In this sense, it acts in synergy with IL-18. With respect to these immunoregulatory influences, IL-12 has been studied in the treatment of parasitic and neoplastic disorders with the advantage of low toxicity and minimal adverse events.

Interleukin 13 (IL-13) An anti-inflammatory cytokine whose gene is localised on chromosome 5 in close proximity to the gene coding for IL-4. It has similar biological effects as IL-4. It is produced predominantly by activated T_H2-lymphocytes. It exerts a regulatory activity on various immune system cells, especially monocytes, macrophages, B-lymphocytes and NK-cells. It is a chemotactic factor for monocytes and macrophages, but inhibits the production of pro-inflammatory cytokines in them. It therefore can be regarded as a significant endogenous anti-inflammatory regulator, similar to IL-10. It inhibits the replication of HIV-1 in macrophages and monocytes, so differs from IL-3 and GM-CSF, which, on the contrary, stimulate the replication of this aetiological agent of AIDS. It also stimulates the proliferation and differentiation of B-lymphocytes, similar to IL-4.

Interleukin 14 (IL-14) A glycoprotein with MW 55 kDa which previously was termed a high-molecular B-cell growth factor. It is secreted mainly by follicular dendritic cells, T-cells of the germinal centres and certain neoplastic cells. Its main function is to increase B-cell proliferation and to induce and maintain the production of memory B-cells. The receptor for IL-14 can be found only on activated B-lymphocytes, not on resting ones. The IL-14 molecule has a similar amino-acid sequence as the Bb factor, present in the alternative pathway of complement activation.

Interleukin 15 (IL-15) A glycoprotein with MW 15 kDa and the function of a pro-inflammatory cytokine. It is produced by multiple cells and tissues, including activated macrophages, fibroblasts, skeletal muscles and the kidneys. It increases the cytotoxicity of CTL (cytotoxic T-lymphocytes) and NK-cells. In this way, it is similar to IL-2 and IL-12. It binds to a receptor consisting of three polypeptide chains, two of which are identical to the receptor for IL-2. IL-15 induces proliferation on mast cells, helper and cytotoxic lymphocytes, including those having the antigen receptor gamma/delta. It stimulates the production of IL-5 by allergen-specific T-cell clones, thereby moving the T_H1/T_H2 balance to favour T_H2-cells, with associated participation in allergic responses mediated by this T-lymphocyte subpopulation. IL-15 is an effective chemotaxin of T-lymphocytes; it suppresses their apoptosis and induces the expression of ligands for leukoadhesive β-integrins. It is hypothesised that it plays a key role in the upkeep of chronic inflammation in diseases such as rheumatoid arthritis, pulmonary sarcoidosis, bronchial asthma and ulcerative colitis.

Interleukin 16 (IL-16) An immunomodulatory and pro-inflammatory cytokine whose structure is much conserved among individual animal species. It is synthesized by cytotoxic (CD8⁺) lymphocytes in the form of a high-molecular precursor (MW 80 kDa), whereby polypeptide chains with a MW 14 kDa emerge in the producing cells. These chains polymerise to tetrameres which are the only biologically effective form of IL-16. They are secreted by CD8$^+$ lymphocytes in response to an antigen, mitogen, histamine or serotonin. IL-16 uses the CD4 molecule as a receptor, which is why it exerts its action not only on helper T-lymphocytes, but also on macrophages and eosinophils which also have this differentiation antigen on their surface. IL-16 is a chemotactic factor for these cells and it induces in them the synthesis of other cytokines and also the expression of HLA-DR histocompatibility antigens. On the other hand, after binding to CD4$^+$ lymphocytes, IL-16 inhibits the ensuing immune response as well as the infectiousness and intracellular replication of HIV-1, the aetiological agent of AIDS. The epithelial cells of the airways of patients with asthma can also release a biologically effective IL-16, while the epithelial cells of healthy individuals can't. This suggests a potential therapeutic effect for IL-16 inhibitors.

Interleukin 17 (IL-17) A glycoprotein containing 155 amino acid units that has been described as recently as 1995. Its amino acid sequence shows a considerable homology with one of the proteins of herpetic lymphotropic virus (HVS13). It is produced as a dimer by activated T-lymphocytes. It stimulates fibroblasts, endothelial and epithelial cells to synthesise IL-6, IL-8 and GM-CSF, which indicates that it could contribute to inflammatory processes involving T-lymphocytes.

Interleukin 18 (IL-18) A pro-inflammatory cytokine which was originally described in 1989 as an inducing factor of IFN-γ (IGIF). However, this activity is performed in conjunction with a secondary stimulus such as IL-12, mitogens or a microbial agent. Both cytokines (IL-18 and IL-12) act in synergy and have a critical role in inducing the production of IFN-γ especially by T$_H$1-lymphocytes. IL-18 is produced predominantly by activated macrophages in the form of an ac-

tive precursor that is cleaved by caspase 1 (formerly this protease was referred to as IL-1β converting enzyme – ICE) to the active cytokine. IL-18 is structurally similar to IL-1β and is coded for by a gene localised on chromosome 9. It acts mainly via a specific receptor, IL-18R, whose soluble form (sIL-18R) is able to neutralise the effects of IL-18. The most significant pro-inflammatory activity of IL-18 is its capability to induce the production of TNF-α, IL-1β, GM-CSF, chemokines CXC and CC, Fas ligands and the nuclear factor κB (NF-κB). The stimulation of Fas ligand expression on NK-cells and T-lymphocytes then leads to an increase in their cytotoxic activity. On the other hand, IL-18 is a very effective activator of HIV-1 (aetiological agent of AIDS) replication in human macrophages. The normal concentration of IL-18 in the blood is 50 to 150 pg/mL, whereas in patients with acute lymphoblastic leukaemia, chronic lymphocytic leukaemia and acute and chronic myeloid leukaemias, it rises to 200 to 1200 pg/mL. The overproduction of IL-18 leads to an increased production of nitric oxide (NO), which then participates instantly in various pathological reactions.

Interleukins Cytokines participating in the regulatory interactions between leukocytes. There are currently 33 known interleukins, which are termed by abbreviations IL-1 to IL-33.

Intermittent hydrarthrosis of the joints (hydrops articulorum intermittens) Characterised by recurrent attacks of a predominantly unilateral and relatively painless, non-inflammatory joint effusion. It is a long-lasting disorder often with life-long persistence. The knee joint is the most frequently affected joint, though rarely it can affect the elbow, hip or shoulder joints.

Clinical symptoms and signs:
periodic recurrent joint effusion,
no apparent radiologic joint damage,
very rarely progresses to rheumatoid arthritis.

International classification of functioning (ICF)

This has replaced the previous IDH classification (impairment–disability–handicap). In 2001, the ICF (international classification of functioning) was issued by the World Health Organisation as an international framework for measuring health and disability at both individual and population levels. It was endorsed by all 191 Member States of the World Health Organisation. The ICF classification replaced the term "disability" by "activity", while a number designate "diminished activity". In place of "handicap" it uses the term "participation" (in social life). A number also designate "restricted participation". In the ICF classification "environment" is a new dimension, where facilitating "F" and barrier "B" factors are also included.

Intraarticular glucocorticoid treatment

The intraarticular injection of glucocorticoids is a useful method for suppressing active synovitis within a joint. Intraarticular injections should not be used too frequently or to joints without signs of actual inflammation. One joint should not be treated more than 3–4 times in a year. Most frequently triamcinolone acetonide (Kenalog) and methylprednisolone (Depomedrone) are used, though hydrocortisone can be used if only a short term effect is required.

Intraarticular treatment

Rheumatoid arthritis in adults and adolescents is probably the disorder in which most intraarticular injections are given by rheumatologists. They are particularly useful when exceptional inflammatory activity is present in one or more joints. They are also used following disease flare to cover the delayed effect of an increase in general systemic treatment (DMARDs). In children with juvenile idiopathic arthritis, the choice of preparations is limited (methylprednisolone is more appropriate) due to potential growth disturbance of the affected joint. The dosing interval between intraarticular injections into the same joint should generally not be less than 3 months.

Potential hazards of intraarticular and intralesional injections of glucocorticoids:

- radiological deterioration of the joints – steroid arthropathy (Charcot-like arthropathy, osteonecrosis – low incidence),
- iatrogenic infection – very rare complication,
- rupture of the tendons,
- tissue atrophy, adipose necrosis, calcifications,
- nerve damage (most frequent after carpal tunnel injection),
- post-injection flare,
- uterine bleeding,
- pancreatitis – rarely,
- erythema and sensation of warmth on the face and body,
- posterior subcapsular cataract (only after many injections).

Iontophoresis

This is a non-invasive method of inserting treatments into the body using a galvanic current. Histamine (muscle relaxant effect), novocaine, lidocaine, dionine (analgesic effect), hyaluronidase (fibrolytic effect) and hydrocortisone (anti-inflammatory effect) are inserted from the anode. Salicylates (anti-inflammatory and fibrolytic effect) and iodine (fibrolytic effect) are inserted from the cathode. When using non-steroidal anti-inflammatory drugs, the active electrode can vary.

Ir genes (immune response genes)

An obsolete term for genes regulating the immune response of an individual to specific antigens, both in a quantitative and qualitative sense (immune response genes). The current view is that these genes are now the class II MHC (major histocompatibility complex) genes.

Isolated vasculitis of the central nervous system (CNS)

A rare disorder occurring in middle age. Headache, nausea and vomiting are the most prominent clinical features. Confusion, dementia and loss of consciousness together with signs of focal ischaemic cerebral event (stroke) can also be seen. The diagnosis is confirmed using cerebral angiography, or a targeted biopsy of the CNS. Aggressive treatment with corticosteroids and cyclophosphamide can reduce the mortality of this, often fatal, disorder.

J

Janda hypermobility test → see Hypermobility test 2 (according to Janda)

Jansen type metaphyseal chondrodysplasia An autosomal dominant hereditary metaphyseal chondrodysplasia with dysproportional nanism (dwarfism) and short and deformed limbs. The metaphyses have a shape resembling rickets. It may be confused with rickets in the neonate and infant. However, X-rays show visible prominent separation between the epiphysis and the metaphysis, especially at the distal end of the femur and proximal end of the tibia. During toddler age, spotty calcifications appear in the metaphysis, formed by a partially calcified cartilage protruding into the diaphysis. Besides long bone involvement, the skull and spine can also be affected. There is usually generalised demineralisation of the skeleton. Laboratory tests show the same as in primary hyperparathyroidism, with increased serum calcium and alkaline phosphatase levels and a low serum phosphate, but the serum concentrations of the parathormone (PTH) or PTHrP (PTH-related protein) are very low. Hypercalciuria and elevated hydroxyprolinuria are present. The aetiology is a mutation of the gene coding for the PTH/PTHrP receptor, which is then capable of self-activation without the presence of bound hormone.

Joint A point of inter-connection of two or more bones that enables movement between them. The degree of movement depends on the type of joint.

The following types of joints are recognised:
Synarthroses – Joints without a cavity. Movement is very limited. The bones are inter-connected by fibrous tissue or cartilage.
- fibrous articulations:
  syndesmosis – the bones are connected by dense fibrous tissue (sutures, distal tibiofibular articulation),

  gomphosis – dental alveoli connection with the help of collagen fibres (teeth in bony sockets),
- cartilaginous articulations:
  synchondrosis – the bones are connected by hyaline cartilage (synchondrosis sphenopetrosa, synchondrosis manubriosternalis and xiphosternalis),
  symphysis – the bones are connected predominantly by a fibrous cartilage and a very small amount of hyaline cartilage (symphysis pubis, symphysis intervertebral). In the course of life a cleft often appears in the fibrous cartilage of the symphysis. This articulation is called hemiarthrosis and is considered to be a transition form of a joint towards diarthrosis (for example the vertical cleft filled with synovial fluid – cavum symphysis in the fibrous cartilage of symphysis pubis – pubic symphysis, the clefts in the intervertebral discs of the cervical spine – uncovertebral clefts). Rigid connection of the bones by bone tissue is called synostosis.

Diarthroses – Joints with a cavity (cavum articulare) containing synovial fluid. The bones touch one another with the contact surfaces covered by a hyaline cartilage, except for the perimeter of contact surfaces where they are connected by fibrous tissue forming a joint capsule composed of dense collagen tissue lined by synovial membrane on the inside and strengthened by ligaments externally. Such joints are called synovial joints. The range of movement in them is substantially greater than with synarthroses.

Diarthroses whose mobility is substantially limited due to the shape of articular surfaces and strong ligaments are referred to as amphiarthroses (for example, the proximal tibiofibular joint and the sacroiliac joint).

Joint and Periarticular structures A complex functional unit consisting of articulating bones, intra-articular structures (menisci), articular capsule, solidifying ligaments, adjacent muscles, tendons, peritendon and bursae. Neuro-regulatory mechanisms from peripheral nerves to central nervous system, and arterial, venous and lymphatic systems, belong to this unit. The basic physical examination consists of five tests:
1. inspection,
2. palpation,
3. active and passive movements examination,
4. examination of physiological movements in the joint,
5. muscle strength testing (ability of muscular resistance).

Joint involvement in syphilis Syphilitic arthropathies are arthritides occurring in syphilis.
Clinical symptoms and signs: Changes in the joints occur at any stage of syphilis, but is commoner in early syphilis. Typically the joints are painless or only mildly painful at night, which is in contrast to the large swelling of the joints. A beneficial response from antiluetic treatment is also typical.

Joint play This is the paraphysiological movement in a joint that can only be elicited passively as a ventro-dorsal or medio-lateral shift, or, for example, a dorsal shift of the tibia and internal rotation of the knee. These are the mutual shifts of articular surfaces, rotation and distractions.

Joint Prosthesis An artificial joint designed from special material (metal, ceramics, polyethylene, etc.) for replacing a joint damaged by trauma, osteoarthrosis, arthritis, tumour, etc. The most frequently used have been hip and knee joint prostheses, but increasingly shoulder, ankle and elbow joints, small joints of the hands and feet and the spine are being used. Prostheses are divided into total joint prostheses – replacement of the whole joint – and hemiprostheses – replacement of a certain part of the joint. De-

pending on the fixation method, they can be subdivided into cemented prostheses – the components are fixed to the bone by bony cement, uncemented – the components are fixed to bone without a cement interlayer, and hybrid – each component is fixed in a different manner. In terms of construction, there are prostheses shaped as a monoblock – the prosthesis is made from one piece of material, or as modular – the prosthesis is made up of multiple components.
Indication for the use of joint prostheses:
• primary – primary treatment of the joint by prosthesis,
• revision – the prosthesis is used after primary implantation failed,
• tumorous (individual) – replacement of a joint and other articular structures affected by a neoplastic disease.

Joint protection The main principles:
• To control and save overall energy output
• Large joints and muscle groups must be involved in each activity
• Limit the influence of gravity during each activity (shuffle objects, do not elevate them)
• Use joints and muscles on those functional levels in which their performance is most effective
• All activities during which the joints are in one particular position for a long time are contraindicated
• Do not attempt any difficult muscle exercise that cannot be immediately terminated if necessary

Juvenile ankylosing spondylitis The rare onset of ankylosing spondylitis in childhood (mainly in pre-pubertal boys) gives a clinical picture in which affection of peripheral joints precedes that of the axial skeleton. The presence of the HLA-B27 antigen in blood tests helps to confirm the diagnosis. Patients usually develop typical features of ankylosing spondylitis after puberty.
Clinical symptoms and signs:
enthesitis of the Achilles tendon insertion on the calcaneus and other enthesopathies, arthritis of the lower limbs.

Juvenile chronic arthritis (JCA) → see Juvenile idiopathic arthritis (JIA)

Juvenile dermatomyositis (JDM) A rare multisystem disorder of autoimmune aetiology manifested by an aseptic inflammation of the skin and striated muscles.

Clinical symptoms and signs:
- *acute type:*
  fever,
  malaise,
  characteristic heliotrope rash on the upper eyelids, an erythematous rash over the dorsal aspects of the MCP joints (Gottron's sign) and an erythematous rash on the chest.
  symmetrically painful/tender muscles with weakness, most marked proximally.
  difficulty swallowing solid food (dysphagia).
- *chronic type:*
  arthralgia, possibly arthritis,
  weakness, falls, stumbling,
  inability to climb stairs and do press-ups
  soft tissue calcification in the limbs.
  The diagnosis is suspected from the clinical picture associated with elevated muscle enzymes, and confirmed by electromyography and muscle biopsy. Treatment usually involves corticosteroids with or without immunosuppressive agents. The prognosis is very variable.

Juvenile idiopathic arthritis (JIA) Previously referred to as juvenile rheumatoid arthritis (JRA) or juvenile chronic arthritis (JCA). It is a chronic inflammatory disorder with onset before 16 years of age which has a prominent manifestation involving the musculoskeletal system, but can also affect various organs and tissues. It is a heterogeneous disease containing several forms (pauciarticular, polyarticular, systemic).

Forms of JIA

Systemic form (Still's disease)

Affects both genders, more frequently boys, with onset usually between 1 and 4 years of age, rarely between 6 and 7.

Clinical symptoms and signs: High temperature (intermittent, can subside during the day and last longer than three months); maculopapular, sometimes confluent non-itching rash that comes and goes; generalised lymphadenopathy (capable of causing abdominal pain); hepatosplenomegaly, serositis, myocarditis; arthralgia – polyarthritis (especially the knees, wrists and ankles are affected); growth disturbances. The mortality rate is 4% (infections and amyloidosis).

Polyarticular form

Affects mostly girls between 8 and 14 years old.

Clinical symptoms and signs: Systemic symptoms and signs are mild or absent. A symmetrical polyarthritis develops acutely or subacutely. It affects especially hands, knees, ankles, cervical spine and temporomandibular joints, potentially leading to severe contractures if untreated. Local changes of bone growth (micrognathia) are frequent features. Not infrequently accompanied by fever and lymphadenopathy. Acute phase reactants (ESR, CRP) are often markedly elevated. Rheumatoid nodules may be present, especially in patients with positive rheumatoid factor. Radiological changes show periarticular osteoporosis and erosions. In severe cases, severe deformities and ankylosis can develop. The prognosis can be poor.

Therapy: Initially, NSAIDs drugs are administered. In actively progressing cases, DMARDs are given, followed by biological treatment (anti-TNF therapy) in unresponsive cases. Continuous exercise (prevention of contractures) and physiotherapy are important; in severe disturbances of function, surgical reconstruction is applicable.

Systematic exercise, positioning and wearing orthoses is important. A multi-disciplinary approach with nurses, physiotherapists, occupational therapists and school tutors is important to ensure a good quality of life.

Pauciarticular form

It occurs in girls before the age of 5.

Clinical symptoms and signs: Four or fewer joints are involved. It usually affects major joints, especially the knees, ankles, wrists or elbows. Fever and other systemic symptoms rarely occur. Typically there is chronic iridocyclitis. The disease goes into remission after 5 years in 30–40% of cases, with the prognosis for joints being very good.

Therapy: NSAIDs are used. DMARDs and glucocorticoids are not indicated in most cases. The intraarticular injection of glucocorticoids is the most appropriate way of suppressing the arthritis. Regular eye review by an ophthalmologist is recommended to detect and treat (topical hydrocortisone) any chronic iridocyclitis to prevent blindness.

Still's disease in adults

The disease resembles the systemic form of JIA but has its onset in adulthood.

Clinical symptoms and signs: Rash, fever, leukocytosis and marked increase in serum ferritin level.

Therapy: Salicylates and NSAIDs are given to reduce fever. In severe disease, glucocorticoids and DMARDs are given. The treatment of choice in adults now is Anakinra 100 mg sc daily.

Juvenile Osteoporosis A very rare disorder (several reported cases). The onset is usually between the 8th and 12th year of age and is manifested by bone pain, kyphosis and fractures. Initially, it is important to exclude osteogenesis imperfecta in the patient or family. Its pathogenesis is unclear and therefore no known treatment modality is recommended.

Juvenile rheumatoid arthritis (JRA) →
see Juvenile idiopathic arthritis (JIA)

Juvenile sclerosis A heterogeneous group of disorders characterised in localised form by induration of the skin and dermis, in the systemic form other organs are also affected due to vasculitis of the capillaries and small vessels.

Clinical symptoms and signs:
- *localised form:*
  morphea,
  linear scleroderma,
- *systemic form:*
  sclerodactyly or scleroderma,
  Raynaud's phenomenon,
  arthritis.
  calcinosis

Juvenile systemic lupus erythematosus A multisystem chronic disorder characterised by inflammation of the connective tissue, immune complex vasculitis and production of antinuclear antibodies.

Clinical symptoms and signs:
- fever,
- weight loss,
- skin signs, especially photosensitive rash
- arthritis/arthralgia,
- butterfly rash,
- anaemia, leukopenia,
- lymphadenopathy,
- pericarditis,
- hepatitis,
- neuropsychiatric disturbances,
- growth retardation,
- pulmonary fibrosis.

Kallikrein A proteolytic enzyme that is a component of the kinin and haemocoagulation systems. It participates in the production of bradykinin, activates Hageman's factor and is able to directly cleave the C5 component of the complement.

Kaltenborn method A set of three exercises mainly used in vertebrogenic syndromes for relaxing the rigidity of the spine at blocked points. The movements can be targeted segmentally at a given section of the spine and with their help release the whole of the spine. In rheumatology, the Kaltenborn method can be utilised in vertebrogenic disorders and the early stages of ankylosing spondylitis.

Kawasaki disease (KD) It is also known as mucocutaneous lymph node syndrome. It is an infantile systemic inflammatory disease with polyarteritis, aseptic lymphadenopathy, and inflammation of the skin and mucous membranes. It is an acute febrile disease of children younger than five years of age that occurs mainly in Japan, but sporadically in other countries. It mainly has a mild course but in approximately 2% of patients, it is fatal due to a necrotising vasculitis or multiple aneurysms of the coronary arteries (detectable by Echocardiography). Laboratory findings include raised acute phase reactants, leucocytosis and often a marked thrombocytosis. Its aetiology is unknown. An infection or a certain toxin produced by infecting microorganisms at the onset is hypothesised, followed by a number of immunological abnormalities such as increased production of IL-1 and TNF-α, as well as immune complexes. These cause damage to the vascular endothelium during the acute stage of the disease. Treatment includes intravenous immunoglobulin (2 g/Kg) and high dose aspirin.
Clinical symptoms and signs: Diagnostic criteria (American Heart Association 2004) comprise a fever lasting longer than 5 days plus 4 of the following: conjunctivitis and ocular erythema, dry red lips and tongue, gingivitis, cervical lymphadenopathy (the size of one node at least 1.5 cm), oedema and erythema on the palms and soles, polymorphous rash on the trunk.

Kegel exercise An exercise developed by American gynaecologist Arnold H. Kegel (1894–1981). The exercises are aimed at strengthening the pelvic floor and should help to prevent stress incontinence (involuntary urine leakage). The exercise system contains 4 phases: visualisation (to perceive with inner vision the region controlled by the muscles), relaxation (to learn how to breath in a comfortable supine position with pillow under the knees), isolation (controlling the vaginal and anal sphincters) and strengthening (isometric contraction of vaginal sphincters).

Kenalog (Triamcinalone) → see Glucocorticoids, Intraarticular glucocorticoid treatment

Kibler's fold A fold of the skin is moved between the thumb and the index finger, for example, on the back. Increased skin resistance (inability to move the fold further) indicates a hyperalgesic cutaneous zone related to a certain section of the spine eliciting a burning pain sensation in the examined patient.

Kienbock's disease Avascular necrosis of the lunate bone in the wrist named after the radiologist Robert Kienböck (Vienna, 1871–1953). The disorder predominantly affects men between 20 and 30 years of age and can develop after strenuous work, for example with a pneumatic hammer. An innate predisposition is also reported.

Kinesiology The scientific study of human movement. It encompasses an understanding of the interaction of anatomy, physiology, biomechanics and psychology in movement. A full understanding of kinesiology is important in the field of physiotherapy, but also in occupational therapy, osteopathy and chiropractic practice.

Kinesiotherapy The main, active component of physiotherapy and a means of restoring the range of movement, improving muscle strength and endurance, improving movement coordination, increasing the aerobic capacity and inducing a global sensation of wellness. In rheumatic disorders, especially in inflammatory forms, therapeutic exercise is governed by the activity of the disease and by the degree of functional impairment, age and endurance of the patient. The passive, active, assisted or anti-gravitational exercises can help to restore the range of movement. Endurance is improved by frequent repeating of exercise with a low load; muscle strength is restored by a small number of exercises with a higher load. It has been demonstrated that this therapeutic exercise has a positive influence on the increase in aerobic capacity, improvement in the rheological properties of synovial fluid and improvement of the overall mobility and skills of the patient. Kinesiotherapy may also have negative effects (theory of hypoxemic reperfusion of reactive oxygen species complexes into the joint cavity during movement; inactivation of α_1-antitrypsin in the synovial fluid; increased degradation of hyaluronic acid due to exercise).

Kininases Enzymes inactivating the kinins. In human plasma, there are two of them, kininase I or carboxy peptidase N, which cleaves the C-terminal arginine from kinins and anaphylatoxins and kininase II which is a peptidyl dipeptidase cleaving the C-terminal dipeptide Phe-Arg from the kinin molecules. In this way angiotensin I is converted to angiotensin II.

Köhler's disease Köhler's disease, first described by the German radiologist Alban Köhler (1874–1947), is an aseptic necrosis of the navicular bone, often in both feet, especially in 3 to 8 years old boys. There is a pressure and after load pain in the anterior part of the foot causing a thickening of the metatarsal part of the foot, gait disturbance and a limp. Radiological findings include widening of the articular cavity between the navicular and surrounding bones with increased density (sclerosis) of the body of the navicular bone.

Köhler's disease II Spontaneous osteonecrosis predominantly in 12 to 18 years old girls. It affects the capitulum of the 2nd or 3rd metatarsals.

König's disease Osteochondritis dissecans (first described 1887 by Franz König, German surgeon, 1832–1910), predominantly affecting elbow or knee, and rarely ankle or hip. It is more frequent in men. In contrast to the Perthe's disease, the necrosis affects the surface of the bone around the joint. Loose bodies may form within the joint on separation of the bone fragments.

Krause-Weber's test Used in the assessment of mobility and especially to monitor changes in mobility following treatment. It consists of five elements, each of which is rated on a scale from 0 to 10, with a maximum score of 50 points.

1. exercise: the patient lies in a supine position with his/her hands behind the head and should sit up without raising the lower limbs from the floor,
2. exercise: the patient lies on the floor with their hands behind the head and should elevate the lower limbs by 25–30° for 10 seconds,
3. exercise: the patient lies in a prone position with their hands behind the head and should elevate the head and the upper part of the thorax off the floor for 10 seconds,
4. exercise: the patient lies prone with hands behind their head and extend the lower limbs off the floor for 10 seconds,
5. exercise: the patient is in a standing position with feet together and should bend

K

forward so that he/she touches the ground with tips of the fingers without bending the knees.

Ku antigen → see Antibodies against Ku antigen

L

Laboratory indicators of the bone turnover In the process of bone remodelling, the crosslink fragments of collagen enter the blood, and then may be detected in the serum or urine.

At the present time their assessment is utilised for:
- monitoring the effect of treatment (a significant change can be seen in 3 to 6 months),
- prediction of bone loss, especially for the identification of so-called fast-losers, i.e. persons with increased bone turnover,
- prediction of fracture risk independently of the bone mineral density scan.

The individual markers differ by their specificity, sensitivity and severity of assessment, and their availability in the routine clinical practice. The significance of individual markers and their combination is still the subject of clinical monitoring.

We subdivide the markers of osteoformation from the markers of osteoresorption.

Markers of osteoresorption:
- crosslink compounds of collagen – deoxy-pyridinoline (DPD),
- C-terminal telopeptide fragment of type I collagen (CTX),
- N-terminal telopeptide fragment of type I collagen (NTX),
- C-telopeptide crosslink domain of type I collagen (ICTP).

Markers of osteoformation:
- Bone specific isoenzyme of alkaline phosphatase (bALP),
- osteocalcin,
- propeptides of type I procollagen (PICP, PINP).

Lactoferrin Protein that contains iron, found in milk and in secondary granules of neutrophils in which it is involved in antimicrobial pathways by absorbing iron from the environment. Iron is crucial for the growth and reproduction of micro-organisms.

LAK cells These are lymphokine (mainly IL-2) activated killer cells. NK cells are most frequently subject to activation, less frequently cytotoxic T-lymphocytes. LAK cells are also able to lyse those target cells that cannot be lysed by less active NK cells. This has recently led to their use in the treatment of certain tumours.

Lambert-Eaton Syndrome A complication of intrathoracic tumours, especially small cell lung cancer. Muscle weakness is the primary manifestation but myalgias and paraesthesiae can occur.

Aetiology – decreased release of acetylcholine in the nerve terminals;

EMG – has differential diagnostic value.

Treatment: Includes tumour excision, glucocorticoids and guanetidine administration.

Laminin Glycoprotein of high molecular weight (MW 900 kDa) comprising three (alpha, beta and gamma) polypeptide chains. Fifteen different forms of laminin have been identified. Laminin belongs to adhesive molecules and is part of the intercellular matrix, where it is bound to collagen type IV, heparan and glycosaminoglycans participating in the formation of the basement membrane of many tissues, including vessels. It is involved in the adhesion and chemotaxis of neutrophils. Laminin is the morphogenic factor of epithelial cells and hepatocytes, and by binding to receptors on the surface of nerve cells it enables mutual aggregation of these cells and the production of dendrites. It is produced by macrophages. The importance of laminins is illustrated by the fact that the dysfunctional structure of laminin-2 is the cause of some types of muscular dystrophy.

Large granular lymphocytes → see LGL (large granular lymphocytes)

Laser (Light Amplification by Stimulated Emission of Radiation) therapy (LT) Utilisation of monochromatic (only one wavelength) polarised (undulation only on one plane) coherent (vibration in one phase) light for medical treatment. Only so-called "low level lasers" with power of 40–200 mW are used in physiotherapy. Depending on the radiation technique, devices are divided into:
1. spot radiation,
2. scanners,
3. clusters; shower of lasers with several infrared diodes in one probe.

Indications in rheumatology are painful damage of soft tissues such as tendinitis, bursitis, epicondylitis, myositis, periarthritis, and osteoarthritic pain. Lasers can also be used for irradiation of acupuncture points referred to as "laser acupuncture". In laser therapy, safety procedures and contraindications (eyes and thyroid gland irradiation in particular) must be respected.

Lazy leukocyte syndrome An older term for unidentified conditions associated with deficient chemotaxis of leukocytes leading to increased risk of pyogenic infections. Nowadays, specific causes of deficient chemotaxis have been identified, so the nomenclature has been modified, e.g. leukocyte adhesion deficiency (LAD) syndrome.

LcSSc → see Systemic sclerosis (SSc)

LE cells The history of antinuclear antibodies (ANA) began in 1948 when Hargreaves described the phenomenon of LE cells. An LE cell is a polymorphonuclear (PMN) leukocyte, which has phagocytosed the released nuclear material of another leukocyte. Antibodies against nucleosomes, which in vitro bind to a released nucleus, are responsible for the LE phenomenon. As a consequence of the binding, complement is activated, with opsonisation of nuclear material, and finally phagocytosis by a PMN leukocyte occurs. This results in the formation of a large lucid

phagocytosed nucleus surrounded by small amounts of cytoplasm. The original nucleus of a phagocytosing leukocyte is compressed to the cell membrane. LE cells are typical for systemic lupus erythematosus, although they may occasionally be present in rheumatoid arthritis and systemic sclerosis. At present the detection of LE cells has been superseded and more sensitive techniques, such as immunofluorescent ANA detection, are used.

Lectins Proteins and glycoproteins which are able to specifically recognise and bind to different mono-, di- and trisaccharides. They activate the agglutination of erythrocytes and other cells, and are polyclonal (non-specific) mitogens of lymphocytes (e.g. phytohaemagglutinin, concanavalin A). This property is enabled by the presence of glycocalyx, which is located on the surface of most of the cells and which contains different oligosaccharide chains. Lectins were originally isolated from plants, but now are also known to be present in animals (so called collectins in human and other mammals) and micro-organisms.

Leflunomide A dihydroorotate dehydrogenase inhibitor which selectively blocks de novo synthesis of pyrimidines in rapidly proliferating activated lymphocytes. This suspends activated autoimmune lymphocytes in the G1/S phase of cell cycle, whilst not affecting other lymphocytes in G0 phase, as long as they are not needed in the immune response. Though primarily acting as an immunomodulating agent with anti-inflammatory activity, leflunomide does not have the property of a non-selective immunosuppressant. It inhibits IL-2 synthesis and the expression of adhesive molecules, decreasing the number of neutrophils that infiltrate the joint cavity.

Leflunomide belongs to the group of disease modifying antirheumatic drugs that have been registered for the treatment of rheumatoid arthritis (RA). Chemically, it is N-(4'-trifluoromethylphenyl)-5-methylisoxazole-4-carboxamide. It is administered orally with a bioavailability of about 80%. An effective therapeutic level is reached approximately 6 to 10 hours after administration. Leflunomide is metabolised in the liver and one of the active metabolites has a very long biological halftime up to 14 days. A higher dose is often administered initially (100 mg a day during the first three days) to ensure more rapid achievement of equilibrium, otherwise it can take up to two months if the maintenance dose (10 to 20 mg daily) is administered initially. Approximately 40% of its metabolites are eliminated via the urine and 50% via the stool.

Clinical efficacy: The efficiency of leflunomide against placebo and other commonly used DMARDs in the treatment of RA has been tested. Clinical studies have proven comparable efficiency of leflunomide to methotrexate (MTX) and sulfasalazine (SSZ) (Strand et al. 1999, Smolen et al. 1999). It was shown that leflunomide improved inflammatory parameters such as the ACR 20 index in patients with RA, improves the quality of the patient's life and delays radiological erosive progress in joints over 6 and 12 months of treatment. Leflunomide is also licensed for treatment of psoriatic arthritis.

Dosage: Leflunomide can be administered at a dose of 100 mg per day for three days (though this is associated with a higher incidence of diarrhoea and so is now avoided), followed by 10 mg or 20 mg over the long term. Its clinical effect is apparent at the end of the first month. Blood count and liver enzymes should be checked on a monthly basis. After discontinuation of leflunomide treatment due to severe toxicity, switching to another DMARD, e.g. MTX, or before conception, the patient must undergo a washout phase based on administration of 8 g of cholestyramine 3 times a day or administration of 50 g of activated charcoal 4 times a day for a period of 11 days.

Adverse effects: Blood cell count disturbances, diarrhoea, increased liver enzymes, leukopenia, anaemia, thrombocytopenia, hair loss, skin rashes. The agent is contraindicated in pregnancy and during breast feeding. Women of a fertile age should be informed that in the case of planned pregnancy, a two year period must elapse between termination of treatment and conception, or confirmation of zero serum levels following washout.

Legg-Calve-Perthes Disease Bone necrosis and necrosis of the bone marrow of the femoral head caused by blood supply impairment. Its aetiology is unknown, but may involve inherited vascularisation impairment. Onset at the age of 2–8 years old, and is more frequent in males (4:1). It lasts for 4 to 4.5 years.

Clinical symptoms: Hip pain, pain could eventually be located in the perineum and thigh or in the limb. Necrosis with fractured and compressed trabeculae leads to deformation of the femoral head and thereby to incongruence of the head and articular cavity (development of coxarthrosis).

Radiologically the disease progresses in three stages:
1. initial stage,
2. stage of fragmentation,
3. stage of re-ossification.

Differential diagnosis: specific and non-specific coxitis.

Treatment: Conservative, avoidance of excessive physical activity, plasters (splints), avoidance of muscle atrophy by active exercise. In mid-life may require hip joint replacement.

Lequesne's algofunctional test and assessment of the severity of hip joint impairment → see Instruments of assessing (health status measurements, outcome measurement)

Lesion of the accessory nerve The cause is most often iatrogenic. As an example, lymph node biopsy in the neck area can lead to atrophy of the trapezius muscle and depression of the shoulder. Electromyographic examination reveals a neurogenic lesion.

Treatment: Exercise, impulse therapy.

Lesion of the axillary nerve This can be caused by trauma, haemorrhage, or pressure in the axilla. Abduction and elevation of the shoulder can be weakened and there is hypoaesthesia in the shoulder area and on the lateral side above the elbow. Electromyographic examination confirms a neurogenic lesion.

Treatment: Physiotherapy.

L

Lesion of the long thoracic nerve The lesion is most frequently caused by nerve compression (e.g. when carrying heavy loads). Hypoaesthesia is not a typical symptom. The serratus muscle becomes atrophic, which results in difficulty or inability to elevate the shoulder above the horizontal line.

Treatment: Physiotherapy.

Lesions and ruptures of the humerus rotator These are frequent after traumas and micro-traumas, mainly in sportsmen but also as a consequence of trophic changes to tendons, especially in the elderly. Painful arc according to lesion localisation is typical. Subsequent atrophy of affected muscles is frequent.

Leukocytes Cells derived from mesenchymal tissue. They are involved in the body's defensive mechanism. They are divided into lymphocytes (B-lymphocytes, T-lymphocytes and natural killer cells, NK cells, also called large granular lymphocytes, LGL), granulocytes (neutrophils, eosinophils, basophils) and mononuclear phagocytes (blood monocytes and tissue macrophages), which represent the mononuclear phagocytic system.

Leukocyte granules The membrane-limited cell organelles found in the cytoplasm of granulocytes, certain lymphocytes (LGL) and mast cells. Some of them are typical lysosomes. The granules contain hydrolytic enzymes, cytotoxic substances, certain receptors, diverse mediators and other substances. There are three types of granules in the neutrophilic granulocytes – azurophilic, specific and small – that differ in their electron microscopic structure and biochemical composition.

Leukocytopenia (leukopenia) A reduced number of leukocytes in peripheral blood. May be inherited, may be present in certain infectious diseases (influenza, atypical pneumonia, infectious mononucleosis, sepsis, miliary tuberculosis, toxoplasmosis, malaria, typhoid fever) may be a symptom of hypersplenism (liver cirrhosis, Felty's syndrome, Gaucher's disease), impaired haematopoiesis (aplastic anaemia, pancytopenia, carcinoma metastasis, malignant lymphomas) or it can be a side effect of certain drugs like analgesics. In rheumatology, it may be disease associated mainly in systemic lupus erythematosus and Felty's syndrome.

Leukocytosis An increased number of leukocytes in peripheral blood. It is physiologically present in newborns, during pregnancy, and after excessive physical activity. With pathological conditions, it most frequently accompanies infectious diseases, malignancies, certain intoxications, metabolic imbalance (diabetes, uraemia, hepatic coma), or traumas (burns, fractures, crush syndrome, surgical interventions). Leukocytosis can be present in polyarteritis nodosa, acute exacerbation of systemic lupus erythematosus, dermatomyositis and in Still's disease.

Leukopenia → see Leukocytopenia (leukopenia)

Leukotrienes (LT) Metabolites of arachidonic acid formed by the action of the 5-lipoxygenase enzyme. The most important are LTB_4 chemotactic factor for neutrophils, monocytes, macrophages and LTC_4, LTD_4, LTE_4 (previously called slow reacting substance of anaphylaxis, SRS-A), which evoke increased vascular permeability and long term contraction of smooth muscles, mainly in the bronchus. They participate in the destruction of joint cartilage.

LFA-1 (lymphocyte function-associated antigen-1) Belongs to leukocyte integrins (CD11a/CD18). It is particularly important during adhesive interactions of leukocytes with endothelial cells during inflammation and adhesive interactions of T-lymphocytes with antigen presenting cells during immune and inflammatory responses.

LFA-3 LFA-3 or CD58 is the ligand for CD2, which is also known as LFA-2. It is a differential mark of T-lymphocytes. LFA-3 is a member of the immunoglobulin superfamily.

LGL (large granular lymphocytes) Large granular lymphocytes are a subpopulation of peripheral lymphocytes with typical granules within the cytoplasm. The granules contain perforins and other cytotoxic substances. LGL possess NK-activity (also called NK cells) and by induction of apoptosis are able to kill malignant cells and cells infected by viruses.

Licofelone Licofelone (LCF) is the first member of a new group of anti-inflammatory drugs. The drug inhibits three major enzymes of the cascade of arachidonic acid – cyclooxygenase 1, cyclooxygenase 2 and lipoxygenase. By inhibiting these three enzymes, licofelone decreases the synthesis of prostaglandins and leukotrienes. LCF has got a good safety profile in terms of gastrointestinal (GIT) side effects. In clinical trials involving 36 patients with osteoarthritis of the hip or knee, LCF had better GIT tolerance when compared with naproxen (500 mg/day) even when a double dose of Licofelone (400 mg) was administered. Symptom relief in patients with knee osteoarthrosis, evaluated using the WOMAC system, was better with LCF than the selective COX-2 inhibitor celecoxib. Further work on the clinical role and licensing of this drug is awaited.

Likert 5-degree scale → see Algometry (evaluation of pain threshold)

Limited cutaneous SSc (lcSSc) → see Systemic sclerosis (SSc)

Limiting factors of rehabilitation
- pain,
- muscle contractures,
- signs of inflammation,
- swelling,
- joint effusion,
- psychological barrier (anxiety, depression).

Local factors Bone remodelling is regulated at a cellular level by local factors. They affect the differentiation of precursor cells, the activity and numbers of osteoblasts and osteoclasts. They modulate the activity of other systemic regulators. They are produced by osteocytes, endothelial cells, blood cells, fibroblasts and chondrocytes. They are represented by growth factors, cytokines and prostaglandins.

Currently, very many local factors have been recognised.

Localised Osteoporosis Besides generalised osteoporosis, there are conditions associated with local bone mineral density loss. Normally referred to as regional or localised osteoporosis, it can be found after a fixation and immobilisation of a limb, after poliomyelitis, at insertions of tendon lesions, and in the area surrounding inflamed joints in active RA. The cause of localised osteoporosis in an immobilised site is mainly due to a decrease of afferent signalling from various receptors, the so-called decrease of a trophic influence of the nervous system. The aetiopathogenesis of periarticular osteoporosis in rheumatoid arthritis is multifactorial and local factors play the key role. They directly regulate bone remodelling at the cellular level. They affect the differentiation of precursor cells, the activity of osteoblasts and osteoclasts and their numbers. They modulate the activity of other systemic regulators. They are represented by growth factors, cytokines and prostaglandins.

Regional osteoporosis may develop due to inadequate osteoblast and osteoclast numbers in a certain region. The complete remodelling cycle requires a sufficient and constant supply of precursor cells from the bone marrow.

Looser zones Poorly defined transparent zones on bone X-rays. They run vertically to the bone surface and are caused by the aggregation of non-mineralized osteoid. They occur symmetrically or asymmetrically in stressed areas of the skeleton, most frequently in the shoulders, tibia, fibula, metatarsal bones and ribs, less frequently in the radius and ulna. They are not considered a fracture but may fracture at any moment. Looser zones are typical of osteomalacia and are its frequent symptom.

Lower limb length An important measurement in prosthetics and physiotherapy for measuring leg length discrepancy. Anatomical – the distance between the greater trochanter and lower margin of the lateral malleolus; functional – the distance from anterior iliac crest to the lower margin of the medial malleolus; umbilico-malleolar – from the umbilicus to lower margin of the medial malleolus.

Lupus anticoagulants These are antibodies directed against β2-glycoprotein-1, prothrombin, or annexin V and others. They are detected by a prolongation of in vitro clotting assays, usually the activated partial thromboplastin time (APTT) is not corrected by 1:1 dilution of patient's plasma with normal plasma. In vivo, however, there is a paradoxical increase in arterial and venous thromboses. These IgG or IgM antibodies occur in patients with primary antiphospholipid antibody syndrome, but also in SLE with antiphospholipid syndrome, in some patients with neoplasms or in patients with drug sensitivity and occasionally in healthy individuals and patients with AIDS and active opportunistic infections.

Lupus – drug induced → see Drug-Induced Lupus

Lyme borreliosis (LB, Lyme disease) A multisystemic inflammatory disease caused by spirochetes belonging to the Borrelia stem (*B. burgdoferi* sensu stricto, *B. garinii, B. afzelii*). It is transmitted to humans after a bite from the Ixodes tick. Skin, neurological and joint symptoms are the most typical clinical symptoms. Clinical symptoms correlate with the occurrence of a particular genospecies and globally it is applicable that *B. burgdoferi* sensu stricto invokes joint defects, whereas *B. garinii* invokes neurological impairment and *B. afzelii* skin diseases (particularly chronic skin diseases). A disease similar to LB associated especially with skin symptoms and caused by a new borrelia species, *B. lonestarii species nova,* has recently been described in the US. Two more genotypes have been described in Europe: *B. valaisiana* and *B. lusitaniae* from which *B. valaisiana* is associated with the development of erythema migrans.

Clinical picture: With LB this can be extremely varied and multisystemic and the overlapping of symptoms are typical. It can be differentiated into:
- *stage of early localised infection:* with typical symptom of erythema migrans (as solitary lesions, but multiple lesions may occur) and systemic symptoms like fatigue, subfebrile body temperatures, headache, myalgia and arthralgia,
- *stage of early disseminated infection:* develops 1 to 9 months after infection and may be characterised by cardiac symptoms (arrhythmias, pericarditis, myocarditis), neurological symptoms (meningitis, cranial neuritis, radiculoneuritis, possibly neuropathy),
- *stage of late infection or chronic stage:* is characterised by arthritis, neurological defects (encephalopathy, axonal polyneuropathy and leukoencephalitis), ophthalmic, muscle (myositis, myopathy), lympho-reticular and skin (acrodermatitis chronica atrophicans) symptoms.

Lyme disease → see Lyme borreliosis (Lyme disease)

Lymphocytes Basic cells of lymphatic tissue, lymph and blood. They are spheroidal with a diameter of 7–12 μm with a large central nucleus, surrounded by a narrow rim of cytoplasm. Larger lymphocytes possess more cytoplasm, which does not usually contain any granules. However, large granular lymphocytes (LGL) do have granules in their cytoplasm. According to their function, surface antigens and ultrastructure, lymphocytes are divided into three main population groups: B lymphocytes (B cells), T lymphocytes (T cells) and NK cells. The NK cells are usually identical with LGL. B lymphocytes are responsible for specific antibody immunity, T lymphocytes are responsible for specific cellular immunity and NK cells for non-specific cellular immunity (particularly against malignant cells and cells infected by viruses).

Particular populations of lymphocytes can be distinguished according to their CD antigens. A calm (metabolically "sleeping") lymphocyte is activated by an antigen or mitogen and becomes a metabolically activated lymphoblast, which in association with cytokines is then subject to division and differentiation, whereby memory and efficient lymphocytes, which are involved in immune responses, develop.

Lymphocytes – circulation The movement of lymphocytes in the body takes place between the blood and lymphatic system, lymph nodes, spleen and tissues. Less than 10% of the total volume of lymphocytes is constantly circulating, while the rest are deposited in tissues and organs. Approximately 70% of circulating lymphocytes have the capability to re-circulate, i.e. they move in a certain cycle during which they leave the systemic circulation and return back to lymph nodes, lymphoid follicles and the spleen, from where the cycle may recommence. These cells are mostly long-life mature T lymphocytes, but also memory B lymphocytes. Approximately 30% of lymphocytes in the vascular space are not subject to re-circulation. These are mostly short-lived immature T and B cells that terminate their life in vessels, or can be activated and then leave the vascular space. The re-circulation enables lymphocytes to perform immune surveillance throughout all of the body, mobilise themselves to localities where immune protection is needed and also reactivate non-functional cells.

Lymphoid organs Organs in which lymphocytes prevail but other cells are also present. They are divided into primary and secondary lymphoid organs. The thymus and bone marrow, which is considered to be the equivalent of the bursa of Fabricius in birds, are amongst the primary lymphoid organs. B lymphocytes (bone marrow) or T lymphocytes (thymus) mature in primary lymphoid organs. Secondary lymphoid organs comprise lymph nodes, the spleen, lymphoid tissue in mucosa, and tonsils. These are the places where, during the initiation of immune responses, B and T lymphocytes react with antigen presenting cells.

Lymphomatoid granulomatosis (LG) A rare multi-systemic disease from the group of vasculitides which is characterised by focal and transmural infiltration of the vascular wall by lymphocytes, plasma cells and histiocytes.

Clinical symptoms: Dependent on the severity of organ impairment. Most frequent are pulmonary symptoms (cough, dyspnoea, chest pain) and skin rashes (erythema, induration). Fever, malaise and weight loss are non-specific symptoms.

Lymphotoxin (LT) One of the tumour necrotizing factors (TNF-β). It is produced mainly by T_H1 lymphocytes after antigen or mitogen stimulation. LT inhibits the growth of tumours both in vivo and in vitro and blocks tumour transformation of cells invoked by carcinogens. LT is also involved in protection against viral and saprophytic infections. It was one of the first lymphokines to be detected and currently is considered to be a member of the cytotoxin group.

Lysosomes They are organelles localised in the cytoplasm of all cells that contain a nucleus. They are notably abundant in the cytoplasm of professional phagocytes (phagolysosome). Typically they contain hydrolytic (lysosomal) enzymes. Lysosomes of phagocytes contain different antimicrobial substances, typical neutral proteases and components of certain receptors (granules of leukocytes). Antibodies against lysosomal enzymes of leukocytes may be produced (ANCA). These antibodies are associated with certain vasculitides and other autoimmune diseases.

Lysozyme An enzyme that lyses the β-1,4-glycosidic linkage of polysaccharides. The older name of this enzyme was muramidase. It occurs in egg white, tears, saliva, nasal secretions, skin, specific granules of leukocytes and in serum. Lysozyme is able to lyse cell membrane glycoproteins of certain gram-positive (mostly non-pathogenic) bacteria and thereby cause their osmotic lysis. It can only destroy other micro-organisms with the interaction of other antimicrobial factors (complement, secretory IgA, leukocyte's proteases etc.).

L

Mab → see Monoclonal antibodies (Mab)

Macrophages Large, mostly single nucleus cells of 16–22 μm in diameter. They are usually formed from blood monocytes after their deposition in different tissues. Some of the normal macrophages deposited in certain organs, such as the lungs, can also directly undergo division. They are a component part of the mononuclear phagocytic system (MPS) and belong to the group of professional phagocytes constituting the basic component of natural (non-specific) immunity against pathogenic microorganisms (phagocytosis). They represent a heterogeneous population of cells in the human body and differ from each other in terms of development, functional activity, anatomical localisation and biological function. They can be divided into normal and inflammatory cells. Macrophages of tissue (histiocytes), the liver (Kupffer's cells), lungs (alveolar macrophages), serum fluid (pleural and peritoneal macrophages), skin (histiocytes, Langerhans' cells) and other tissues belong to the group of normal macrophages. Inflammatory macrophages occur in inflammatory exudates where they have important effector (cell-killing, matrix destroying) and regulatory (matrix regenerating) functions. They originate almost exclusively from blood monocytes.

From a functional aspect, macrophages occur in the three stages: silent (non-reactive), pre-activated and activated. Activation is due to cytokines (MAF, MIF, interferon-gamma) or due to some components of micro-organisms. In terms of function, only activated macrophages are fully competent, these being of principal importance in natural immunity against intracellular parasites and malignant cells. Apart from antimicrobial and tumorocidal effect, macrophages act in the early phase of the specific immune response as antigen presenting cells and as K cells, where in the presence of antibodies they can kill cells that have their specific antigens on their surface. This is possible due to the presence of Fc-receptors (FcR). The antibody binds through the Fc-component of its molecule to FcR on the surface of the macrophage and to the binding site on the antigen determinant on the surface of the target cell. Such contact of two cells leads to the killing of the target cell by the mechanism of antibody-dependant cellular cytotoxicity (ADCC).

Apart from immune system functions, macrophages are involved in certain metabolic reactions, e.g. cholesterol metabolism, metabolism of vitamin D and arachidonic acid. They are also important secretory cells. They release various antimicrobial and cytotoxic substances, bioactive lipids, complement components, certain factors of haemocoagulation, cytokines, proteolytic and other enzymes, as well as inhibitors of enzymes, stress proteins and factors involved in tissue reorganisation. They thereby significantly interfere with various physiological and pathophysiological processes in the body.

Magnesium (Mg) The fourth commonest cation in the human body and the second commonest intracellular cation. Magnesium is essential for the function of approximately 300 enzyme systems, transcription of deoxyribonucleic acid and proteosynthesis, and is a natural antagonist of the calcium channels as well as being essential for bone mineralisation.

Magnetic Resonance Imaging MRI is a medical imaging technique based on the effect that hydrogen protons in tissues exposed to an external magnetic field produce a rotating magnetic field (so called spin) detectable by the scanner. Externally, tissues show different sizes of magnetic torque, the vector of which is oriented identically with the vector of the magnetic field. To measure this magnetic torque, it must be diverted by magnetic impulse, the energy of which is absorbed by protons and a resonance can be detected. Thereby the longitudinal tissue resonance decreases and transverse tissue resonance increases. When the electrical impulse is discontinued, relaxation occurs (T1 longitudinal relaxation time, T2 transverse relaxation time). Imaging of tissues is based on the difference of these times in tissues and assigned intensity of grey (black/white scale). It does not use a noxious ionizing radiation for imaging.

Magnetic resonance imaging in rheumatology enables excellent imaging of soft tissues like cartilage, synovial tissue, ligaments, and tendons along with bone structure imaging. The picture can be obtained in different planes and sections. This is the advantage of MRI over standard X-ray and CT (computed tomography). MRI compared to X-ray is more sensitive in terms of capturing early changes in the inflammatory arthropathies; it is also able to capture defects of the cartilage and bone that are not visible on X-ray pictures. MRI enables better monitoring of tissue response to treatment than standard radiography and is free of radiation.

For musculoskeletal system imaging by MRI, the T-1 spin echo (SE) sequences are usually used due to their relatively short imaging time and the well detailed anatomic picture they provide. T2 SE sequences make it possible to view processes with higher water content but their disadvantage is the longer imaging time. Newer modern sequences that shorten the imaging time are now employed like gradient echo sequence and turbo spin (fat suppression); they provide more significant contrast between synovia and the surrounding tissues on post-contrast scans.

It is important to image synovial proliferation and fluid that occur long before destructive bone changes and develop in the early stage of rheumatoid arthritis. Inflamed synovia and pannus absorb the contrast after IV injection. Enhancement of proliferated synovia is rapid, with the maximum reached within 0.5 to 1.5 minutes after IV injection of the contrast. Saturation of synovial fluid is slower. In clinical practice, Gd-DTPA (gadolinium chelate with diethylenetriaminepentaacetic acid also called gadopentate dimeglumine) is used as the contrast substance. It is a paramagnetic substance which by shortening the T1 in T1 measured images gives a stronger signal from the tissues to which it penetrates.

MRI is of major importance in the diagnostics of vertebral column impairment associated with rheumatic diseases, particularly cervical spine impairment in rheumatoid arthritis. In atlantoaxial subluxation, not only is pannus invading the ligamentous apparatus of this segment captured, but possible erosions of the dens of the axis, compression of spinal canal and the level of myelopathy can be identified.

Magnetic therapy Utilisation of magnetic fields for therapeutic purposes. There are three types of magnetic field:

1. *static magnetic field* Occurs around permanent magnets or conductors and coils through which direct current flows. The magnetic field is constant.
2. *alternating magnetic field* Occurs around conductors and coils supplied by alternating electrical current. Its parameters change smoothly in form of a curve from a zero value to a maximum value, back to zero and onwards to minimum value etc.
3. *pulsatile magnetic field* Occurs around conductors and coils supplied by pulsatile electrical current. It is similar to alternating magnetic field, forming a curve from zero to maximum, back to zero and to minimum, but in jumps.

The intensity of the magnetic field is directly proportionate to the flowing electrical current and indirectly proportionate to the distance from the conductor (in metres). The intensity of the magnetic field is measured in ampere/metre (A/m). The unit is defined as the intensity of the magnetic field at a distance of $r' = 1/2 \pi$ (m) from the conductor through which electrical current of 1 ampere flows. The unit of magnetic field induction is 1 T (tesla).

Therapeutic utilisation of magnetic fields results from its physiological effect on the body. It particularly possesses analgesic, anti-inflammatory and anti-oedematous properties and also induces myorelaxation and vasodilatation. The least efficient is a static magnetic field, with a stronger effect produced by an alternating magnetic field and the strongest effect by a pulsatile magnetic field. A static magnetic field activates exclusively the vagus nerve, while alternating and pulsatile magnetic fields also partially activate the sympathetic nervous system. Importantly, metal implants are not a contraindication for this treatment. Recently the TAMMEF system (therapeutic application of a musically modulated electromagnetic field) has been employed. The electromagnetic field reacts to musical impulses in a pulsatile way.

Major histocompatibility complex (MHC) One of many histocompatibility systems, it holds a dominant position among the given animal species. It is a system of genes whose products are strong transplant antigens. Typical features of MHC are its complexity and polymorphism, the ability of its molecules to regulate the immune response and induce a reaction in mixed lymphocyte cultures (MLC), with membership of the immunoglobulin superfamily and responsibility for the immunochemical uniqueness of every individual in the population. The human MHC is referred to as the HLA complex.

Mantoux test (Charles Mantoux, French physician, 1877–1947)
A test in which 0.1 ml of tuberculin (1 in 1,000 strength) is injected intradermally and the reaction is read at 72 hours. A positive reaction (induration >10 mm in diameter) indicates delayed sensitivity (immunopathology) to *Mycobacterium tuberculosis,* indicating that an individual has previously been exposed to this microbe or is now infected.

Marfan's syndrome (Antoine Marfan, French paediatrician, 1858–1942)
An autosomal dominant disorder affecting the bones and connective tissue. The genetic defect is localised on chromosome 15 resulting in impairment of collagen and glycoprotein synthesis. In the clinical picture, affected individuals are tall and very slim with thin extremities (dolichostenomely) and typical prolonged lower part of the body and fingers (arachnodactyly). Hyperextensibility of the fingers and high arched palate are typical. Pectus excavatum or pectus carinatum may be present. Component parts of the clinical picture include ophthalmic and cardiovascular complications. Ophthalmic complications include lens ectopy, myopia and iris vibration. Cardiovascular complications include dilatation of the aorta and aortal valve insufficiency, as well as mitral valve prolapse, dissection of the aorta, pulmonary artery dilatation, arrhythmias and even heart failure. Genetic counselling is important as there is a 50% risk of inheritance of the disease to any offspring and pregnancy in patients with Marfan's syndrome is a high risk due to cardiac complications.

Markers of osteoformation Biosynthesis of bone takes place in two steps. The first is mediated by osteoblasts and consists of the intracellular synthesis of precursors of the bone matrix components (type I collagen, osteocalcin, sialoproteins, proteoglycans, and alkaline phosphatase). These are secreted into the extracellular space where composition of collagen fibrils and organisation of collagen and associated molecules into a lamellar osteoid occurs. In this phase, mature interfibrillar bonds (crosslinks) are then formed extracellularly. This so-called maturation phase of bone matrix formation will have been concluded in the course of 5–10 days before the course of the second phase (mineralisation) of bone growth. Some of them, especially serum osteocalcin and alkaline phosphatase, are used practically for the evaluation of osteoformation following treatment of osteoporosis or Paget's disease.

Markers of osteoresorption The process of bone resorption is mediated by osteoclasts that dissolve the mineral component and break down the bone matrix. This leads to the

M

release of calcium, phosphate, a number of enzymes and degradation products of the matrix, which can then be measured in the blood or urine with variable bone specificity. However, the most popularly used are several degradation products of collagen such as serum or urinary excretion of N-telopeptide (NTX) or carboxy-terminal collagen cross-links (CTX). These are helpful in monitoring the effectiveness of anti-resorptive treatment in osteoporosis, where a fall of greater than 40% in urinary NTX excretion or serum CTX at six months of treatment compared to baseline correlates with subsequent improvement in measured BMD.

Maroteaux-Lamy disease → see Mucopolysaccharidosis (MPS)

Massage We distinguish the following types of massage:
- hand massage (standard massage, reflex massage, sports massage, cosmetic massage),
- apparatus-assisted massage (massage under water, vibratory massage, vacuum massage, syncardial massage). Massage of the internal organs (vagina, prostate, soft palate and cardiac massage) also belongs to this type of massage.

The aim of the massage is to positively influence the general condition, problems and changes due to disease, trauma or excessive physical effort. The general effect of massage is in the influence on the autonomic nervous system, circulation, local influence on the skin, muscles, extra-articular structures, blood and lymphatic system.

Mast Cells A heterogeneous population of cells varying in shape and size (diameter 10–30 μm) and containing numerous characteristic electron-microscopic dense granules in their cytoplasm. They occur predominantly in connective tissue, mucosa, skin and around vessels. They have high affinity receptors for the Fc domains of IgE that result in their involvement in early type allergic reactions (IgE mediated). Specific IgE, arising after the first contact of the individual with a certain aller-

gen, binds to these receptors. During the second or subsequent contact, the allergen can bypass the IgE molecules and directly bind to mast cells, causing degranulation with release of histamine and other mediators of anaphylaxis. These mediators can also be released by anti-IgE antibodies, and anaphylatoxins C3 and C5a for which there are specific receptors on the surface of mast cells.

M-cells (microfold cells) Specialised cells of the intestinal epithelium. They transport microorganisms and macromolecular components of food from the intestinal lumen to Peyer's patches (aggregations of lymphoid tissue) where they present these components to antigen-presenting cells found on the basolateral side. M-cells have a filtering function for the presentation of intra-intestinal antigens and thereby are involved in the regulation of immune response induction at the level of mucosal immunity.

McCune-Albright syndrome (polyostotic fibrous dysplasia) A complex of polyostotic (rarely also monoostotic) fibrous dysplasia, pigmented skin macules of "café au lait" type and overactivity of one or more endocrine glands constitute the McCune-Albright syndrome (Donovan James McCune, American paediatrician, 1902–1976, and Fuller Albright, American physician, 1900–1969). In a typical case, the endocrinopathy is represented by precocious puberty but can also include acromegaly, thyrotoxicosis, Cushing syndrome, hyperprolactinaemia, or hyperparathyroidism. The loss of phosphate may then result in hypophosphataemic disease reminiscent of oncologic rickets, but unlike it, the disease is caused by inhibition of phosphate transport by intestinal mucosa cells, not by the renal tubules. Endocrine hyperfunction is basically caused by overactivity of the target organ. An aromatase inhibitor and testosterone were used to suppress early puberty in females; treatment with medroxyprogesterone has also been reported. Calcitriol and phosphate supplementation in associated hypophosphataemic bone disease may eventually improve the X-ray picture of rickets, but it is not routine practice. Administration of pamidronate in McCune-Albright syndrome improved clinical symptoms, particularly pain and associated gait disturbance.

McMaster Toronto arthritis patient preference disability index (MACTAR)
→ see Instruments of assessing (health status measurements, outcome measurement)

MCTD → see Mixed connective tissue disease (MCTD)

Mechanical therapy Utilisation of mechanical instruments and appliances for medical treatment. These include certain active and passive body movements or parts of the body with traction, extension, massage, stationary bicycle, walking machine etc.

Melsack's questionnaire → see Algometry (evaluation of pain threshold)

Membrane immunoglobulin The molecule of immunoglobulin whose C-ends of heavy chains are prolonged by a hydrophobic tail consisting of 20 amino-acid units. Thereby the molecule is embodied in the cytoplasmic membrane of B lymphocytes, where it becomes a component of the B cell antigen receptor complex (Ig-α/Ig-β antigen receptor). Particularly IgD and IgM monomers possess this attribute.

Mesna → see Cyclophosphamide

Methotrexate As a medical agent, methotrexate was first described in 1946 and then administered in children with leukaemia in 1948. It was first successfully used in rheumatoid arthritis (RA) and psoriatic arthritis (PsA) in 1951, but the FDA only approved MTX for PsA treatment in 1971 and for RA treatment even later in 1988. However, the eighties was a period of increased concerns over MTX, which resulted in a large number of publications.

Mechanisms of action Methotrexate is a typical antimetabolite. After entry into target cells, it acts as a competitive and reversible inhibitor of the enzyme dihydrofolate reductase (DHFR) leading to reduced production of tetrahydrofolate. Its mode of action in rheumatoid arthritis and other autoimmune diseases remains unclear.

Pharmacokinetics: Methotrexate is usually well absorbed after oral administration. Major differences have been found with regard to biological availability after oral administration, 33% (range 13–76%) of MTX in particular patients when compared with intravenous administration. Differences in an individual patient on repeated testing were considerably smaller. The biological availability after intramuscular injection is better (76%) and more consistent. Therefore, better long-term clinical results are achieved by parenteral administration, though disadvantages include higher costs and inconvenience to the patient. Nowadays subcutaneous is the application of choice. In active cases with an induction phase, intravenous administration may also be preferable. Absorption is rapid, with maximum concentration achieved in an average of 83 minutes, serum elimination half-life is 6 to 7 hours. MTX is metabolized predominantly in the liver, 30 to 80% is eliminated via the kidney and 3 to 23% via bile.

Administration

The initial oral dose varies between 10–15 mg weekly, often given at once or spread over 24 hours in divided doses. Folic acid (5 mg daily) is given on the other days to reduce toxicity either 5 mg once weekly or 1 mg daily. Dosage escalation of MTX can occur at 2 to 6 weekly intervals to a maximum of 25 to 30 mg weekly. Subcutaneous MTX is often given in a similar regime. Blood count and liver function should be monitored one month after initiation, but then every three months when on a stable regime.

Clinical efficacy: A large number of clinical trials over the last 15 years have confirmed methotrexate as one of the most effective DMARDs for RA. Considering efficiency versus toxicity, methotrexate is now preferred to oral or parenteral gold, sulfasalazine, azathioprine and cyclosporin. It has been shown to retard the radiological progression of bone erosions.

M

Adverse effects of methotrexate treatment in autoimmune disease:

- gastrointestinal: nausea, dyspepsia, stomatitis, mouth ulceration
- bone marrow depression: leukopenia, thrombocytopenia, aplastic anaemia, pancytopenia,
- liver impairment: hepatosplenomegaly, liver fibrosis, liver cirrhosis,
- lung impairment: acute interstitial pneumonitis, interstitial lung fibrosis, dry/exudative pleuritis, lung oedema, pulmonary nodules,
- infections and malignancies: cell immunity defects, non-specific and specific infections.

Methotrexate as a component of DMARDs combination treatment (disease-modifying anti-rheumatic drugs)

Methotrexate (MTX) theoretically has good eligibility to become a suitable component of combination treatment of rheumatoid arthritis (RA). It has rapid onset of action, acceptable long-term toxicity and presumably a different mechanism of action than other immunomodulating drugs. The treatment combination of MTX, sulfasalazine and hydroxychloroquine (O'Dell regime) is more effective than a combination of only sulfasalazine + hydroxychloroquine or MTX monotherapy. Other combinations include MTX and cyclosporin. The trial showed that, compared to a control group of MTX monotherapy (32% of patients), better disease control occurred in patients receiving combination treatment. Another study compared combination treatment with MTX, sulfasalazine and a high dose of prednisolone (60 mg a day) with sequential reduction, against classic sulfasalazine monotherapy. Again, this combination treatment produced better disease control than monotherapy. A lower radiological disease progression was achieved and this effect persisted even one year after termination of treatment. However, sulfasalazine monotherapy did not retain a beneficial clinical effect after withdrawal of MTX and prednisolone. Recently, in order to suppress very severe RA activity (clinical and radiological), MTX has been successfully combined with anti TNF therapy (infliximab, entanercept or adalimumab), rituximab and abatacept.

Clinical efficacy: A large number of clinical trials over the last 15 years have confirmed methotrexate as one of the most effective DMARDs for RA. It has been shown to retard the radiological progression of bone erosions.

Contra-indication:

- pregnancy: methotrexate is highly teratogenic so should not be administered for at least three months before conceiving and during pregnancy.
- interactions: avoid trimethoprim and trimethoprim including antibiotics as increased risk of severe toxicity (bone marrow aplasia, desquamation of oesophagus)

Methylprednisolone → see Glucocorticoids, Intraarticular glucocorticoid treatment

Metric measurement of vertebral column in spondyloarthritis (SpA)

Schober's test: From the junction of both posterior superior iliac spines, measure 10 cm cranially and mark both points. During the maximum forward flexion to touch the toes, both points move more than 13 cm apart (3 to 5 cm movement). This distance is reduced in patients with limited flexion of the lumbar spine (Paul Schober, German physician, 1865–1943).

Schober's test modified: From the anal cleft, measure 15 cm up the spine and mark each point. During the maximum forward flexion to touch the toes, both points move more than 20 cm apart (>5 cm movement).

Ott's sign: Mark the spinal process of C7 and then another point 30 cm caudally. The distance between both points increases at least by 3 to 4 cm during maximum forward flexion (Viktor Rudolf Ott, German physician, 1914–1986).

Rotation of cervical spine: Using a tape measure note the distance from the spinal process of C7 to the centre of the jaw. Then ask the examined individual to rotate the head towards the measured side. The difference between the central position and maximum rotation should be 8 to 10 cms. This is markedly reduced in the elderly. Measure the opposite side in the same way.

Rotation of thorax and lumbar spine: With the individual in the standing position, mark the spinal process of L5 and the point on the jugular notch. Ask the patient to rotate towards the opposite side. The range of movement should be 8 cm. Measure the opposite side in the same way.

Rotation of lumbar area: Marks are made at the level of L5 and the xiphoid process. The examined individual rotates maximally and the distance between both marks is measured. The distance during rotation to the opposite side is measured in the same way.

Finger floor distance: The distance between the fingers and the floor during maximum forward bend is measured with the knees straight. This is a good measure of overall progress of ankylosing spondylitis.

Measurement of bend to side (lateral deviation): The examined individual stands with their legs together, arms by their sides, and slides their hands along the lateral side of the thigh. Normally the movement on the thigh is 20 cm. Care must be taken in performing the test that subjects don't leave the frontal plane by bending forward or backward.

Chest expansion: Measurement of the distance between complete exhalation and complete inspiration. The normal range in healthy individuals is >5 cm.

Special tests of Bath Ankylosing Spondylitis and Dougados functional index provide a complex functional evaluation.

MGUS (monoclonal gammopathy of unknown significance) Monoclonal gammopathies often do not manifest themselves clinically (often discovered incidentally on blood tests including serum protein electrophoresis). MGUS does not have direct aggressive potential, does not require treatment but is supposed potentially to progress to multiple myeloma or other blood malignancies. The portion of actively proliferating plasma cells can be determined by analysing bone marrow. Patients with MGUS will need

regular (annual) monitoring of their immunoglobulins as a small number will progress to myeloma with time.

MHC → see Major histocompatibility complex (MHC)

Microfold cells → see M-cells (microfold cells)

Microscopic polyangiitis Necrotising vasculitis that affects small vessels in the kidneys, skin and lungs. p-ANCA (MPO-ANCA) is present in 70% on laboratory testing. The most severe organ involvement is kidney, leading to impairment with microscopic haematuria and mild proteinuria. Lung involvement is less common than in Wegener's granulomatosis. High dose glucocorticoids (up to 60 mg per day) and cyclophosphamide are used in treatment, often in pulse intravenous form.

Microscopic polyarteritis → see Microscopic polyangiitis, Polyarteritis nodosa (PAN)

Migration Tight adhesion of leukocytes to vascular endothelium (inflammation).

Mixed connective tissue disease (MCTD) An overlap syndrome characterised by the presence of symptoms of systemic lupus erythematosus (SLE), systemic sclerosis (SSc) and polymyositis (PM). It was first described by Sharp in 1972. The presence of Raynaud's phenomenon, diffuse 'sausage-like' swelling of the fingers and high titre autoantibodies against small nuclear ribonucleoprotein, which is sensitive to ribonuclease, referred to as U1RNP, are typical for the syndrome. U1RNP is a polypeptide complex with molecular weight of 68 kDa. High titre of anti-U1RNP autoantibodies is a permanent finding in certain patients; sometimes these antibodies disappear with time.

Clinical symptoms: Various clinical symptoms are present in MCTD. Scleroderma, diffuse swelling of the fingers, arthritis, myositis, leukopenia, serositis, interstitial pneumonia, are among the most frequent symptoms. Clinically MCTD suggests PM, SLE, rheumatoid arthritis and SSc in the early oedematous phase.

MLC (mixed-lymphocyte culture) A test prepared by mixing lymphocytes isolated from two different individuals whereby one of them is usually the potential donor and the other one is the potential recipient of a transplant. As the two individuals (except monozygotic twins) are not genetically identical, different histocompatibility antigens on the surface of donor lymphocytes will activate the recipient lymphocytes and vice versa. The result is activation of DNA synthesis (the measurement is based on incorporation of tritium labelled thymidine) and the proliferation of lymphocytes. This is called mixed-lymphocyte reaction (MLR). The test is important for determining histocompatibility between donor and recipient in the transplantation of bone marrow and organs.

MLC Test Mixed-lymphocyte culture test.

Monoclonal antibodies (Mab) Identical copies of immunoglobulin molecules that are of the same primary structure, identical specificity of binding sites and identical functions as they are products of one particular clone of plasma cells. Monoclonal antibody concentrations rise spontaneously during malignant growth of plasma cells, or of their precursors (gammopathy) or artificially in laboratory conditions by hybridoma technology. Monoclonal antibodies are specific against a particular determinant (epitope) of a certain antigen. The properties of monoclonal antibodies do not essentially differ from conventional antibodies. However, they possess certain important advantages. Mabs are chemically identical which is why they are monospecific and effective. It is possible to produce Mabs in unlimited quantities, even when using impure antigens. They are used predominantly in analytic and isolating immunochemical laboratory methods, and in the differential diagnosis of viral, bacterial and parasitic infectious diseases. Trials of their utilisation

with in vivo diagnosis of malignancies (radioimmunoscintigraphy) and treatment using immunotoxins are being carried out. Humanised monoclonal antibodies are now most commonly used. Biologic agents based on Mabs include these three letters mab in their generic name like infliximab, adalimumab, certolizumab, golilumab or rituximab.

Monoclonal gammopathy of unknown significance → see MGUS (monoclonal gammopathy of unknown significance)

Monocyte Large cell (diameter 16 to 22 µm) with kidney-shaped nucleus and an abundance of organelles in their cytoplasm (lysosomes, mitochondria and pinocyte vacuoles). Monocytes are present in peripheral blood (2 to 10% of leukocytes in humans). After migration into tissues, they transform into tissue macrophages. Macrophages are part of the mononuclear phagocyte system (MPS) and belong to professional phagocytes.

Monokines Cytokines that are produced mainly by mononuclear phagocytes – macrophages and monocytes. Typical representatives are IL-1 and TNF-α.

Mononuclear phagocyte system Consists of blood monocytes, tissue macrophages and their precursor cells in bone marrow. Their common property is active phagocytosis, pinocytosis and the ability to adhere to various surfaces. On their surface, monocytes and macrophages possess receptors for the Fc domains of immunoglobulins and for the C3b fragment of complement. This enables them to perform very effective phagocytosis. They express class II MHC (major histocompatibility complex) antigens on their surface, enabling them to perform the function of antigen presenting cells. The term MPS (mononuclear phagocyte system) has recently been substituted by the previously used term "reticuloendothelial system" (RES).

Morquio-Brailsford's disease → see Mucopolysaccharidosis (MPS)

Morton's metatarsalgia → see Tunnel syndromes of foot

MOS-SF – medical outcome study – short form 36 → see Instruments of assessing (health status measurements, outcome measurement)

Movement Passive movement is a movement in which the patient does not actively participate. However, even passive movement is basically active muscle exercise as the change of muscle length and the realisation of the motion activates a sensitive component of motion regulation. It is used for maintaining the range of motion (ROM), stimulating proprioceptive signalisation from proprioreceptors (muscle spindle, muscle and ligament proprioreceptors), improving the circulation. It helps to prevent muscle atrophy and the development of contractures.

Active movement is performed by a patient using his own strength. If the physiotherapist assists or the movement is performed without gravity, it is referred to as active assisted movement. If resistance is applied to the movement, it is referred to as resisted movement; if maximal resistance is applied, it is referred to as absolute resisted movement. Isokinetic (machine) movement is performed at a constant speed and resistance in the whole range.

M-protein Can have two meanings:
- complete or incomplete molecule of monoclonal immunoglobulin which is produced in multiple myeloma,
- type specific surface antigens of group A beta-hemolytic streptococci.

Mucocutaneous lymph node syndrome → see Kawasaki disease (KD)

Mucopolysaccharidosis (MPS) A complex of diseases whose common attribute is an inherited lysosomal defect for deficient degradation of glycosaminoglycans (muco-polysaccharides) leading to lysosomal storage diseases. MPS typically leads to multiple organ impairment with a variable clinical picture. Most are inherited as autosomal recessive, except Hunter's disease which is an X-linked recessive.

Mucopolysaccharidosis Type IH (Hurler's disease) This is the most typical and most frequent form of MPS. The incidence of the syndrome is estimated at 1:100,000 newborns. The lysosomal enzyme deficiency is l-iduronidase. The disease can manifest itself biochemically as early as at birth, with clinical symptoms developing in the second year of life. Typical features are growth retardation, facial dysmorphism with wide flat nose, exophthalmos, thick lips, macroglossia and macrocephaly. Gradually, articular contractures of fingers cause claw hands. The clinical picture also includes corneal opacities, skin defects (dry skin, acanthosis, and hirsutism) and cardiovascular symptoms. A protuberant abdomen due to hepatosplenomegaly is often a significant sign. Although early mental development can be normal, later signs of mental retardation appear. The prognosis is extremely severe, as the disease leads in most cases to death in childhood. The disease has a typical X-ray picture with progressive changes of bone structures such as multiple dysostosis imaging as skull coarsening, extended ribs and clavicles, coarser shoulder blades, ovoid and partly hook-shaped vertebral bodies, dysplasia of pelvis bones. Phalangeal and metacarpal bones are widened and shortened, the pointed proximal ends of the metacarpal bones have a characteristic 'sugar loaf' appearance (Gertrud Hurler, German paediatrician, 1889–1965).

Mucopolysaccharidosis Type IS (Scheie's disease) This disease has a slower progression though the clinical symptoms develop in childhood. Articular stiffness, claw hands and corneal opacities are the principal symptoms of the disease. The lysosomal enzyme deficiency is the same as Hurler's disease (Harold Glendon Scheie, American ophthalmologist, 1909–1990).

M

Mucopolysaccharidosis Type II (Hunter's disease)

Hunter's disease only affects males, as it is X-linked recessive. Clinical and radiological symptoms are similar to type IH but the disease has a milder course and slower progression. Corneal opacity is not present. The lysosomal enzyme deficiency is iduronate-2-sulphatase (Charles A. Hunter, Scottish-Canadian physician, 1873–1955).

Mucopolysaccharidosis Type III (Sanfilippo's disease)

The facial and skeletal symptoms are less distinct, but the mental and motor deterioration are particularly severe. Several lysosomal enzyme deficiencies have been described (Sylvester Sanfilippo, American pediatrician).

Mucopolysaccharidosis Type IV (Morquio-Brailsford's disease syndrome)

Characterised by severe dwarfism with short trunk, pectus carinatum, kyphoscoliosis (gibbus) and coxa valga, but with normal mental function. Radiological changes are similar to type I with changes in the areas of the epiphyses and universal platyspondyly are more distinct. Compression of the spinal cord due to atlantoaxial dislocation can occur (needs surgical intervention). Progression of hearing impairment may lead to complete deafness. Aortic valve insufficiency is a frequent finding. At least two lysosomal enzyme deficiencies have been described.

Mucopolysaccharidosis Type VI (Maroteaux-Lamy disease)

Characterised by normal intellect and skeletal symptoms which are the same as in type IH, but progression is slower. Growth retardation develops at the age of 2 to 3 years old. The disease is often accompanied by corneal opacity. The lysosomal enzyme deficiency is arylsulphatase B.

Mucopolysaccharidosis Type VII (Sly's disease)

Very rare, the picture is similar to Hurler's disease. The lysosomal enzyme deficiency is β-glucuronidase.

Multicentric reticulohistiocytosis

A rare systemic disease of unknown aetiology whose manifestation includes skin, mucosal and synovial nodular lesions, potentially destructive symmetric polyarthritis, with a tendency towards multiple organ impairment. Histopathologically, it is characterised by typical infiltrations of large multinucleated giant cells and lipid-laden histiocytes in skin and synovia. Large cells may be of asymmetric shape and 50 to 100 μm in size on average and may contain up to 20 nuclei.

Clinical symptoms: Arthritic changes are the initial features of the disease in 2/3 of cases. Eruption of skin nodules occurs within several months to years (3 years on average). They can occur as the first sign in 18 to 20% of cases. In other cases, skin nodules may develop simultaneously with arthritis. Systemic symptoms such as intermittent fever, fatigue, tiredness, nausea, or weight loss may occur in the course of the disease. In some patients, the disease has a tendency towards spontaneous remission of active inflammation after several years. However, the disease leads to a mutilating form of arthritis in 12 to 45% of cases. Treatment can vary from NSAIDs, steroids, and alkylating agents.

Multiple myeloma

→ see Plasmocytoma and its musculoskeletal symptoms (MM; multiple myeloma)

Muscle activation

The property of muscle fibres – shortening of the fibres during muscle contraction. Muscle activation can be divided into following types:
- Isotonic – muscle contraction leading to movement
- Isometric – muscle contraction without movement
- Isokinetic – the muscle performs a movement of a certain force balanced with equal resistance.

Muscle atrophy

A decrease in the volume of muscles due to various reasons (denervation, inactivity). This results in the muscle becoming weaker, as strength is related to muscle mass.

Muscle contracture A pathological condition characterised by muscle shortening in the absence of the activated contractile mechanism, with standstill action potential. The causes can be neurogenic, myogenic, reflex, functional or fibrous.

Muscle disequilibrium A condition in which one group of muscles predominates over another group, e.g. flexors over extensors (iliopsoas muscle versus gluteus maximus muscle, hip flexors over hip extensors etc.).

Muscle hypertonia Increased muscle tone.

Muscle hypotonia Decreased muscle tone.

Muscle spindle A sensory organ present within skeletal muscles, which acts as a permanent detector (proprioception) of inner muscle tone.

Muscle strength The ability of muscle fibre to respond to a stimulus by contraction. It is proportional to the number of muscle fibres.

Muscle synkinesis Involuntary muscle activity accompanying voluntary muscle movements of other muscles, usually due to miswiring of nerves following injury (e.g. neck tightness on smiling after facial nerve (Bell's palsy).

Muscle testing Muscle strength is assessed by muscle testing. The results are divided into six grades:

Grade 0: no signs of contraction, despite maximum attempt to make the movement

Grade 1: flicker of contraction, the muscle is able to perform a contraction but the strength is insufficient to activate much movement; it correlates to 10% of normal muscle strength,

Grade 2: the active movement is only possible when gravity is eliminated; it correlates to 20% of normal muscle strength,

Grade 3: the active movement is performed to the full range against gravity (the limb weight) alone; it correlates to approximately 50% of normal muscle strength,

Grade 4: the active movement is performed to the full range and is able to overcome medium resistance; it correlates to 70% of normal muscle strength,

Grade 5: normal power within the full range when the muscle is able to overcome intensive external resistance; it correlates to 100% of normal muscle strength.

Muscle tone (tonus) Residual muscle tension is reflectively maintained muscle tone, which depends on impulses from peripheral receptors and is also subject to supraspinal regulation. The loss of tonus (hypotonia) develops in peripheral motor nerve palsy or central nervous system (CNS) malfunction. Generally reduced tonus is usually associated with laxity. Increased tonus (hypertonia) occurs in CNS dysfunction (e.g. hypertonus in patients with spastic hemiparesis). A general decrease or increase in muscle tone originates from subcortical structures (reticular formation, basal ganglions, and cerebellum). Relaxing techniques are used in the treatment of hypertonic syndrome.

M

Muscle weakness A decrease in muscle strength less than would be expected given the person's general physical fitness. It depends on energy source depletion, lack of oxygen and inhibition of the area of the cerebral cortex, from which the impulses that promote muscle function originate.

Muscles Muscle tissue consists of muscle cells and muscle fibres (fibrils) and is derived from mesenchyme. There are three types of muscles: skeletal (striated muscle – free), cardiac muscle (striated muscle – involuntary) and smooth muscles (visceral – involuntary). Skeletal muscle is further divided into type I fibres (slow twitch) and type II fibres (fast twitch). The human body possesses more than 600 muscles (40% of body mass). Muscle function: kinetic, thermogenic, postural.

Muscle impairment in rheumatoid arthritis (RA) – causes:
• *Myositis* – non-specific myositis associated with RA; plasma cell and lymphocytic infiltration and atrophy of type IIa myofibrils

occur in muscles surrounding the affected joint, as well as in remote muscles,

- *Arthritis* – nociceptive irritation with inflammation of affected joint reflexively inhibits active muscle contraction,
- *Inactivity* – many muscles become functionless due to long-term reduction in joint mobility,
- *Vasculopathy* – narrowing of arterioles and venules due to inflammation causes decreased blood perfusion to the muscles with reduced metabolism leading to muscle weakness and atrophy,
- *Iatrogenic* – drug induced myopathy (penicillamine, chloroquine, glucocorticoids),
- *Sensory neuropathy* – infiltrates in peripheral nerves secondary to rheumatoid arthritis,
- *Changes of muscle spindles* – degeneration of extrafusal muscle fibres.

Musculoskeletal complication in rare inherited haemorrhagic diatheses

Haemophilia is defined as a qualitative or quantitative defect of factor VIII (haemophilia A), factor IX (haemophilia B or Christmas disease) or factor XI (haemophilia C).

Clinical symptoms
repeated intra-articular haemorrhage, haemophilic arthropathy, secondary destructive arthropathy due to repeated intra-articular bleeding.

Musculoskeletal manifestations of sarcoidosis

Sarcoidosis is a multisystem granulomatous disease of unknown aetiology characterised by the presence of non-caseating granulomas in various organs.

Clinical symptoms: Depend on severity of organ involvement. Typical features of the disease are musculoskeletal symptoms involving the joints, bones and skeletal muscles.

Musculoskeletal symptoms in parasitic diseases

The manifestation of parasitic diseases rarely involves the musculoskeletal system. These are acute, sub-acute and chronic diseases occurring mainly in tropical and subtropical areas. They originate on the basis of an immune defect or by infiltration of a parasite into musculoskeletal system structures.

Clinical symptoms: Arthralgia, myalgia, arthritis, myositis and vasculitis occur in parasitic diseases. The condition improves following eradication of the parasite.

Musculoskeletal symptoms in primary hyperlipidaemias

Diseases characterised by a defect of the lipoprotein metabolism due to increased synthesis or impaired degradation of lipoproteins, which are involved in transporting cholesterol and triglycerides in plasma. Pathologically, elevated concentrations of lipoprotein particles play a causal role in the development of atherosclerosis and pancreatitis. Joint symptoms may be the clue to the diagnosis long before xanthomas and ischemic heart disease (IHD) develop.

Clinical symptoms: Ophthalmic, dermatologic, musculoskeletal, cardiovascular and abdominal symptoms indicate the possibility of lipid metabolism defect:

- *ophthalmic:* corneal arcus lipidis, retinal lipidaemia,
- *dermatologic*: xanthomas, can be clinically devided into xanthelasma palpebrarum, tuberous, tuberoeruptive and eruptive xanthomas, xanthoma striatum palmare,
- *musculoskeletal:* xanthomas on tendons and in periosteal areas (Achilles tendon, tendons of extensors of fingers to hand and foot), arthralgia, arthritis, tendinitis, less often myalgia,
- *cardiovascular:* ischaemic heart disease, myocardial infarction, hypertension, aortal stenosis (xanthoma of aortal valve), arteriosclerosis of lower extremities – claudication,
- *abdominal:* pancreatitis, cholelithiasis hepatosplenomegaly, liver steatosis, abdominal pain.

Musculoskeletal symptoms in scurvy

Scurvy is a disease caused by deficiency of vitamin C, characterised by purpura, gingival bleeding, tooth loss and pallor.

Clinical symptoms: Vitamin C deficiency manifests in skin and mucosal affections with folliculitis, skin haemorrhages ranging from purpura to ecchymoses, mucosal fragility, hypertrophic gingivitis, septic complications and thrombophlebitis. In terms of musculoskeletal system impairment, haemarthrosis into major joints and osteoporosis may occur in adults, whereas in children growth impairment due to metaphyseal defects of long bones develops.

Mutation Changes of the nucleotide sequence of the DNA molecule in an organism during cell division, either spontaneously or due to effects of chemical mutagens or ionizing radiation. They can be divided into point mutations (change, exchange, deletion or insertion of only one nucleotide) and group mutations (several nucleotides are affected). They do not have to be functionally manifested and may cause one or possibly more gene defect.

Myasthenia gravis A neuromuscular disease leading to fluctuating weakness of muscles and fatiguability. Muscle weakness increases during the day and after repeated nerve stimulation of muscles.

Aetiology Autoimmune blockade of the neuromuscular junction is caused by antibodies against acetylcholine receptors. Hyperplasia of the thymus is frequent. The disease moderates or remits after thymectomy.

Typical symptoms Initially, after prolonged activity, weakness of the proximal muscles occurs. Weakness of the upper eyelid elevator leads to ptosis, which is a common sign and may be accompanied by diplopia. The patient can experience difficulties with mastication, swallowing (dysphagia) and speech (dysarthria). Eventually, symptoms are present without any physical activity. In severe long-term cases, progressive muscle atrophy may develop. Clinically it is literally life saving to recognize impairment of the respiratory muscles (especially the diaphragm).

Myasthenic crisis Significant worsening of muscle weakness, and paresis of respiratory muscles is characteristic (check peak expiratory flow rate!). It may be caused by intercurrent diseases, pregnancy and mental stress.

Cholinergic crisis
Develops due to an overdose of cholinesterase inhibitors. Symptoms include vomiting, abdominal cramps, increased salivation, muscle cramps and mental symptoms (disorientation).

Swallowing and respiratory muscles impairment may be present during both a myasthenic and cholinergic crisis.

Diagnostic test Edrophonium chloride (Tensilon®) is used by slow IV administration (edrophonium chloride 10 mg/mL), with immediate relief of the symptoms. Atropine is administered in cholinergic crisis.

Treatment: Cholinesterase can be blocked by the following drugs: neostigmine, prostigmine, pyridostigmine bromide (Mestinon®), edrophonium chloride. Other options are thymectomy, or irradiation of the thymus. Myasthenia can be induced by D-penicillamine and chloroquine; aminoglycoside antibiotics can induce myasthenia by blocking the neuromuscular transfer. Miosis (small pupils) is the major sign in cholinesterase inhibitors overdose.

Myasthenic crisis → see Myasthenia gravis

Mycobacterial, mycotic and parasitic infections of musculoskeletal system
Most frequently these are infections caused by the direct presence of infectious agents in the articular cavity or tissue; agents can reach these structures by various routes (via blood, lymph or direct entry following injury etc.).

Mycotic arthritis Granulomatous arthritis caused by certain fungal species. They occur in patients who suffer from serious diseases such as malignancy or haematological disorders or in patients taking glucocorticoids or immunosuppressants.

Clinical picture: An inflammatory arthritis can occur in the course of mycotic diseases following haematogenous spread of infection from its primary focus, or after trauma, skin and mucosal defects. A regional lymph node reaction occurs and in more severe cases all internal organs can be involved, including the central nervous system.

Myeloperoxidase (MPO) An enzyme of peroxidases located in azurophilic granules of neutrophils. Together with hydrogen peroxide and an oxidative cofactor (Cl^- or I^-) they form the myeloperoxidase system, the most effective antimicrobial and cytotoxic mechanism of human and other mammalian leukocytes. Patients with MPO deficiency are particularly liable to infectious diseases caused by *Candida albicans*.

Myeloperoxidase system The most effective antimicrobial and cytotoxic system of leukocytes. It consists of myeloperoxidase (MPO), hydrogen peroxide and an oxidative cofactor. It acts in two forms:
1. $MPO + H_2O_2 + Cl^- \rightarrow H_2O + OCl^-$
2. $MPO + H_2O_2 + I^- \rightarrow H_2O + OI^-$
The products of the first form are hypochlorites, even free chlorine, which are direct toxic agents. Hypochlorites are a thousand times more toxic for target cells than hydrogen peroxide. A product of the second form is free iodine which binds to proteins of target cells and thereby kills their biological activities.

Myocrisin → see Gold salts

Myofibrils These are cylindrical organelles found within muscle cells, consisting of bundles of actomyosin filaments attached to the cell membrane at each end. They can be subdivided into different types depending on their properties:
- type I – slow red fibres – SO (slow oxidative).
  properties: abundance of mitochondria and myoglobin, many capillaries, slow contraction, low fatigability, static function, "tonic fibres" (slow fibres),
- type II A – fast, white fibres – FOG (fast oxidative and glycolytic).
  properties: more myofibrils, fewer mitochondria, fast and very strong contraction, rapid movement, "twitch fibres"
- type II B – fast red fibres – FG (fast glycolytic).
  properties: few capillaries and myoglobin, fast contraction with maximal strength, rapid fatigability,

- type III intermediate – intermediate, undifferentiated, potential source of three previous types.

Myoglobin A single chain globular protein containing haeme which is the primary oxygen binding protein of skeletal and cardiac muscle. Unlike haemoglobin, myoglobin binds only one molecule of oxygen. The serum concentration of myoglobin is an index of damage to the myocardium and striated muscles. Myoglobin is not present in smooth muscle. Raised levels of serum myoglobin are found in the active phase of polymyositis and dermatomyositis, as well as following myocardial infarction, crush syndrome, blast syndrome and in thermal damage. Moreover, increased myoglobin levels are present in muscular dystrophy, skeletal muscle ischemia (cardioversion, post-infectious myoglobinuria), in rhabdomyolysis (Conn syndrome, crush syndrome, tetanus, typhoid fever, trauma and skeletal muscle inflammation).

Myositis → see Idiopathic inflammatory myopathies (IIM)

Myositis ossificans progressive → see Fibrodysplasia ossificans progressive, Progressive type of myositis ossificans (myositis ossificans progressiva)

Myotonia A symptom manifesting after nerve impulse or as a result of artificial muscle stimulus (electric or by tapping) in which muscle contraction lasts longer than normal and muscle relaxation is slow. Persisting muscle contractions have a typical electromyographic (EMG) picture. Myotonia occurs in certain inherited diseases: myotonia congenita Thomsen, myotonia congenita Becker, paramyotonia congenita Eulenburg, dystrophia myotonica Curshman-Steinert, but can also develop after administration of certain substances having rather an experimental significance. The diagnosis is established from the clinical picture and typical EMG findings. All forms of myotonia are incurable.

Nailfold Capillaroscopy An examination using widefield microscopy of the nailfold capillary bed 10 to 200-point zoom. It has been useful in diagnosing and observing the progress of systemic connective tissue diseases, especially systemic sclerosis. Changes in capillaries can also be detected in diabetes mellitus, arterial hypertension, atherosclerosis and other disorders. The simplicity, noninvasiveness and affordability are all advantageous.

The capillaries of the finger nail folds on the hands are the most appropriate for monitoring microvasculature in vivo as they run parallel to the surface of the skin. The skin transparency can be increased by local application of an immersion oil. A capillaroscope or videocapillaroscope capable of scanning and recording the capillaroscopic picture by a camera can be used to record the picture. Alternatively, a stereomicroscope, a modified standard microscope or an ophthalmoscope can be used.

A microvasculature, including arterioles, precapillaries, capillaries and venules, are all viewed by nailfold capillaroscopy. The shape of the capillaries is evaluated in the morphology assessment. The capillaries may be dilated, coiled and branched or have the shape of a bush. Dilatation of the capillaries may be graded in a qualitative or quantitative way. Concurrent elongation and dilatation of the capillaries is referred to as capillary enlargement.

Subpapillary venous plexus A reticular plexus visible proximally from the edge of the nailfold.

Microhaemorrhage Leaking of erythrocytes from capillaries, often visible with the naked eye, growing out of the nailfold.

Avascular regions Areas lacking capillaries on the distal edge of the nailfold. Their size is expressed in mm².

Decreased number of capillaries This is evaluated by counting the number of capillaries per 1 mm² at the edge of the nailfold and/or per l mm² from its proximal edge. The capillary count varies between 9 and 13 per 1 mm.

Variability of the capillaroscopic picture and morphology changes to capillaries can also occur in healthy individuals, but are usually mild in degree, and between different fingers. They are often due to microtrauma (manual work, influence of chemical agents, etc.). A normal capillaroscopic finding is found in approximately 80%. In healthy individuals, the microvasculature in the nailfold does not change greatly over long-term observation. Nailfold capillaroscopy can assess functional disturbances in microcirculation in vivo using a higher magnification, thus monitoring of the flow of erythrocyte aggregates and plasma gaps in the arterial and venous arm of the capillary loop. The examination should be performed under resting conditions, because the flow velocity varies with temperature and mental status, even during the examination.

Naive lymphocytes Lymphocytes which have not met a specific antigen and therefore did not have the opportunity to be activated by the antigen and subsequently be differentiated into memory and efficient cells. All lymphocytes that leave the pivotal (central) lymphoid organs are naïve. Those leaving bone marrow are naive B lymphocytes and those leaving the thymus are naive T lymphocytes.

Necrosis The local death of cells or tissues due to chemical or physical damage, or after complete interruption of blood supply to the affected tissue. It differs from apoptosis (biologically programmed death of cell). After necrosis an inflammatory response develops, not after apoptosis. Migration of the inflammatory response to the area of necrosis is mediated by necrotaxis.

Necrosis of tibial tuberosity of the femur in children → see Osgood-Schlatter disease

Negative thermal therapy Local cryotherapy is used in inflammatory rheumatic diseases in order to suppress inflammatory symptoms, provide pain relief, muscle relaxation, and reduce swelling. Systemic application of coldness is used in cases of hyperpyrexia and in cryochambers for the purpose of managing inflammation, e.g. in rheumatoid arthritis. Cryotherapy has similar effects to thermal therapy (pain relief, muscle relaxation).

Neonatal Lupus A syndrome of dermal lupus and inherited complete heart block in the newborn of some mothers with SLE, Sjögren's syndrome or other connective tissue inflammatory diseases caused by the transplacental passage of maternal IgG antibodies against anti-Ro (SSA). Anti-La (SSB) antibodies and rarely also anti-U1RNP may also be present. Anti-Ro (SS-A) antibodies are not only an important marker, but play a significant role in the pathogenesis of the disease. Using an indirect immunofluorescent technique, deposits of immunoglobulins can be found in the conduction system of the heart in the week 9 to 10 of pregnancy. Apart from the above mentioned clinical symptoms, inherited heart defects, cardiomyopathies and myocarditis may also be present as part of neonatal lupus. Other symptoms include haematological disorders (haemolytic anaemia, leukopenia, and thrombocytopenia), hepatosplenomegaly, and occasionally pulmonary and neurological symptoms. Clinical symptoms, except for complete heart block, usually disappear within one year of birth with the disappearance of the antibodies.

Neopterin A metabolite of guanosine triphosphate (GTP) produced by macrophages after IFN-γ stimulation. The level of neopterin in serum and urine of HIV-1 infected individuals increases in proportion to the progression of AIDS. An increased level of neopterin along with a decreased number of T-helper-lymphocytes (CD4$^+$) are among the major indicators of the initial conversion from the asymptomatic phase of HIV-1 infection to the clinical symptoms of AIDS.

Nerve A bundle of nerve fibres (axons) forming part of the peripheral nervous system. The majority of nerves consist of motor and sensory fibres (mixed nerve). Certain cranial nerves contain only sensory fibres and serve for specific purposes like smell, vision, hearing and vestibular function.

Nervous system A complicated system of nerve cells whose primary function is to monitor, protect and respond to changes in the internal and external environment. The system is divided into the central nervous system (CNS; brain and spinal cord); peripheral nervous system (PNS; cranial and spinal nerves) and autonomous nervous system (ANS), which is a subdivision of spinal motor nerves. The ANS is subdivided into the sympathetic system (prepares the organism for extreme situations) and the parasympathetic system (restores and preserves physical energy during rest periods).

Neuralgia Pain localised in the area supplied by one or more nerves.

Neurogenic pain Pain caused by damage or intermittent impairment of the peripheral or central nervous system. The term is mainly used as a general name for peripheral or central nervous system lesions of various aetiologies. For more specific determination, the term peripheral and central neurogenic pain may be used.

Neuron The neuron is an electrically excitable cell forming the basic structural and functional unit (nerve cell) of the nervous system. It consists of a cell body, dendrites and axon. Functionally neurons can be divided into sensory, motor or combined neurons. From a structural point of view, the neuron can be pseudo-unipolar, bipolar and multipolar (most of them). The afferent neuron carries impulses from sensory receptors to the central nervous system. Efferent neurons carry impulses from the central nervous system to effector organs (muscles and glands).

Neuropathic arthropathy → see Charcot's joint (neuropathic arthropathy)

Neuropathic pain Pain caused by damage to the peripheral or central nervous system. Pain due to peripheral nervous system lesions (neuropathy) is usually burning or an electric shock-like pain, due to firing of pain and non-pain sensory nerve fibres.

Neurotransmitters Chemicals localised in nerve axon terminals that are released into the synaptic gap where they induce excitatory or inhibitory postsynaptic potentials. Acetylcholine, dopamine, noradrenaline, glutaminic acid, serotonin, endorphin, encephalin, substance P and others belong to this group.

Neutrophils Belongs to granulocytes and also called neutrophil granulocytes or polymorphonuclear neutrophils (PMN). They are present in peripheral blood (45 to 70% of circulating leukocytes) or are either tethered to the endothelium of blood vessels (so called marginal pool) or deposited in tissues where they move particularly during inflammatory reactions (inflammation). They are typical professional phagocytes as they have immunoadherent receptors on their surface through which they are effectively able to perform the phagocytosis of particles (including pathogenic microorganisms) opsonised by antibodies or by the iC3 fragment of complement. The enzyme NADPH-oxidase, which initiates the production of oxygen dependent antimicrobial and cytotoxic substances (reactive oxygen intermediates [ROI]), is activated in their cytoplasmic membrane during contact of the neutrophils with the particle or by chemotactic factors. ROIs along with oxygen independent factors (defensin, lactoferrin, neutral proteinases) kill phagocytosed cells. Oxygen independent antimicrobial substances are present in their progenitor forms in the granules (granule of leukocytes). Neutrophil granulocytes are paramount in the defence

against extracellular pathogenic parasites and are the first cells to appear in the area of inflammation. As with macrophages, neutrophils can also be present in the three stages: quiescent (resting), pre-activated and activated. Activated neutrophils possess the most efficient antimicrobial and cytotoxic activity, which can also cause damage to their own tissues.

Neutrophilic dermatoses A group of non-infective diseases characterized by skin lesions which on histopathological examination show intense inflammatory infiltrates of mainly neutrophils. The term neutrophilic dermatosis is sometimes associated with a good response of these diseases to glucocorticoids and immunosuppressive agents.

Nitric oxide (NO) A mediator of immune, nervous and the cardiovascular system. NO is a product of NO synthase activity and a free radical containing one disparate electron.

NO synthase (nitric oxide synthase, NOS) Synthase of NO, an enzyme that removes NO in the form of a free radical (NO·) from the guanidine group of L-arginine, leading to L-citrulline production. Subsequently other reactive products derived from nitrogen (reactive nitrogen intermediates [RNI]) develop. In the human body, the enzyme is present in three isoforms: constitutive neurogenic NO synthase (nNOS), constitutive endothelial synthase (eNOS) and inducible synthase (iNOS). nNOS is present in neurons and skeletal muscles, eNOS in endothelial cells and iNOS mostly in macrophages, but also in a number of cells of epithelial, myeloid or mesenchymal origin. NO has a number of physiological functions (involvement in defensive inflammation, immune responses, cardiovascular and nervous system regulations) and pathological functions (injurious inflammation, direct toxic damage of tissues). In immune responses, it acts as a regulator and an effector (injurious) molecule. NO synthesised by eNOS is involved in the regulation of blood pressure, causing relaxation of smooth muscles of vessels, whereas in the nervous system NO plays the role of neu-

N

rotransmitter of nitrergic (non-adrenergic and non-cholinergic) neurons.

Nociception All processes due to nociceptor activation. Nociception does not always lead to painful sensation, and vice versa. The pain does not always have to be caused by nociception (pain without nociception like psychogenic pain).

Nociceptive pain → see Types of pain

Non-inflammatory myopathies A group of muscular diseases in which muscle fibres are subject to damage and necrosis. Electromyographic examination confirms myogenic lesions. Serum muscle enzymes become raised during degradation of a large number of muscle fibres. Biopsy of muscle confirms muscle fibre atrophy which is non-neurogenic in origin, and the necrosis of muscle cells without inflammatory changes. Some myopathies are hereditary, whereas the remainder are of toxic origin (drugs).

Drug induced muscular diseases
Myopathies are caused by:
glucocorticoids (particularly fluoroglucocorticoids)
chloroquine, hydroxychloroquine, cyclosporin, colchicine, ipecacuanha,
quinolones, aminocaproic acid (Amicar®),
beta-blockers,
cimetidine, clofibrate, etrenitate, Sodium cromoglycate.
Polymyositis may be caused by:
• D-penicillamine, penicillin, sulfonamides,
• Cimetidine,
• Phenylbutazone, niflumic acid,
• Propylthiouracil.
Myasthenia may be caused by:
• D-penicillamine,
Chloroquine, hydroxychloroquine

Non-steroidal anti-inflammatory drugs (NSAIDs) They represent a heterogeneous group of drugs with anti-inflammatory, antipyretic and analgesic effects. They act by non-selective inhibition of the enzyme cyclooxygenase. They differ from each other in their chemical structure, certain pharmaco-kinetic properties, efficacy and adverse effects.

Non-steroidal anti-iflammatory drugs (NSAIDs) – advice for treatment in rheumatic disease The aim of NSAID medication is pain relief and reducing the period of morning stiffness, leading to relief of symptoms and improvement in the patient's quality of life.
Advice for NSAID medication
• the onset of analgesic effect is within several minutes or hours,
• the onset of anti-inflammatory effect during continual administration is up to 7 days,
• strong COX-1 inhibitors have the most significant anti-aggregate effect,
• the minimum effective dose is recommended,
• the length of treatment should be as short as possible,
• two orally administered NSAIDs should not be combined (increased gastrotoxicity),
• NSAIDs with selective COX-2 inhibition have less gastro-intestinal toxicity, but have a higher cardiovascular risk. The latter should be borne in mind when prescribing them in the elderly.

Non-steroidal anti-inflammatory drugs (NSAIDs) – classification Commonly, they are classified according to their chemical structure, their pharmacodynamic effect according to the degree of inhibition of both isoenzymes of cyclooxygenase (COX-1 and COX-2) and their biological half-life. A large group of NSAIDs can be easily divided into acids and neutral substances. The group of neutral NSAIDs contains only nabumetone, which as a pro-drug is metabolised in the liver into its effective substance of 6-methoxy-2-naphthyl acetoacetic acid. Acid forms of NSAIDs include most known agents and are divided into derivates of enol acids like pyrazolones and oxicams, which are commonly characterised by long plasma elimination half-life and frequently used derivates of carboxyl acids.

Classification of NSAIDs according to chemical structure

Acid NSAIDs:
- Derivates of enol acids:
  - pyrazolones – azapropazone, oxyphenyl-butazone, phenylbutazone, sulfinpyrazone.
  - oxicams –isoxicam, lornoxicam, meloxi-cam, piroxicam, tenoxicam,
- Derivates of carboxyl acids:
  - salicylic acid – acetylsalicyclic acid (Aspirin®), aloxiprin, diflunisal, lysinsalicy-late, salsalate.
  - acetoacetic acid – aceclofenac, acemeta-cin, diclofenac, etodolac, indomethacin, sulindac, tolmetin.
  - anthranilic acid –mefenamic acid, niflu-mic acid.
  - propionic acid – fenbufen, fenoprofen, flurbiprofen, ibuprofen, ketoprofen, naproxen, pirprofen, tiaprofenic acid.

Neutral NSAIDs:
- alkanone – nabumetone.
- coxibs – celecoxib, etoricoxib, lumiracoxib, parecoxib.

Non-steroidal anti-inflammatory drugs (NSAIDs) – clinical effect and indication

They are subject to common properties and these properties are very similar among different NSAIDs. After NSAID administration, relief of pain, stiffness and other symptoms occurs. Individual variations in the effectiveness of a particular NSAID can be explained by the pharmacokinetics of the drug

Table 6. Variability of NSAID effectiveness

Physical and chemical properties	Lipid solubility
Pharmacokinetics	plasma half-life
Pharmacodynamics	selectivity of COX-2 inhibition
Dose selection and application period	chronopharmacology
Variability of disease	elimination organ disorders
Adverse effects, pharmacogenetic differences	idiosyncrasy

at the cellular level. Various factors such as physical and chemical properties of the drug, pharmacokinetic parameters, the ability to inhibit a particular isoform of cyclooxyge-nase, selection of the form of application and the variability of the treated disease or symptom, all affect the variability of NSAID effectiveness (see table 6).

In clinical practice, the selection of a NSAID is subject to basic pharmacokinetic properties. Absorption of the majority of NSAIDs is rapid after oral administration (0.5 to 1.5 hours) unless it is an enteric-coated or slow release form of the drug. The time of clinical effectiveness is usually determined by the plasma elimination half-life. Particular NSAID groups have different plasma elimination half-life (table 7).

Table 7. Classification of NSAIDs based on plasma elimination half-life (Pavelka and Štolfa 2005)

Plasma elimination half-life of NSAIDs			
short (to medium-long) < 6 h		long > 10 h	
aspirin	0.25	fenbufen	10
tolmetin	1.0	diflunisal	13
diclofenac	1.1	naproxen	14
flufenamic acid	1.4	sulindac	14
ketoprofen	1.8	azapropazone	15
ibuprofen	2.1	nabumetone	26
fenprofen	2.5	piroxicam	57
etodolac	3.0	tenoxicam	60
tiaprofenic acid	3.0	phenylbutazone	68
flurbiprofen	3.8		
indomethacin	4.6		

N

NSAID groups have a broad range of indications, due to their anti-inflammatory, analgesic, anti-aggregation and antipyretic effects.

Indications of NSAID treatment:
- arthritic diseases including inflammatory rheumatic diseases, systemic connective tissues diseases, reactive arthritis, irritative synovitis, metabolic arthropathy (gout, chondrocalcinosis), osteoarthrosis, traumatic synovitis, tenosynovitis, bursitis in extra-articular rheumatism, and acute lumbosacral disease.
- acute and chronic nociceptive (somatic and/or visceral) pain and malignancy associated pain.
- prevention of ectopic calcification development after total hip joint replacement.
- acute pain conditions, renal and biliary colic, migraine, toothache (pulpitis), postoperative pain, trauma pain;
- dysmenorrhoea, premature labour reversal;
- fever;
- cardiovascular indications;
- other: Bartter syndrome, juvenile idiopathic arthritis, closure of patent ductus arteriosus.

Non-steroidal anti-inflammatory drugs (NSAIDs) – common properties
- anti-inflammatory effect,
- analgesic effect,
- antipyretic effect,
- acid character,*
- fat soluble,
- strong binding to plasma proteins,
- inhibition of prostaglandin synthesis in macrophages and fibroblasts,
- inhibition of thromboxane synthesis in thrombocytes, *
- inhibition of prostacyclin synthesis in endothelial cells, *
- induction of apoptosis.

* *selective COX-2 inhibitors and coxibs do not have significant effects*

Non-steroidal anti-inflammatory drugs (NSAIDs) – mechanisms of action
The NSAID group includes approximately 200 active substances originating from about 20 chemically different groups. Their common property is the blockade of the cyclooxygenase enzyme (COX) in a metabolic cascade of arachidonic acid (figure 2) through unstable

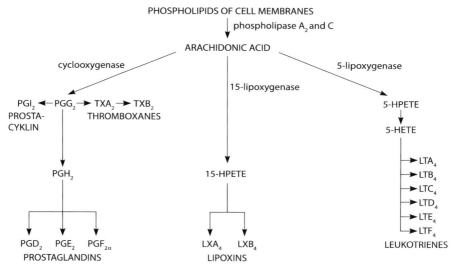

Figure 2. Metabolic pathways of arachidonic acid
HPETE – hydroperoxyeicosatetraenoic acid
HETE – hydroxyeicosatetraenoic acid
HPETE and HETE are abbreviations in the table.

endoperoxides to prostaglandins, thromboxanes and prostacyclins. The anti-inflammatory effect of NSAIDs is explained by inhibition of the cyclooxygenase enzyme and subsequent blockade of prostaglandin synthesis. The majority of NSAIDs inhibit transformation of arachidonic acid into thromboxane (TXA_2), prostaglandins (PGE_2) and prostacyclins (PGI_2). However, the mechanism of NSAIDs anti-inflammatory action is more complicated and includes the inhibition of the transcription of a number of pro-inflammatory genes, the products of which are significant mediators of inflammation, e.g. the pro-inflammatory cytokines TNF, IL-1 and IL-6.

NSAID mechanisms of action:

- membrane enzymes inhibition:
  - NADPH-oxidases of neutrophils (and superoxide production), phospholipase C of macrophages,
  - Peroxidases of 12-hydroperoxyeicosatetraenoic acid of thrombocytes;
- entrapment of precursors of arachidonic acid and its establishment to membranes of macrophages;
- inhibition of transmembrane transport of ions in erythrocytes and in the cells of renal tubules;
- inhibition of oxidative phosphorylation in mitochondria;
- inhibition of aggregation and adhesion of neutrophils;
- inhibition of lysosomal enzymes release;
- inhibition of pro-inflammatory cytokines;
- inhibition of NO synthase, particularly in endothelial cells;

NSAIDs interfere with pathways of inflammation even more significantly than has been reported. It has been confirmed that low doses of aspirin and newer forms of NSAIDs inhibit the biosynthesis of prostaglandins from arachidonic acid. Higher anti-inflammatory doses of aspirin (> 3.0 g/day) and sodium salicylate that do not inhibit cyclooxygenase and other NSAIDs act as anti-inflammatory agents by inhibiting reactions that are not mediated by prostaglandins (NADPH-oxidase inhibition, inhibition of phospholipase C and peroxidase of 12-hydroperoxyeicosatetraenoic acid). At the same time they block synthesis of proteoglycans in chondrocytes, the production of superoxide radicals, the transmembrane transport of anions, and inhibit aggregation and adhesion of neutrophils, the production of pro-inflammatory cytokines and synthesis of NO.

Classification of NSAIDs based on pharmacodynamic effect:

- selective inhibitors of COX-1 such as aspirin (doses up to 300 mg/day),
- non-selective inhibitors of COX-1 and COX-2 such as aspirin (doses >500 mg/day), ibuprofen, diclofenac, ketoprofen, tiaprofenic acid, indomethacin and others,
- selective inhibitors of COX-2 such as etodolac, meloxicam.

Gastrointestinal complications are among the most frequent adverse effects of NSAIDs and along with renal complications are prostaglandin-dependent. In the group of typical NSAIDs (such as non-selective COX-2 and COX-1 inhibitors) the two mechanisms cannot be separated from each other. New groups of selective COX-2 inhibitors (etodolac, meloxicam) and specific COX-2 inhibitors (celecoxib, etoricoxib, lumiracoxib, parecoxib) have reduced the risk of gastrointestinal complications while preserving their anti-inflammatory and analgesic effects. The risk of gastrointestinal complications is lower in drugs with higher selectivity for COX-2. Selectivity for COX-2 is assessed by a IC_{50} COX-2/COX-1 ratio (ratio of half inhibitory concentrations of COX-2/COX-1). Therefore all NSAID groups have been tested and high selectivity for COX-2 is the criterion for the development of new anti-inflammatory drugs.

Selectivity of particular NSAID groups and other new anti-inflammatory drugs blocking COX-2

- less than 5 times more selective for COX-2: acetylsalicylic acid, flurbiprofen, naproxen, piroxicam, indomethacin, nabumetone, ketoprofen, diclofenac, ibuprofen, tenoxicam, mefenamic acid.
- 5 – 50 times more selective for COX-2: meloxicam, celecoxib, etodolac;
- More than 50 times more selective for COX-2: etoricoxib, lumiracoxib.

Adverse effects of NSAID's

Gastrointestinal symptoms

Prolonged administration of NSAIDs is associated with a higher incidence of gastric ulcer and subsequent tendency towards its complications such as gastrointestinal bleeding and perforation. A higher risk of gastrointestinal complications associated with NSAID administration is seen in elderly patients (>60 years of age), patients with a history of peptic ulcers or its complications, and patients taking glucocorticoids, anticoagulant or antiaggregate medication.

Cardiovascular effects of NSAID and COX-2 inhibitors

NSAIDs and COX-2 inhibitors increase blood pressure (BP) or may de-stabilise BP. This has a clinical impact particularly in older individuals among whom the prevalence of hypertension and osteoarthrosis is high. The BP should be regularly checked in patients with arterial hypertension and diabetes during treatment with NSAIDs and COX-2 inhibitors. NSAIDs and COX-2 inhibitors also increase the risk of congestive heart failure, particularly in older individuals with ischaemic heart disease. There are differences within the group of NSAIDs and COX-2 inhibitors. A higher incidence of cardiovascular complications (myocardial infarction) has been confirmed, which is probably due to the imbalance between inhibition of vascular prostacyclin synthesis and the absence of the impact on thrombocyte thromboxane synthesis. The thrombotic potential of COX-2 inhibitors depends on the cardiovascular profile of the particular patient, particular drug, its dose and the duration of treatment. The risk of cardiovascular complications is also present among non-selective NSAIDs.

Renal complications

Inhibition of renal prostaglandins by NSAIDs leads to oedema, hyponatraemia and impaired effect of diuretics and beta-blockers. The incidence of kidney disease depends on the length of NSAID administration. However, functional renal impairment may occur after only a couple of days or weeks of NSAID administration, whereas interstitial nephritis after weeks to months of NSAID administration. Analgesic nephropathy can develop after a couple of years of regular NSAID medication. Elderly patients (>60 years old) are at higher risk as mild renal impairment may already by present due to a physiological decrease in glomerular filtration from nephrosclerosis accompanying hypertension or diabetes.

Bone marrow inhibition has been reported mainly in association with pyrazolones administration.

Central nervous system symptoms include tinnitus during salicylate medication and chronic fatigue and headache after indomethacin administration (especially in females). Increased bronchospasm can occur with most NSAIDs, which is important in patients with asthma. The list of adverse effects is given in table 8.

Adverse effects are relatively frequent and serious in combination with anticoagulant treatment (table 9).

Nottingham health profile → see Instruments of assessing (health status measurements, outcome measurement)

NSAIDs → see Non-steroidal anti-inflammatory drugs (NSAIDs)

NTX → see Crosslinked telopeptides of type I collagen, Markers of osteoresorption, Peptide fragments of collagen type I (NTX, CTX)

Nuclear factors Proteins also referred to as transcription factors because they bind to the promoter location (regulation units) of various genes and thereby stimulate (sometimes also inhibit) transcription (transcription to mRNA). Some of them are able to activate other genes, the products of which are involved in various physiological or pathological reactions. A number of them are in an inactive phase under physiological conditions and can be activated directly (viruses, various inflammatory stimuli produced in tissue or cell damage) or by various extra-cellular stimuli that act through receptors (e.g. antigens, hormones, cytokines). The transcription factors can therefore be regarded as nuclear messengers transforming external signals into long-term

Table 8. Adverse effects of NSAIDs

Disease	Mechanism	Frequency	Note
Gastrointestinal			
Dyspepsia	local irritation, ↓ synthesis of PG	Frequent	Differences among NSAIDs
Erosion, ulcer	Local irritation, ↓ synthesis of PG	2 to 10%	
Bleeding, perforation	↓ synthesis of PG, thromboxane		More factors
Hepatopathy	dose-dependent or idiosyncratic	Rare	Differences
Renal			
H_2O and sodium retention	↓ synthesis of PG	Dose	
↓ renal perfusion	↓ synthesis of PG	depen-	
acute renal insufficiency	↓ synthesis of PG	dent	
interstitial nephritis	dose-dependent, or idiosyncratic		
papillary necrosis	dose-dependent or, idiosyncratic	Rare	
Haematological			
Bone marrow inhibition	dose-dependent or idiosyncratic	Rare	More frequently after pyrazolones
Dermal			
Allergic reactions	Multifactor origin	Relatively frequent	Differences
Central Nervous System			
Fatigue, headache, vertigo, tinnitus (unknown origin, probably PG?), direct effect, e.g. indomethacin			
Increased bronchospasm (salicylates)			

Table 9. NSAID interactions

Agent	Result of interaction	Mechanism
Warfarin	Serious bleeding	Summation of effect on various receptors, release from plasma proteins binding, high levels of free agent
Warfarin and other drugs	bleeding	complex – PG effect
Oral hypoglycaemic agents	hypoglycaemia	
Antihypertensive drugs	reduced effect	

changes in gene transcription. 'Alert' cytokines (IL-1, TNF-α) and other chemotactic factors that act via receptors as well as certain bacterial products (e.g. LPS) belong to the group of inflammatory stimuli. They are associated with activation of transcription factors such as the nuclear factor kappa B (NF-κB), activator protein-1 (AP-1), nuclear factor of activated T cells (NF-AT) and signal transduction activating transcription factors (STAT). A synergic relationship has been observed among certain transcription factors. For example, during inflammation that is the cause of bronchial asthma, NF-κB and AP-1 act synergistically. Glucocorticoid receptors in the cytoplasm of cells belong to transcription factors. Activated glucocorticoid receptors inhibit the activity of other transcription factors and so inhibit the initiation or potentiation of the inflammatory process. Traditional aspirin acts mostly through inhibition of NF-κB. That is why the transcription factors have been used as a target for novel anti-inflammatory agents. The nomenclature of transcription factors is trivial and is derived from a particular function. Basically they can be divided into two large groups: the group of factors that are present in a number of cells and the group of factors that are specific to a certain type of cells.

Nuclear Scintigraphy of the skeleton (bone scintigraphy or bone scan) This

non-invasive method of nuclear medicine consists of the intravenous injection of a radiopharmaceutical agent where its increased (rarely decreased) accumulation in certain regions of the body can be detected through its emission of gamma rays by radiation detectors (gamma camera). The distribution of these tracers is dependent on the rate of bone turnover and blood flow

Technetium-99m Tc is used in the investigation of soft tissues. Hyperaemia and increased permeability of the vessel walls during inflammation of the synovial membrane can be detected by increased accumulation of the radiopharmaceutical agent in the inflamed joint. Methylene diphosphonate labelled by 99m Tc (osteotropic radiopharmaceutical agent) is used for investigating bony structures, with increased activity in the skeleton such as primary or metastatic tumours, Paget's disease, or healing fractures.

NZB/NZW mice (New Zealand black/ New Zealand white mice) F1-hybrid

mice in which a disease similar to human systemic lupus erythematosus develops spontaneously. The disease is of genetic origin; antinuclear antibodies and immune complexes develop, subsequently causing glomerulonephritis (membrane glomerulonephritis) and shortening the life of these animals.

N

Ochronosis → see Alkaptonuria and Ochronosis, Arthropathy in ochronosis

Oestrogens These female sex steroids are more important to bone than the classical calcitropic molecules (PTH, 1,25(OH)2 vitamin D and somatotropin-IGF-1). The primary importance of oestrogens for bone integrity in both genders is likely to be associated with the early development of specific intracellular (cytosol) receptors during evolution.

The effect of oestrogens on bone and calcium homeostasis is complex. They have an inhibitory influence on bone resorption – they protect against a proresorptive effect mediated by hormones and molecules (e.g. parathyroid hormone, thyroid hormones and heavy metals) and inhibit the release of cytokines from osteoblasts and peripheral monocytes. An effect on calcitonin and calcitriol regulation is exerted via specific oestrogen receptors on osteocytes. The absence of oestrogens causes an overproduction of interleukin (IL)-1 by peripheral monocytes. Tumour necrosis factor (TNF) alpha also increases bone resorption. IL-1 and TNF alpha play a critical role in the pathogenesis of bone loss in the absence of oestrogens. Oestrogens also suppress the production of IL-6, which is induced by IL-1 and TNF alpha. IL-6 is an important stimulator of osteoclast production. Oestrogen receptors are present on the surface of mononuclear cells, osteoblast precursors, osteoblasts and osteoclasts. At the same time, oestrogens stimulate the gene expression of the growth factor TGF beta, which is an anabolic factor inhibiting the production of osteoclasts. Oestrogens also regulate the production of prostaglandins (PG) which influence the production and effectiveness of cytokines. Except the afore-mentioned direct effect on bone, the absence of oestrogens leads to alterations of the calcium–phosphate metabolism. Oestrogen deficiency causes escalation of osteoresorption; calcium excretion by the kidneys is decreased and calcium absorption in the gut via parathormone (PTH) production of 1,25(OH)2D3 is increased. The following rise of serum calcium causes a drop in PTH secretion and an increase in calcitonin secretion. This process leads to decreased osteoresorption, decreased intestinal absorption and increased calcium excretion. A decrease in serum calcium occurs, though within the physiological range. Oestrogen deficiency causes, via PTH effect, an increase of phosphate concentration in the blood. The decrease of PTH and increase of phosphate lead to a decrease in the production of 1,25(OH)2D3. All these adaptive mechanisms contribute to the deepening of the primary disturbance of bone in oestrogen-deficient conditions. An early menarche, the number of pregnancies and hormonal contraception all have a protective influence against the occurrence of osteoporosis. As the pathophysiological overview shows, there is an acceleration of bone loss after the menopause. The yearly bone turnover in the premenopausal women affects approximately 2–5% of cortical bone and 15–25% of trabecular bone.

Orthoses Orthopaedic devices that help locomotive system function. They hold body parts in their correct position or move them into the correct position. Sometimes they compensate for lost function, or correct a deficit to a manageable level.

Depending on their purpose, orthoses are divided into:
- *Therapeutic* – can be used as temporary therapeutic or physiotherapeutic devices.
- *Compensatory* – they permanently compensate a particular defect of the locomotive system, e.g. different length of limbs.
- *Prophylactic* – used, for example, in sport to avoid unfavourable injury.

Static orthoses (stability)
- *Supportive* – they compensate for loss of load capacity.
- *Fixative* – they maintain stability where there is pathologic damage to the locomotive system; temporary (compensative) orthoses help, for example, during sequential therapy of fractures (plaster fixation), permanent orthoses are used when the muscle system does not hold the joint in the required position as a consequence of a permanent defect.

Dynamic orthoses
- *Correct defective posture* – e.g. corsets in the treatment of pathological curvature of the spine.
- *Movement control orthosis* – e.g. orthosis used with knee instability where the orthosis prevents mediolateral movement, but anteroposterior movement can occur.

Orthoses influencing muscle work

These are orthoses with dynamic functions. The function of weak muscles is taken over by the orthosis, which utilises:
- the transfer of work from healthy muscle
- springs and rubber tension apparatus
- the elasticity of material from which the orthoses are made
- hydraulic or electric drive

Orthoses of fingers

Can be divided into fixative, redressive, retentive, substitute and movement regulating orthoses. A fixative or retentive orthosis is used in the rupture of the extensor pollicis longus muscle; the PIP (proximal interphalageal) joint remains free. An extensive dynamic PIP orthosis enables the movement of the joint against resistance (flexion or extension). The three-point correction principle is used in Boutonniere deformity (correction of flexion deformity in PIP and extension deformity in DIP – distal interphalangeal joint). In Swan neck type deformity, the orthosis corrects extension deformity in the PIP joint and the flexion position in the MCP (metacarpophalangeal) and DIP joint.

A fixative thermoplastic splinter avoids ulnar or possibly radial deviation in the MCP joints. Spring extension splints of the fingers are used after orthopaedic hand operations in patients with hands affected by a rheumatologic process.

Orthopaedic shoes Suitable for individuals who owing to foot deformity (often in rheumatological diseases) cannot wear ordinary shoes. They are made for the purpose of foot deformity correction, pain relief and gait support, progression prevention and for cosmetic cover for a deformed foot.

Orthopaedic shoe inserts Orthoses that are inserted into shoes in order to correct certain less serious foot defects. Correction inserts help actively or passively correct flattening of the arch of the foot. Relieving inserts contain holes for relieving the pain arising from sore areas (callosities). Correction inserts are used to correct different lengths of limbs.

Oscar (OsteoClastS-Associated Receptor) A product of gene coding for the leukocyte receptor complex. It is specifically expressed in preosteoclasts and mature osteoclasts. OSCAR-L exprimed by osteoblast/stromal cells is its ligand. The presence of a soluble form of OSCAR in the co-culture of osteoblasts and bone marrow cells inhibits the formation of osteoclasts. OSCAR is therefore a specific regulator of osteoclastic differentiation.

Osgood-Schlatter disease Necrosis of tibial tuberosity of the tibia in children, especially in 8 to 14 year old boys. The defect is frequently bilateral. Patients complain of pain, particularly when climbing stairs. The pain is located in the area of the tibial tuberosity, which is swollen and tender to pressure. X-ray shows irregularity and calcification around the insertion of the patellar tendon.

Treatment heat, rest, a protective plaster is necessary in more serious cases. Improvement may take two or more years.

Osteitis deformans → see Paget's disease

Osteoarthritis (OA) A very common degenerative joint disease which progresses with age and characteristically affects the

small joints of the hand, lower limb joints and the vertebral column. OA embraces heterogeneous diseases of different aetiological origin, but with a similar biological, pathological, radiological and clinical picture. It manifests itself by joint dysfunction due to dysregulation of cartilage metabolism, which leads to changes in the mechanical properties of cartilage. The pathological picture includes focal destruction of the cartilage as well as areas of remodelling in the form of osteosclerosis and osteophyte formation. OA can be primary or secondary (e.g. due to metabolic, endocrine, haematological diseases).

Risk factors of OA:

- Heredity, particularly in the polyarticular form of small joints of the hands,
- Obesity, where it is associated with knee osteoarthritis,
- Hypermobility accompanying collagen abnormalities,
- Post-traumatic conditions,
- Sports with risk for joint injuries,
- Posture at work.

Clinical symptoms: Pain is typically associated with exercise, and is associated with brief morning and inactivity stiffness. Gradually reduced function and immobility develop.

The X-ray picture shows loss of joint space, the development of sub-articular cysts, subchondral sclerosis, osteophyte formation, and deformities. The course of OA is very variable and in most cases progresses very slowly. However, very rapid progression can occur.

Osteoarthritis – hands (Heberden and Bouchard type)

A hereditary disease especially affecting women. The DIP (distal interphalangeal) joints are affected producing Heberden's nodes whilst involvement of the PIP (proximal interphalangeal) joints cause Bouchard's nodes. It commonly manifests itself between 40 to 60 years of age (menopausal).

Clinical symptoms: Cartilaginous stiff nodes gradually grow on the opposite articular surfaces on the dorsal articular margins. The nodes are sore in the course of growth with intermittent inflammatory erythema and swelling. Deviation of the distal and mid-

dle phalanges is frequent. Once growth of the nodes stops, the affected joints become pain-free. Compared with rheumatoid arthritis, hand function usually remains good, though may be a problem in certain jobs or pastimes (e.g. pianist). More often, it only causes cosmetic problems (knobbly looking hands). Initially, the radiographs are normal, but later show unequal narrowing of the articular cavity and osteophyte formation. It is very important to emphasise to the patient that it is not rheumatoid arthritis or gout.

Treatment: Non-steroidal anti-inflammatory drugs, or intra-articular glucocorticoids, are administered during inflammatory episodes. The use of SYSADOA are other options in more stubborn cases. Treatment may be supplemented by ultrasound administration, thermotherapy (wax, mud) and therapeutic exercise.

Osteoarthritis (OA) of the first carpometacarpal (CMC) joint (Rhizarthrosis)

OA may occur only in the first CMC (OA of the thumb) and the trapeziometacarpal joint. Rhizarthosis is a common problem that affects mainly women in their 50s. The affection may be uni- or bilateral, with different clinical and radiological stages. As the cause is generally unknown it is referred to as idiopathic. The most common symptom is pain, particularly in everyday movements at using the pinch function (touch the thumb with another finger) to turn keys, open a jar, a window, turn a knob. Little by little the joint deteriorates and later it subluxes. The result is then a characteristic deformation at the base of the thumb. Treatment is the same as in all other forms of OA but if conservative treatment is insufficient, surgery may be indicated.

Osteoarthritis (OA) – pharmacological treatment

The pharmacological treatment of OA is represented by two large groups of drugs:

1. SYRADOA (symptomatic rapid-acting drugs of osteoarthritis) can be simple analgesics such as paracetamol, aspirin, NSAIDs (non-steroidal anti-inflammato-

ry drugs), opioids or intra-articular gluco-corticoids;
2. SYSADOA (symptomatic slow-acting drugs of osteoarthritis) such as intraartic-ular hyaluronate or oral glucosamine sul-phate, chondroitin sulphate, diacerein, etc. (so-called chondroprotective agents).

Initially, simple analgesics usually provide satisfactory pain relief. In advanced disease, in order to suppress the inflammation and ease pain, NSAIDs are prescribed. Treatment with standard NSAIDs is associated with a number of adverse effects, particularly gas-tropathy (gastric ulcer, bleeding). The risk of gastrointestinal complications is increased in elderly patients who often suffer from OA.

In terms of these complications, NSAIDs with strong selectivity to cyclooxygenase 2 (COX-2) have a significantly lower incidence of adverse gastrointestinal effects. In terms of biological and biochemical properties, low dose meloxicam belongs to this group. At the stage of painful OA, it is administered orally in a daily dose of 7.5 mg, but can be increased to 15 mg daily if required.

Another specific COX 2 inhibitor is cele-coxib. Studies have shown that celecoxib is as effective as non-selective NSAIDs, when ad-ministered in a single daily dose of 100–200 mg (Bensen et al. 1999, Pavelka and Štolfa 2005). The safety profile of celecoxib has been extensively tested in comparative trial with diclofenac, ibuprofen and naproxen. These trials confirmed the favourable safety of cele-coxib with less renal adverse effects and no increased cardiovascular risk.

Osteoarthritis – primary generalised nodal osteoarthritis (GNOA)
Initially, it manifests by inflammatory episodes of the DIP (distal interphalangeal) and PIP (proxi-mal interphalangeal) joints of the hand in rela-tively young women (around 40 years old), often peri-menopausal. Familial incidence is frequent. It never affects the MCP (metacar-pophalangeal) joints but often affects the knees, hips and intervertebral (facetal) joints. Initially, radiological changes are not visible, but typical osteoarthritic changes develop lat-er. Deviation of the phalanges occurs.

Treatment: Non-steroidal anti-inflamma-tory drugs are administered during inflam-matory episodes. Afterwards, treatment is the same as in other forms of osteoarthrosis.

Osteoarthritis (OA) – surgical treatment
Surgical procedures play a key role in the treat-ment of OA. They are indicated when pharma-cological and non-pharmacological treatment fails especially in severe hip and knee arthritis. The indications for surgical treatment include permanent severe pain (including night pain) and greatly reduced function of the affected joint with very limited mobility. At present, to-tal hip or knee joint replacements are the most effective and frequently used procedure. Most patients are able to return to their normal daily activities after surgery. An improvement in the materials used in the development of the pros-theses guarantees their longer durability up to 10 to 15 years.

Osteoblasts
Uninuclear cells whose main function is the production of bone tissue (os-teoformation). They develop from a pluripo-tent mesenchymal cell that gradually matures to preosteoblasts and osteoblasts. From a morphological point of view, they have a rounded nucleus localised in the basal part of the cell. In the nucleus, receptors for oestro-gens, vitamin D3, integrins and cytokines can be found. The nucleus is localised on the op-posite side to the position of contact between the osteoblast and the bone surface. The cyto-plasm is heavily basophilic; the Golgi appara-tus lies between the nucleus and the apical part of the cell. The endoplasmic reticulum is pronounced. The plasma membrane of active osteoblasts contains a high concentration of alkaline phosphatase and receptors for para-thormone. Osteoblasts are localised on the surface of trabeculae and in the osteons of compact bone where they are capable of pro-ducing osteoid in the places of active osteo-formation. After completion of the osteofor-mation phase, osteoblasts are transformed into lining cells or osteocytes.

Osteocalcin
Osteocalcin, also known as bone Gla-protein (BGP), is a small non-colla-

gen protein (MW 58 kDa) specific for bone and dentin. It forms 1–2% of bone proteins. Osteocalcin is preferentially synthesised in osteoblasts under the control of 1,25-dihydroxyvitamin D3, and is then incorporated into the extracellular bone. A portion of newly-synthesised osteocalcin is released into the circulation and reflects the intensity of osteoformation.

At present, osteocalcin, together with the bone isoenzyme of alkaline phosphatase, is the most utilised marker of osteoformation. In the most frequently used method, the intact molecule is determined by a method using two monoclonal antibodies detecting the intact molecule together with its N-terminal peptide.

Serum osteocalcin correlates with the increased skeletal growth during puberty and is elevated in various disturbances of bone metabolism associated with increased bone turnover (e.g. primary and iatrogenic hyperthyroidism, hyperparathyroidism, acromegaly and renal osteodystrophy). Likewise, the level of osteocalcin is decreased in hypothyroidism, hypoparathyroidism, in glucocorticoid-treated patients, in the osteoporosis induced by hepatic disorders, diabetes, in some patients with multiple myeloma and malignant hypercalcaemia. In hypercorticism, the synthesis of osteocalcin in osteoblasts is suppressed. Decreased levels have a diagnostic value and an increase of its level is a marker of successful treatment. Interestingly, in Paget's disease, the concentration of osteocalcin rises far less than the value of the bone isoenzyme of alkaline phosphatase. Generally, osteocalcin reacts very sensitively to disturbances of bone metabolism associated with the endocrine disorders.

The serum osteocalcin level is also raised in certain forms of osteoporosis. Pathologically increased values are found in postmenopausal women with rapid bone loss (fast-losers). Measurement of decarboxylated osteocalcin may be useful in determining the prognosis following hip fracture in elderly women.

Osteochondritis dissecans → see König's disease

Osteoclasts Large multicellular cells containing 4–20 nuclei. The main function of osteoclasts is the resorption of mineralised bone matrix. Osteoclasts are formed by a fusion of unicellular phagocytic cells (monocytes) following development from preosteoclasts. There are receptors for calcitonin and integrin in their cytoplasm. Osteoclasts contain esterases and produce enzymes such as tartrate resistant acid phosphatase, glucuronidase and carboanhydrase. They also possess colony stimulating factor (CSF-1).

The nuclei of osteoclasts have no uniform appearance. There are numerous Golgi apparatuses, mitochondria and transport vesicles filled with lysosomal enzymes around the nuclei. Once activated, osteoclasts move to areas of microfracture by chemotaxis and come to lie in Howship's lacuna and osteons of compact bone. The osteoclast resorption area is increased by a ruffled border from which is secretes hydrogen ions and several hydrolytic enzymes including cathepsin and matrix metalloprotease groups into the subosteoclastic space. As a consequence of the low pH, hydroxyapatite crystals dissolve allowing exposure of the bone matrix to the lytic enzymes and its resorption. Osteoclast activity is regulated by several hormones including parathormone, calcitonin and interleukin 6 (IL-6) and by osteoprotegerin and RANK ligand produced by osteoblasts.

OsteoClastS-Associated Receptor →
see Oscar (OsteoClastS-Associated Receptor)

Osteocytes These develop from osteoblasts and accumulate in the lacunae between the lamellae of compact bone and inside trabeculae. These cells were originally osteoblasts entrapped in the bone matrix that they produced and which was consequently calcified. The shape of osteocytes depends on their age and activity. A young osteocyte has many features in common with its precursor – the osteoblast, but is smaller with a smaller Golgi apparatus and endoplasmic reticulum. These changes are substantially more pronounced in older osteocytes with glycogen accumula-

O

tion within the cytoplasm. Osteocytes possess cytoplasmic processes that form a net of cells in the bone channels. These processes facilitate the transport of cytokines, hormones, growth factors as well as signal transmission. Osteocytes work as sensors reacting to changes in the flow of fluids in bone channels. They react to these stimuli, induced by mechanical and environmental changes, by synthesis of active substances influencing the process of bone remodelling by gentle adjustments of osteoblastic and osteoclastic activity. The other function of these stimuli is the nutrition of bone tissue. During osteoclastic resorption of bone, osteocytes undergo phagocytosis.

Osteogenesis imperfecta (OI) This represents a group of hereditary connective tissue diseases characterised by a qualitative or quantitative defect of type I collagen. William Vrolik (physician working in anatomy and pathology, The Netherlands, 1801 1863) first described the symptoms of the disease in the *Pathological anatomy handbook* in 1844. There are 8 main types of osteogenesis imperfecta People with type I tending to have mild symptoms.. People with types IV, V, and VI tend to have more moderate symptoms. People with types II, III, VII, and VIII tend to have severe symptoms, with type II being lethal in the perinatal period. Osteopenia and osteoporosis occurs to varying degrees. In the differential diagnosis, children with juvenile osteoporosis, secondary osteoporosis associated with other diseases and, last but not least, child abuse must all be taken into consideration. Personal and family history, thorough physical examination, X-ray review and bone densitometry lead to the diagnosis.

Pathogenesis: Synthesis or structured defects of pro-α1 and pro-α2 chains of type I collagen (encoded by the COL1A1, COL1A2, CRTAP and LEPRE1 genes on chromosomes 7, 17, 1 and 3 respectively) occur. Currently, more than 200 mutations of these genes have been recognised.

Clinical symptoms: Osteopenia or osteoporosis with repeated fractures, mainly af-

fecting cortical bone, and bone deformity are among the main symptoms. Callus formation after fractures is normal and bone remodelling is rapid. Every tissue containing type I collagen may be affected, i.e. teeth, ligaments, skin, sclera etc. Therefore, teeth development may be defective – dentinogenesis imperfecta. The teeth have a greyish even brownish-yellow colour, short and narrow roots, and tooth enamel is fragile. Occasionally, in some families patients present only with the teeth defects (no fractures). Joint hypermobility with lax ligaments can lead to repeated dislocation. Conductive hearing impairment may occur in early middle age. Decreased synthesis or impaired quality of collagen is reflected by increased capillary fragility associated with bruising, haematomas and frequent epistaxes. Patients are prone to develop hernias. The sclera of a number of patients have various shades of blue to greyish colour, may be very slight. Bone deformities are represented by curvature of long bones after repeated fractures and various degrees of thorax deformity (most frequently kyphoscoliosis). Individuals with severe forms of the disease also have a disproportionately large head and triangular-shaped face. A squeaky voice, excessive perspiration, constipation, mitral valve defects and aortal insufficiency are among other variable symptoms. Intelligence is always normal, even in the most severely affected patients.

Diagnosis: A skin biopsy for fibroblast culture to analyse the type I collegen genes and white blood cell DNA testing for mutations in COL1A1 and COL1A2 can be helpful, but may not be conclusive.

Treatment: Although there are no curative specific treatments, administration of bisphosphonates appears to offer the best outlook.

Osteokines in Osteoporosis Interleukins (IL) IL-1, IL-4, IL-6 and IL-11, macrophage and granulocyte/macrophage (GM) colony stimulating factor (CSF) and tumour necrosis factors (TNFs) belong to cytokines with important effects in the pathogenesis of osteoporosis. These cytokines stimulate osteoresorption.

IL-1 has a complex impact on osteoporosis. Elevated concentrations of IL-1 are found in patients with severe osteoporosis. IL-1 stimulates the synthesis of IL-6 which increases the osteoclast count. Oestrogens decrease the synthesis of both IL-1 and IL-6. TNF alpha stimulates osteoresorption and replication of osteocytes. CSF plays a role in the maturing of osteoclasts and deficiency of GM-CSF-1 leads to osteoporosis.

Bone remodelling is a complex process regulated by systemic hormones and local factors that have an important position in the maintenance of the dynamic balance (coupling) between the processes of osteoformation and osteoresorption. The actual influence of the individual factors on bone continues to be studied. Understanding their mechanisms of action is the key to the development of new, more preventative and therapeutic measures in fighting osteoporosis.

Osteomalacia The essence of osteomalacia is deficient mineralisation of bone tissue in adults. Consequently, the bone tissue is softer and bones are prone to deformities. In contrast, rickets is a defective mineralisation of the epiphyseal plates in children leading to growth retardation and skeletal deformities. The low concentration of minerals in bone tissue in osteomalacia is caused by deficient mineralisation of newly formed bone so that this condition may be considered as "minor-mineralisation", and not as demineralisation, which is the term often used incorrectly for this condition. In the histological picture, the affected bone shows non-mineralised bone matrix (osteoid) visible as concentric layers in Haversian canals of compact bone and as a wide margin on the trabeculae of bone. The total number of Haversian canals and trabeculae as well as their size remain (in contrast to osteoporosis) normal. Symptoms can be minimal, but include muscle weakness, bone pain due to micro-fractures (looser zones on X-rays) in weight bearing areas and fractures following little or no trauma. The main cause is calcium and vitamin D deficiency due to poor diet or various malabsorption diseases, rarely hereditary causes of osteomalacia appear during childhood. Biochemically, patients have a raised serum alkaline phosphatase and low or normal calcium. Treatment is directed at the cause, and correction will often markedly improve the patient's quality of life.

Osteomyelitis A bacterial infection of bone. Infectious agents include pyogenic bacteria such as cocci (staphylococci, streptococci, pneumococci), *Escherichia coli*, salmonella, *Proteus* and myobacteria. Infectious agents usually reach the bone via blood spread during bacteraemia from a purulent focus elsewhere the body, or they may directly invade the bone during open fractures or operations. The course of osteomyelitis can be acute, sub-acute or chronic. Usually a fever up to 40°C with significant localised pain and decreased mobility occurs. Osteomyelitis is mainly located in the areas of the most rapid enchondral growth with increased blood supply, thus in the metaphyses of long bones. Depending on age, the infection can spread into the joint (pyarthrosis) in children up to 1 year old in whom epiphysis and metaphysis have a common blood supply, whereas this is less likely in children over 12 months old when the blood supply mentioned above is separated. The growth cavity forms a certain barrier so the infection may expand under the periosteum and fistulate externally (sub-periosteal abscess). Another form of abscess is the Brodie abscess (Sir Benjamin Brodie, surgeon in London, 1783–1862), which manifests itself by pain, with the X-ray showing a clear round lesion with a sclerotic margin located in the diaphysis and metaphysis. In osteomyelitis, sclerotising bony enlargement with periosteal apposition occurs predominantly.

A suspected diagnosis of osteomyelitis is confirmed by the clinical picture, X-rays, bone puncture biopsy and cultivation to determine the pathogenic agent. Treatment consists of long-term antibiotics administration and immobilisation of the affected limb. In the chronic stage, treatment includes the debridement of necrotic tissue, removal of bone sequestrae, lavage and local administra-

O

tion of antibiotics. Subsequently, covering of the defect with transfer of vascularised bone, skin and muscle flaps may be necessary.

Osteonecrosis (ON) Cell death involving both the mineralised bone and bone marrow based on loss of bone's blood supply. Osteonecrosis is not a specific clinical entity. It is a common final pathway of numerous diseases.

Clinical symptoms: The most frequent (and most serious) localisation of ON affects the femoral head but it may also occur at other sites (humeral head, femoral condyles, small bones of wrist and foot) and bilateral disease is common. Clinical symptoms are non-specific and particularly include persistent pain of varying intensity, though sometimes the patients may be asymptomatic.

Early X-ray changes of ON are not well recognised, with typical changes becoming visible subsequently. An excellent method of detecting progressive change is the use of magnetic resonance imaging (MRI). Whereas early disease may be curative, established disease is irreversible and requires surgical intervention.

Osteonecrosis of the jaw (ONJ) A very rare complication following administration of bisphosphonates, most commonly in high doses parenterally, in the setting of poor dental hygiene with or without dental procedures. The risk with oral treatment is low. It presents with infection and necrosis of bone in the mandible or maxilla. It is important to check for good dental hygiene before administration of bisphosphonates, as treatment is difficult. Conservative management with limited debridement, antibiotics and mouth rinses assist healing.

Osteopathies – Laboratory investigations The aim of the biochemical examination is the differential diagnosis of other osteopathies, the evaluation of phosphate – calcium metabolism, and the evaluation of bone metabolism activity (it means differentiation of fast-loser and slow-loser osteoporosis).

Routine laboratory examinations:
- blood count, erythrocyte sedimentation rate,
- serum calcium, albumin, phosphate and alkaline phosphatase,
- liver transaminases, creatinine, protein electrophoresis,
- chemical analysis of the urine,
- 24 hour urinary calcium and phosphate excretion.

Specialised laboratory examinations:
- serum and urinary bone markers,
- tests for a diagnosis of secondary osteoporosis: serum PTH, 25-OH Vitamin D, TSH, fT4, STH, IGF1, gonadotrophins (LH, FSH), prolactin, free cortisol in the urine, serum CTH, sex hormones (oestradiol, testosterone), bone biopsy, biopsy of the small intestine and specific antigliadin antibodies, oncomarkers.

Osteopetrosis Belongs to skeletal diseases associated with hyperostosis or osteosclerosis also known as Albers-Schönberg Disease (Heinrich Ernst Albers-Schönberg, German radiologist, 1865–1921). Osteopetrosis causes bones that appear dense and cavities for bone marrow do not form. At present, several forms of osteopetrosis can be distinguished. A 'benign' autosomal dominant adult type with only mild symptoms, a 'malignant' autosomal recessive infantile type which, if not treated, leads to death in infancy, and an 'intermediate' autosomal recessive type which, in childhood, has many symptoms similar to those of malignant osteopetrosis but patients survive. Other types include carbonic anhydrase II deficiency previously described as osteopetrosis with renal tubular acidosis and cerebral calcifications and certain extremely rare types such as neuronal recurrent disease with malignant osteopetrosis, lethal or infantile transitory osteopetrosis.

Pathogenesis: The gene for the adult type of osteopetrosis has been localised on chromosome 1p21. The basic defect is similar in all forms of disease with failure of osteoclasts to resorb bone. It results in a persistently calcified matrix, which was formed by chondroblasts during enchondral ossification. Defective transformation of fibrous bone into compact bone, which is associated with defective bone resorption, contributes significantly to increased bone fragility. Carbonic anhydrase is vital for acid-base homeostasis. Its isoenzymes speed up the reaction of carbon dioxide and water leading to carbonic acid production and subsequent release of hydrogen cation and bicarbonate. Carbonic anhydrase II is missing in erythrocytes in cases of osteopetrosis with renal tubular acidosis and calcification in the brain. Rarely, osteopetrosis can be associated with a neuronal degenerative disease due to accumulation of ceroid lipofuscin secondary to a lysosomal defect.

Clinical symptoms: Infantile osteopetrosis manifests in early childhood. Chronic nasal obstruction due to malformation of paranasal sinuses and mastoid is among the first symptoms. It is not rare for the disease to manifest in infancy with clinical hypocalcaemia. Narrowing of the cranial foramens through which the nerves run leads to visual impairment and paresis of oculomotor and facial nerves. The child often suffers from floating eye movement and/or strabismus, is generally unwell, and teething is delayed. The skeleton looks dense on X-ray picture but bones are very fragile. In certain patients hydrocephalus develops, and sleep apnoea syndrome may occur. Apart from optic nerve palsy, retinal degeneration contributes to visual loss. The bone marrow cavities apart from an abundance of osteoclasts, contain fibrous tissue so the child has a tendency towards spontaneous bleeding and the development of bruises, and suffers from frequent infections. Severe anaemia occurs if hypersplenism and haemolysis are present. The necessity for blood transfusion before the third month of age is a sign of poor prognosis. On physical examination the child is generally unwell and macrocephaly, frontal bossing, and nystagmus are found. The child has an adenoid facies, hepatosplenomegaly (compensatory extramedullary haematopoiesis) and genu valgum. Peripheral leukocytes are unable to perform their immune functions, and therefore untreated patients usually die during the first decade of their life from sepsis accompanied by severe anaemia and haemorrhagic diathesis.

Autosomal recessive deficit of carbonic anhydrase II is accompanied by renal tubular acidosis and cerebral calcification. The neuronal form is a combination of severe skeletal defect, epilepsy and neurodegenerative changes.

Osteopontin (OPN) Also known as ETA-1 (early T lymphocyte activator 1). OPN is a human gene expressed in bone. It is an extracellular structural protein. OPN also has the property of a cytokine, which regulates cell-mediated immune reactions. The expression of osteopontin is located in bone and on the epithelial surface, but also occasionally on the endothelium, smooth muscle cells and on the surface of mononuclear cells during the course of pathological inflammation. They support Th1 and inhibit Th2 expression of cytokines. Osteopontin is a regulating factor of calcium deposition in bone and in areas of pathological inflammation (dystrophic calcification) and is also involved in the pathogenesis of atherosclerosis and tumour growth.

Osteoporosis (OP) Skeleton disease characterised by decreased bone strength with a subsequent increased risk of fractures. Bone strength is determined by the density of bone mineral and the quality of bone tissue, i.e. by the architecture of bone trabeculae, the intensity of bone turnover and the accumulation of microfractures (NIH consensus conference 2000).

Osteoporosis is usually diffuse. Based on aetiology, it can be classified as primary, which is present without a known disease or condition leading to structural or functional defects of bones, or secondary, when it is invoked by a known disease, or by external factors. Primary OP includes postmenopausal OP (type I), senile OP (type II) and juvenile OP (rare). Secondary OP caused by genetic abnormalities, endocrine disorders, nutritional disorders, renal diseases, inactivity, inflammation, tumours or certain drugs. Decreased bone formation and increased bone resorption occur in glucocorticoid induced OP, leading to a rapid reduction in bone substance and increased risk of fractures.

Osteoporosis – Definition A number of diverse definitions of osteoporosis exist based

O

on specific diagnostic criteria. At present, the WHO definition (1994) has usually been used as it takes into account the morphological, as well as the clinical aspect. Osteoporosis is defined as a metabolic disorder of bone characterised by a low bone mineral density and disturbance of microarchitecture with a consequent increase of fragility and risk of fracture.

Osteoporosis – Diagnosis The aim of diagnosis is to define the group of patients with a low bone mineral density, in which the risk of fracture is high enough for antiosteoporotic treatment to be considered.

The T-score reflects the number of standard deviations (SD) compared with the bone mineral density in young healthy individuals of the same gender. This assessment of bone density applies only to postmenopausal women and men over 50 years of age (see table 10). In premenopausal women, children and men under 65 years of age the International Society for Clinical Densitometry (ISCD) recommends the use of the Z-score (Z-score reflects the number of standard deviations compared with the bone mineral density in healthy age, gender and ethnicity matched individuals) to assess low bone mineral density, with a reasonable working definition of "low BMD" as a Z-score -2.0.

Diagnosis of osteoporosis may be established by measurements in the following regions: lumbar spine in the AP projection, femoral neck, greater trochanter and a region referred to as total femur. Bone mineral density measured in other regions may not be used for diagnosing osteoporosis, according to the WHO criteria. Forearm measurements may be accepted in patients where the other sites are non-measurable or uninterpretable

Table 10. WHO classification of bone density

Classification of decreased bone density	T-score
Normal	more than –1.0
Osteopenia	–1.0 to – 2.5
Osteoporosis	less than – 2.5

(due to osteoarthritis, joint prosthesis, etc). Only a region of the forearm referred to as 33% radius may then be used for diagnosing osteoporosis. The peripheral bone mineral densitometry at the heel is unsuitable for diagnosing osteoporosis according to WHO. However it is still applicable as a method of identifying patients at high risk.

A low bone mineral density does not confirm the diagnosis of primary postmenopausal osteoporosis even in a woman after menopause. Likewise, normal values of the bone mineral density measured at a single skeletal site by one method of measurement do not exclude osteoporosis in a given patient. It is important to exclude other relevant disorders where a low bone mineral density and secondary osteoporosis may occur.

Osteoporosis – Epidemiology The contemporary definition only allows indirect measurement of the epidemiology of osteoporosis either on the basis of the prevalence of osteoporotic-related fractures or osteoporosis defined by bone mineral densitometry. The risk of fracture, however, is determined not only by bone mineral density, but also a whole range of other indicators within the bone (quantity of bone mineral, microarchitectural structure, properties of the material, dynamics of the bone turnover, etc.).

The most frequent sites of osteoporotic fractures are the forearm, vertebrae and hip. The life-long risk for any osteoporotic fracture in a 50-year old woman is approximately 39% and in a man approximately 13%.

Hip fracture is the most serious complication of osteoporosis and is associated with high morbidity and mortality. Worldwide an increase in number of these fractures from 1.6 million in 1990 to 6.26 million in 2050 can be expected (Marcus et al. 2008). The 5-year survival is only 82% of the total population survival with mortality at its highest in the first 6 months. The lifetime risk of death following a hip fracture is comparable to that of breast cancer and 4-times higher than uterine cancer.

The epidemiology of vertebral fractures is less well understood due to the lack of a universally accepted diagnostic criterion and a high portion of asymptomatic fractures. Only about one third of vertebral fractures are seen in the outpatient clinic and only 2–8% require hospitalisation. The prevalence of radiological fractures in people >50 years old is between 8–25%, depending on the definition. Vertebral fractures are associated with a similar increase in 5-year mortality as hip fractures.

Fractures of the distal forearm, most of them of Colles type, differ from the epidemiological view from hip and vertebral fractures. There is a significant predominance of women (up to 4:1) with the incidence up to 85%. The distal forearm fractures are not associated with increased mortality or with a long-term disability.

Osteoporosis is socially the most severe locomotor system disorder due to its high incidence and mortality.

Osteoporosis – Fracture risk estimation There is a close correlation between the bone mineral density and the risk of fracture. A decrease by 1 SD represents 1.5–2.5 times higher risk of fracture. This correlation, however, has not been documented in premenopausal women. It is known that many fractures occur in the patients with osteopenia. In deciding whether to start anti-osteoporotic treatment, an assessment of risk is important.

A prevalent vertebral fracture following inadequate trauma is the most significant factor. These patients have up to 5-times higher risk of another fracture and approximately 2-times higher risk of hip fracture. A second vertebral fracture appears within one year in 20% of patients.

Bone turnover is another significant factor. A high bone turnover doubles the risk of fracture, independent of bone mineral density.

The length of the femoral neck is directly proportional to the risk of fracture in this area as well. Evaluating the tendency to falls is important as non-vertebral fractures, which quantitatively dominate, occur almost exclusively after trauma.

Osteoporosis – Genetic factors Genes participate in influencing the maximum peak bone density and in affecting bone remodelling. Knowledge and practical application of genetics in osteoporosis are hampered by its obvious polygenic inheritance. Two types of research studies are involved; association studies searching for links between individual genes or their clusters and incidence of osteoporosis, and the description of definite genetic abnormalities in individual patients or families (Marcus et al. 2008).There are typical descriptions of changes in the genes for Osterix, Sclerostin, LRP5 and others. A strong genetic component is confirmed by studies on identical twin and daughters of osteoporotic mothers (Marcus et al. 2008). The inheritance is strongest in the lumbar spinal region. The collagen synthesising gene type I (COL1A1 gene), oestrogen receptor genes, cytokines and growth factors are considered to be potentially responsible for influencing bone turnover. Changes found in the allele for the vitamin D receptor correlate with calcium absorption from the gastrointestinal tract, the level of peak bone mass (PBM), as well as with bone turnover. Similar variability have been assumed for the oestrogen receptor gene and procollagen type I gene. These hypotheses could explain the great variability of PBM in healthy subjects as well as differences in response to treatment with vitamin D. However, further prospective studies are needed. The gene coding for CaSR may also influence calcium and parathormone levels, and thus bone mineral density.

Osteoporosis in men The lower incidence of osteoporosis in men compared to women is caused by:
- a higher maximum BMD in adolescent males (thicker bones),
- slower and more uniform resorption of BMD with age (no accelerated postmenopausal loss),
- shorter mean life expectancy in men.

However, the difference in the incidence of fractures between women and men significantly decreases with age. The aetiopathogenesis of osteoporosis in men is multifactoral and in contrast to women is secondary in nature in more than 50%. Therefore, a secondary cause should be sort especially in younger men.

Osteoporosis (OP) in rheumatoid arthritis (RA)
Diffuse osteoporosis is very frequent, even in patients who have never been treated with steroids, which has been proved by recent trials of monozygotic twins, from which only one suffered from RA. It is commonly present in patients treated with glucocorticoids.

Possible mechanisms of secondary OP are:
- Systemic effect of inflammatory mediators associated with disease activity (IL-1, IL-6, TNF etc.),
- Changes in circulating hormone concentrations,
- Changes in calcium metabolism,
- Changes in skeletal load,
- Influence of drugs used in RA treatment.

Clinical symptoms:
- Fractures of vertebrae, neck of femur, forearm bones,
- Chronic static pain in the spine, most frequently between scapulae and in the lumbosacral area,
- Acute sharp localised pain to the spine, occasionally radiating to the front of the thorax and abdomen,
- Kyphosis of the thoracic spine,
- Decrease in body height.

Osteoporosis – Indications for treatment
Antiresorptive treatment (except of calcium and vitamin D) is indicated:
- in patients where bone mineral densitometry has verified osteoporosis,
- in patients with an osteoporotic related fracture (in sites where osteoporosis-based fractures occur following low energy trauma).

Osteoporosis – Medical treatments
Drugs used in the treatment of osteoporosis
Bone turnover inhibitors:
- calcium,
- vitamin D and its active metabolites,
- oestrogens,

- synthetic oestrogen derivatives with combined properties of oestrogens, gestagens and androgens (Tibolone) – STEAR,
- selective oestrogen receptor modulators (SERM),
- calcitonin
- bisphosphonates

Stimulation of osteoformation:
- anabolic steroids,
- parathormone,
- fluoride salts.

Drugs with a dual mechanism of action (inhibition of the osteoresorption and stimulation of the osteoformation):
- strontium ranelate,

Drug decreasing the elimination of calcium in the urine:
- thiazide diuretics.

Osteoporosis – Non-medical treatment
Nutritional factors
An adequate supply of nutritional elements is one of the decisive factors in the prevention and treatment of osteoporosis which becomes even more significant in the postmenopausal period. The intake of calcium is of key importance. Calcium has a beneficial influence on maximising bone mass in children and adolescents. An abundance of vitamin D, adequate supply of proteins (too high supply causes an increase of calciuria), phosphates (too high supply stimulates secretion of PTH) and vitamins C and K (necessary for collagen synthesis) are also essential. An excessive supply on sodium (calciuria), proteins, magnesium, zinc, copper and manganese should be avoided, which is usually no problem with a normal dietary regime. An excessive supply of substances forming insoluble salts with calcium, such as oxalic acid, phytic acid, lactose and certain proteins, is inadvisable. Sodium and glucose cause calciuria. Exposure to aluminium, sulphur dioxide and other toxic waste products may worsen the status of bones.

Smoking
Nicotine, similar to other components of cigarettes, has a negative effect on the differentiation of osteoblasts. It is an important risk factor, especially in slender women.

Smoking influences the bone via the following mechanisms:

- a negative influence on the protective effect of oestrogens,
- earlier menopause,
- malnutrition due to anorexia,
- increased sensitivity to parathormone,
- acidosis due to toxic concentrations of carbon dioxide (CO_2),

increased rate of respiratory infections and facilitation of acidosis.

Alcohol

Alcohol also has a direct toxic influence on bone. An increased amount of alcohol has a negative influence on the synthesis and differentiation of osteocytes.

Alcohol influences the bone density by the following mechanisms:

- Malnutrition – lack of proteins and vitamins,
- Malabsorption of calcium,
- Hepatopathy (through disturbance of vitamin D hydroxylation in the liver)
- Increased secretion of cortisol.

However, several observations have also shown a reduction of fracture risk in persons with a low alcohol intake compared with nondrinkers. Due to the difficulty in defining the exact protective dose of alcohol, osteoporotic patients are advised to abstain from alcohol completely.

Physical activity

Physical activity has a positive influence on the increase in bone mineral density. Exercise facilitates activation of remodelling processes and increases in certain hormones (for example oestrogens, gestagens, testosterone and growth hormone). It is hypothesised that pressure caused by a load causes a piezoelectric event change to the transmembrane potential and leads to the stimulation of osteoblasts. On the other hand, a loss of mechanical stimulation of bone (physical inactivity) is associated with a significant decrease in bone mass. A beneficial effect of regular exercise on bone mineral density, however, persists only during the activity. Swimming and gymnastics are reported as the most appropriate sports. Exercising at the same time improves locomotor coordination, which can reduce the incidence of falls and thus reduces the risk of fractures independent of bone mineral density. During excessive exercise, especially in athletes, the development of amenorrhoea with its associated hormonal changes will accelerate osteoporosis in spite of the physical activity.

Osteoporosis – Physical examination

The findings on physical examination that should make one suspicious of a diagnosis of osteoporosis include: a loss in height, enhancement of the thoracic kyphosis, bulging of the abdomen, low body weight (BMI under 19), thin stature and a reduced distance between the iliac crest and the last rib (less than 3 fingers). In addition, there may be physical finding indicating diseases leading to secondary osteoporosis (joint deformities in RA, cushignoid habitus, etc).

The physical findings may be typical of other metabolic osteopathies including the bone deformities in Paget disease, blue sclera in osteogenesis imperfecta, etc. None of the above-mentioned parameters themselves or their combination are able to unambiguously establish the diagnosis of osteoporosis, but should alert the physician's attention to its possibility.

Osteoporosis – Prevention of Fractures

Osteoporosis prevention involves methods aimed to increase the activity of osteoblasts and prevent osteoresorption. The most important factors are the following: adequate intake of calcium, vitamins D and C, exercise, a well-balanced diet, and exclusion of toxic influences (smoking, excessive alcohol intake, heavy metals and excessive supply of phosphates). At the same time, the use of good fitting footwear, correction of vision and prevention of falls (obstacles on floors, elimination of vertigo, etc.) are important in reducing the incidence of fractures.

Osteoporosis – Risk factors

A meta-analysis of large clinical studies by the WHO affiliated working group has considered the following as the most significant risk factors: age, previous fracture after an inadequate

O

trauma (the so-called low-energy trauma), a family history of fractures, corticosteroid treatment, smoking, excessive alcohol intake and rheumatoid arthritis (WHO Scientific Group 2007).

Osteoporosis Risk factors – modifiable
- physical activity,
- physical inactivity – inactivity-induced osteoporosis develops during complete immobilisation. Depending of the intensity of bone metabolism in an individual patient, significant loss of bone mineral density occurs over weeks to months.
- Dietary supply of calcium – insufficient supply of calcium, a disturbance of its absorption from the gastrointestinal tract and increased excretion in the kidneys may lead to a negative calcium balance and increased bone loss.
- Body weight – Reduced body weight, often combined with other risk factors, increases the risk of postmenopausal osteoporosis. A BMI < 19 kg/m^2 is an important risk factor for fractures.

Osteoporosis Risk factors – unmodifiable
- genetic predisposition – higher risk in Caucasians and patients with a family history of osteoporotic fractures and thin stature,
- age,
- gender – more significant risk in women compared to men.

Osteoprotegerin (OPG) Alkaline glycoprotein with four potential N-glycoside bonds. It is released as glycoprotein (Mw 55 kDa), which is intracellularly transformed by disulphide bonds into a dimer with (Mw 110 kDa). It may also exist as a trimer but the prevailing extracellular form is a dimer. Osteoprotegerin is produced by osteoblasts. It is a soluble substance that acts as a receptor blocker binding to RANKL (receptor-activator of nuclear factor κB ligand) and thereby preventing its action on osteoclasts and their precursors. In the past RANKL was known as osteoclastogenesis inhibiting factor, which defined one of his properties. It belongs to the family of TNF-receptors, but does not have a transmembranous domain or sequence that allows signal transduction and therefore is denoted as a blocking receptor. By blocking the differentiation and activation of osteoclasts it prevents, for example, parathormone or vitamin D$_3$ induced hypercalcaemia.

Ott's sign → see Metric measurement of vertebral column in spondyloarthritis (SpA)

Overall status in rheumatoid arthritis (OSRA) → see Instruments of assessing (health status measurements, outcome measurement)

Overlap syndromes A term used to label patients with the diagnostic criteria of two or more systemic connective tissue diseases, but now more commonly called undifferentiated connective tissue diseases (UCTD). Polymyositis (PM), dermatomyositis (DM), systemic sclerosis (SSc), and less frequently rheumatoid arthritis (RA) and systemic lupus erythematosus (SLE) are the most frequent components of overlap syndromes.

Clinical symptoms: Depend on nosological units that form the overlap syndrome. The most frequent symptoms are:
- Raynaud's phenomenon, arthralgia, arthritis, myositis, serositis, interstitial pneumonia,
- Antinuclear antibodies, antibodies against ribonucleoproteins referred to as U1RNP.

P

Paget's disease A progressive disorder affecting a limited number of bones. It is characterised by progressive hypertrophy and osteosclerosis of bone tissue. It leads to an abnormal increased bone turnover causing changes to bone formation. Its prevalence increases with age and in certain countries (especially the Anglo-Saxon population) it affects up to 3% of the population over 40 years of age. Men and women are affected equally. The aetiopathogenesis is unknown, but there has been speculation that a viral (parvo-virus) infection may be implicated. The majority of osteoclasts contain intracellular particles resembling paramyxoviral nucleocapsids. Other possible causes are an inborn error of metabolism or vascular abnormalities. Paget's disease may be inherited in an autosomal dominant trait, with the genetic abnormality localised to chromosome 18.

Many patients remain asymptomatic. The most frequent symptom is bone pain at rest or on weight bearing. The skin over the affected limb is usually warm. Enhanced vascularisation, mechanical stress and irritation of the periosteum by disturbed remodelling are the reasons for pain. Secondary osteoarthritis, especially in the hip or knee may occur if the bone around the joint is affected. Other typical findings include deformities of the femur, tibia (sabre) and forearm. These late onset deformities are asymmetrical and often easy to diagnose. Pathological fractures can occur after minimal trauma. Deformities of the skull cause changes to its shape resulting in a lion face (leontiasis ossea), basilar invagination, hydrocephalus and compression neuropathies leading to hearing and visual loss. Other complications include compression of the spinal cord and nerve roots, compression of the posterior fossa, osteosarcoma and giant-cell tumours, heart failure and hypercalcaemia during immobilisation.

The diagnosis of Paget's disease may follow the typical clinical picture, characteristic radiographic findings and laboratory investigations, though sometimes is only determined in the differential diagnosis of an elevated alkaline phosphatase. Even in the early stages, there are localised areas of osteolysis on X-ray. This finding in the skull is called osteoporosis circumscripta. Later, enlargement of bones, thickening of the cortex, sclerotic changes and other findings appear. Increased uptake on bone scintigraphy is highly sensitive, but a nonspecific method of detecting the regions of skeletal abnormalities. In the blood tests, there is a typical (often very high) elevation of serum alkaline phosphatase level, especially of its bone isoenzyme. Osteoresorption products are also increased.

Treatment of Paget's disease is aimed at suppression of bone pain (short-term) and preventing the progression and complications (long-term).

The following are the indication for medical treatment:

- bone pain,
- prior to orthopaedic surgery,
- hypercalcaemia caused by immobilisation,
- symptomatic heart failure,
- neurological deficit,
- prevention of future complications.

Modern treatment involves the administration of a bisphosphonate (etidronate in a dose 5 mg/kg/day for up to 6 months or risedronate 30 mg/day for up to 2 months) are now considered more effective than calcitonin. More recent data on suppression of disease activity and prevention of recurrence have indicated better results with either tiludronic acid (skelid) 400mg daily orally for 12 weeks or administration of zolendronic acid in a single dose of 5 mg in a slow intravenous infusion over 15 minutes.

A surgical operation is reserved mainly for:

- total hip or knee joint prosthesis,
- tibial osteotomy,

- occipital craniotomy for the decompression of posterior fossa,
- decompression of the spinal cord and nerve roots.

Paget-Schroetter syndrome → see Acute shoulder pain

Pain It is a fundamental component of human life. Despite its aversive character, the perception of pain is a basic condition for human survival. In an acute state, it serves as a positive warning signal for the body, indicating actual or potential tissue damage. Intensive and prolonged pain, however, loses its biological significance and protective function. The pain itself becomes a source of further, often more severe damage to the body. It has a negative influence on the physical condition of the patient, disturbing his mental balance, leading to decompensation and disturbance of social communication. Persistent pain is the reason for repeated seeking of medical help and excessive use of medicaments, especially analgesics. The drop in physical activity and mental decompensation cause gradual isolation of the patient and development of abnormal, often purposeful, painful behaviour. Behavioural and psychosocial influences play an important role in the processing of pain of whatever origin; however, their importance rises with chronicity. Chronic pain is therefore considered a complex bio-psycho-social phenomenon.

Pain has four components:

1. *sensory-discriminative* Most information is available about this component; when and where the pain arises, how it is transmitted and how it is processed in the central nervous system (CNS).
2. *affective-emotional* Less knowledge is known on this though the tracts transmitting it to the brain are understood. This component determines interindividual variability (one is a coward, another a hero). It is genetically determined, but anything can be substantially influenced by education.
3. *vegetative (autonomic)* This is very important in visceral pain. Any kind of pain, especially visceral pain, is accompanied by vegetative changes. This is mainly because of a number of vegetative system fibres, mainly sympathetic, inside the body that influence pain.
4. *motor* It enables the avoidance of painful stimuli or fighting against it: "fight or flight".

Types of pain
By time course:

Acute pain This is subject to actual or developing tissue or organ damage. It has a protective function and is time-limited. Acute pain has a sudden onset and subsides rapidly after withdrawing. It provokes a number of reflex responses such as muscle contraction or activation of the autonomic nervous system (tachycardia, increased cardiac output, hypertension, increased gastrointestinal tract motility, vasoconstriction, hyperventilation, diaphoresis, etc.). Mental changes are minimal (anxiety, insomnia) and transient. Acute pain responds well to opioid and non-opioid analgesics. Insufficient control of pain can lead to the prolonged course of the morbid state (or postoperative state) and to undesirable emotional stress, which has a negative influence on haemocoagulation, immune system activity, cardiovascular and gastrointestinal function.

Chronic pain This is pain defined as follows:

- pain lasting longer than expected healing time,
- pain associated with a chronic disorder, where the aetiology has not been ascertained,
- pain related to neoplastic disease – this is assigned as a separate type of pain.

Chronic pain is not strictly time-limited, with as much as 1/3 of patients not expressing signs of somatic disease. The activity of the autonomic nervous system decreases gradually with the duration of pain. Mental changes, such as sleep disturbance, anxiety and depression, become prominent. Behaviour and personality changes appear. The physical status deteriorates – muscle hypotrophy and atrophy, contractures, weakness, reduction of mobility and immobilisation. The patient is gradually isolated from working, social and family life. Approximately 20% of patients try to commit suicide.

The treatment of chronic pain is more complex than acute pain. The aim is to interfere with all basic pain mechanisms – physiological, behavioural, as well as cognitive. In addition to drug therapy, which by itself is not so effective, psychotherapy and other non-pharmacological procedures, such as acupuncture, rehabilitation, transcutaneous electrostimulation etc, play an important role. The multidisciplinary approach of healthcare and non-healthcare professionals is required.

Chronic pain is not a uniform group. It is often categorised according to length of time and pattern such as permanent, progressive, recurrent or cyclic pain, etc.

The term "benign chronic pain" was introduced in 1970 to distinguish a non-neoplastic pain. It should be considered of less severity with a view of intensity, course and prognosis. Malignant pain is pain associated with oncological disease

From a neurophysiological perspective (pain classification according to Lindblom):

Nociceptive pain This is elicited by stimulation of nociceptors in the somatic and visceral organs.

Somatic pain The result of activation of nociceptors in somatic organs (tendons, muscles, capsule, periosteum). It is mostly well localised, dull, but occasionally sharp. It responds well to all analgesics.

Visceral pain The perception of pain is deep, prickly, gripping, or possibly spasmodic. Unlike somatic pain it is more diffuse – likely as a consequence of the prevalence of C-fibres over A-delta fibres in the visceral afferent nerves. It has a prominent autonomic component – sweating, nausea and hypotension. It is associated with reflex muscle cramps and a secondary hyperalgesic phenomenon due to sensitisation of dorsal horn neurons. Often it is transmitted to cutaneous regions innervated by the same nerve roots as the affected organs. The propagation of pain can be explained by a convergence of cutaneous and visceral afferent horn ganglia, where

one branch goes to the skin and the other to visceral organs or muscles. The nociceptors in the internal organs are activated by different stimuli (traction, ischaemia, distension, etc.). The visceral pain responds poorly to analgesics.

Neuropathic pain This results from damage of the peripheral or central nervous system (somatosensory tracts). It can be associated with nerve dysfunction followed by disturbance of sensitivity or weakening of muscles innervated by a damaged nerve. Absence of afferent inputs in the disrupted nerve causes the reorganisation of central circuits. Tasker introduced the term "de-afferentation pain" for states characterised by neuropathic pain. Interruption of the afferent nerve may cause peripheral and central de-afferentations on all levels of the CNS (dorsal horns, thalamus, and cortex). As a consequence of a lesion in sensory tracts, the central inhibitory control, activated by stimuli from the periphery, is often decreased. It manifests by an increased response to afferent stimuli as hyperesthesia, hyperalgesia and allodynia. It is mostly unpleasant, burning, and often transposed. Neuropathic pain responds weakly to analgesics, while adjuvant treatment is more effective (tricyclic antidepressants, anticonvulsants, NMDA receptor blockers). According to the location of damage, it can be divided into central and peripheral.

Psychogenic pain It may have a psychogenic cause (anxiety), can be related to a psychosomatic disease, or may be an associated sign of a mental disorder (schizophrenia).

Painful arc Shoulder pain elicited on abduction of the arm between 60 and 120°. Pain occurring in this range is typical of supraspinatus tendon or subacromial bursa involvement. Pain at the end of the arc between 160 and 180° indicates an affection of the acromioclavicular joint.

Palindromic rheumatism Characterised by recurrent attacks of painful oedema around the joints and soft periarticular structures. The disease occurs mainly between the third and sixth decade and equally affects both males and females. Attacks of palindromic rheumatism start suddenly, usually involve one to three joints and last for hours or days before spontaneous remission occurs. Prognosis is good, joint damage does not occur.

Clinical symptoms:
- Short course of arthritis,
- Recurrent episodes of disease,
- Joints remain radiologically normal (non-destructive).

Panniculitis Inflammation of subcutaneous fatty tissue manifesting by the formation of inflamed nodules, particularly in the lower extremities, thorax and gluteal area. It mainly affects women in early and middle age. Many forms of panniculitis with or without vasculitis are described, including acute lobular panniculitis without vasculitis (Weber-Christian disease), and panniculitis associated with a connective tissue disease, pancreatic disease (pancreatitis or pancreatic carcinoma) or lymphoma. It consists of a heterogeneous group of symptoms, in which inflammation in fatty tissue occurs, particularly in subcutaneous fatty tissue. The histopathologic picture shows infiltration of neutrophils or lymphocytes, later followed by histiocytic infiltration, and possibly large cell infiltration. Lesions settle by fibrosis formation. In the phase of histiocytic infiltration, panniculitis can have the property of granulomatous inflammation. Subcutaneous fatty tissue has a lobular structure. Central arteries pass through the fatty lobules forming branches of arterioles and capillaries, from which the blood is conducted through venules located in septa between particular lobules. Panniculitis affecting venules in the septum between lobules can be schematically classified as septal (non-necrotizing) panniculitis and lobular (necrotizing) panniculitis, which affects the artery passing through the centre of the lobule.

Panniculosis A non-inflammatory disease of subcutaneous tissue incorrectly known as cellulitis. It is a constitutional disorder of fatty tissue deposit predominantly occurring in women during the menopause.

Pannus Proliferating synovial tissue with activated fibroblasts and inflammatory cell infiltration (lymphocytes, plasma cells, activated macrophages and dendritic cells) which intensively grows into the surrounding bone on the joint margin causing local osteolysis. The typical picture of bone erosion therefore develops. A frequent finding of multi-nucleated cells with phenotypic characteristics of osteoclasts in the interface between bone and pannus led to the presumption of direct involvement of the cells derived from the pannus in bone resorption. The focal inflammation in rheumatoid arthritis affects subchondral and juxta-articular bone, where pannus development begins.

Paracetamol One of the most frequently used non-opioid analgesics. Missing an anti-inflammatory effect, it cannot be included in the group of non-steroidal drugs (NSAIDs), even though recently published trials suggest that paracetamol, particularly in the central nervous system, inhibits the COX-3 isoenzyme. It does not affect the production of physiologically important prostaglandins in the stomach, bowel or platelets and therefore there are none of the typical adverse effects observed when using NSAIDs such as increased risk of gastrointestinal bleeding or an acute decrease in renal function. A daily dose higher than 5 g/day may cause fatal liver impairment. The analgesic and antipyretic effect is comparable to that of aspirin. Paracetamol has neither an anti-inflammatory nor anti-aggregate effect. The analgesic properties of paracetamol will last for around four hours due its short half-life of about two hours. Administration of higher doses (more than 2 grams a day) may cause prolongation of the prothrombin time. Compared to aspirin, paracetamol has a lower ceiling effect. It can pass through the blood brain barrier and only a small amount is bound to plasma proteins (approximately 10%). It is metabolised in the liver and is eliminated via the kidneys in the form of glucuronides and sulphates.

Paraesthesia Decreased or tingling sensation of skin in particular dermatome.

Paraffin Wax A mixture with approximately 5% of paraffin oil, heated to 55 to 60°C, is used for therapeutic purposes. The heat that is released during transformation from a liquid to a solid state is utilised. The manner of use includes soaking the limbs in paraffin wax, transferring the paraffin wax using a paintbrush or suitable tissue soaked several times in the paraffin wax and, most favourably, using plastics. It is necessary to keep the skin dry in the area of paraffin wax administration as different tolerability of the skin to paraffin wax (60°C) and water (46°C) may cause burns. The mixture of paraffin with peloid sheets, so-called parafango, is also frequently used. They are indicated for chronic pain of the musculoskeletal system, non-inflammatory arthrosis, extra-articular rheumatism, vertebrogenic pain syndrome, spondyloarthropathies, and rarely also for inactive ankylosing spondylitis as a form of pre-heating before exercise.

Paraproteins Monoclonal immunoglobulins present in the plasma of patients with multiple myeloma or Waldenström's macroglobulinaemia (gammopathy), monoclonal gammopathy of undetermined significance, cryoglobulinaemia, plasmacytoma, amyloidosis, heavy chain disease, lymphomas, leukaemias and some other diseases.

Parathormone The most important regulator of extracellular calcium, but also has a direct effect on bone. It influences the hydroxylation of vitamin D and reabsorption of calcium in the kidneys. The effect of PTH on bowels is indirect via calcitriol (increase of calcium resorption from the bowel).

Parathormone affects calcium and phosphate metabolism via several mechanisms:
- it stimulates the release of calcium and phosphate from bone,
- it stimulates the reabsorption of calcium from the glomerular filtrate and loss of phosphate to urine,
- it stimulates the renal synthesis of 1,25-(OH)2 vitamin D3 and thus the gastrointestinal absorption of calcium and phosphate.

A prolonged overproduction of parathormone leads to an increase in the number and activity of osteoclasts. The release of calcium is associated with the release of phosphate, bone matrix and collagen. The changes in bone with primary hyperparathyroidism are complex and include a subperiostal osteoresorption, osseous cysts, bone demineralisation and acroosteolysis. Spontaneous fractures are frequent complications.

Parathormone Drug – Teriparatide The only pure osteoanabolic drug indicated for the treatment of severe postmenopausal osteoporosis (previous fracture and T score <2.5 on BMD scan). A synthetic recombinant aminoterminal fragment (1–34) of parathormone is used. When used in a therapeutic dose of 20 micrograms/day subcutaneously, it does not produce osteoporosis as occurs in hyperparathyroidism, but instead the osteoblastic production of growth factors IGF-1 and TGF-β increases, without reducing the production of osteoprotegerin. Teriparatide reduces the risk of vertebral and nonvertebral fractures and greatly increases BMD in the most at-risk groups of patients. Treatment significantly improves pain and quality of life. It is administrated for 18 months.

Paroxysmal nocturnal haemoglobinuria A rare form of haemolytic anaemia with intravascular haemolysis during sleep due to a greater sensitivity of the erythrocytes to haemolysis by an autologous complement. As well as affecting erythrocytes, neutrophils and thrombocytes also have a higher sensitivity to the haemolysis. The cytoplasmic membranes of these cells are deficient in DAF, the decay-accelerating factor that protects against damage after spontaneous activation of complement. The disorder is characterised by leukocytopenia, thrombocytopenia, and iron deficiency and often by the presence of blood (haemoglobin) in the urine

Parvo virus arthritis Parvo virus B19 was associated with clinical disease in the early 1980's. In children, it produces slapped-cheek disease (fifth's disease, erythema infectiosum) but in female adults, it can produce an acute arthralgia/arthritis mimicking rheumatoid arthritis. Symptoms usually settle within three weeks, though occasionally last up to six months. The diagnosis can be confirmed by IgM antibodies to parvo virus within the serum. Only symptomatic treatment and reassurance is required, though rarely it can produce a transient aplastic anaemia and miscarriage in pregnancy.

Pathergy phenomenon Scratching the skin using a sterile needle evokes a strong erythematous reaction with induration. The test is positive in active Behcet's disease as a sign of skin impairment (vasculitis). It is present more frequently in the Turkish population than in Europeans and Americans.

Pauciarticular juvenile idiopathic arthritis → see Juvenile idiopathic arthritis (JIA)

PCR (polymerase chain reaction) A laboratory technique that makes it possible in an automated way to gain millions of copies of a fragment of a DNA molecule by in vitro enzymatic replication. The segment of double-chain DNA isolated from, for example, lymphocytes and containing the required gene is marked by complementary oligonucleotides (primers). The segment undergoes amplification by repeated cycles of denaturation, cooling and primer attachments and their subsequent prolongation using thermostable DNA-polymerase. One cycle takes approximately 3 minutes and results in duplication of a DNA fragment. This means that within 60 minutes thousands of copies of one DNA fragment can be produced. PCR can be used in medical and biological research for prenatal and common diagnostics of genetic, infectious and other diseases, in determining their pathogenesis, in the genetic determination of individuals and populations, and in resolving the most fundamental problems of contemporary molecular biology and medicine.

PEG Abbreviation for polyethylene glycol; a synthetic molecule with variable relative molecular weight. It is used for precipitation of soluble proteins including circulating immune complexes and as a fusogen in hybridoma technology of monoclonal antibod production.

Peptide fragments of collagen type I (NTX, CTX) NTX and CTX are peptide fragments of type I collagen from the telopeptide region of the collagen molecule used as a measure to assess bone loss.

Perforins Glycoproteins with cytolytic properties are located in the granules of cytotoxic T lymphocytes and NK cells. After release to the surface of target cells, perforins undergo polymerisation to form polyperforins which perforate the phospholipid double layer of the cytoplasmic membrane. The damaged membrane causes cell death and lysis. The C9 component of complement, defensins of neutrophils, cytolysins of eosinophils as well as certain viruses, microbial toxins (e.g. streptolysin O) and insect toxins (e.g. mellitin of bees and wasps) or cation detergents act by a similar mechanism.

Peripheral Quantitative Computerised Tomography (pQCT) The measurement of peripherally localised bones without a superposition of the soft tissues. It is measured in the area of forearm. Although a relatively simple method allowing the separate evaluation of trabecular and cortical bone as well as the examination of certain morphological parameters it is, however, currently (due to expense and high dose radiation) infrequently used in the clinical practice.

Personage-Turner syndrome An acute neuropathy of the brachial plexus of unknown origin, which particularly affects young men. The pain radiates into the shoulder and scapula. Hyperaesthesia may develop in the arm and shoulder area. Passive ranges of movements of the shoulder are normal but often paresis of shoulder muscles develops. Depending on the particular muscles affected, active movements of the shoulder are limited. EMG confirms a neurogenic lesion. The disease recovers spontaneously over several months.

Treatment: Bed rest, analgesics, gradually increased doses of oral glucocorticoids, vitamin B1, therapeutic exercise and physical therapy.

Perthes Disease → see Legg-Calve-Perthes Disease

Pes equinus The foot is in a vertical position, with toe tip towards the ground. If the condition is caused by paresis, it can be corrected by a peroneal splints or orthosis. Fixed pes equinus (with shortened Achilles tendon) usually requires surgical intervention.

Pes excavatum (cavus) The longitudinal arc is significantly elevated, the plantar aponeurosis is shortened, and dorsal flexion at the ankle is limited. It is usually combined with mallet toes. Treatment consists of arch underpacking, which allows the aponeurosis to stretch.

Pes varus The opposite of pes planovalgus or flat feet. The ankle is in a varus position with supination and adduction of the anterior part of the foot. An external wing heel is applied as a treatment.

PET → see Positron emission tomography (PET)

Pfeiffer's disease → see Infectious mononucleosis

Phagocytosis A protective mechanism that belongs to the fundamental elements of natural immunity when phagocytes ingest microorganisms and other particles with a diameter greater than 0.5 μm. It is a complex process consisting of several concurring intermediate steps. The disturbance of one of them leads to a deficiency of phagocytosis. The ability to phagocytose is possessed by all nuclear cells in the human body, but protective phagocytosis is performed mainly by professional phagocytes. If particles from the intercellular environment are ingested, the process is referred to as heterophagia; if the ingested material comes from surrounding cells (dam-

aged cell organelles), the process is referred to as autophagia.

Phalen's test Maximal forced flexion of the wrist evokes paraesthesia in fingers on the radial aspect of the hand. Along with Tinel's sign, it is positive in carpal tunnel syndrome.

Pharmacorehabilitation A model of the synergic effect of two therapeutic procedures – rehabilitation and pharmacotherapy. The principle lies in relieving the patient of resting pain and reducing exertional pain to a bearable level. It plays an important role in chronic disorders such as rheumatic diseases. For example, rehabilitation in acute or chronic rheumatoid arthritis should be performed despite the presence of certain limiting factors, while respecting the diurnal variation of symptoms, such as pain, stiffness and fatigue. Analgesic treatment is adjusted so that the therapeutic maximum is reached at the time set for rehabilitation.

Phosphate → see Phosphorus

Phosphorus The sixth most frequent element of the human body and is present as phosphate in biologic systems. An adult body contains approximately 600 mg of phosphorus. The distribution of phosphate in the individual tissues differs substantially from that of calcium. Approximately 85% of phosphorus is deposited in crystalline form in the skeleton. The other 15% is found in the soft tissues and extracellular fluid. 90% (55% in ionised form + 35% in complexes) of plasma phosphate is ultra filtratable and only 10% is protein bound. The serum phosphate level varies more than the serum calcium level with a circadian rhythm leading to 50% of the value during the day.

Phosphate, similarly to calcium, plays a structural role in the skeleton, except that it is also contained in membrane phospholipids, nucleic acids, phosphoproteins, energy-rich compounds (ATP, creatine-phosphate) and in the co-factors of some enzymes (NADP, phosphoinositides). Basic physiological processes such as gene regulation, modulation of

P

enzymatic activities and maintenance of the integrity of cellular membranes are amongst its functions. Phosphate is irreplaceable in buffering systems to provide stability of the acid base balance. It also plays an important role in the metabolic processes of intermediary metabolism and in energy transmission.

Physiatrics A field of medicine engaged in utilising various physical agents for the diagnosis, treatment and rehabilitation of various disorders, or in the prevention of physical deformities and disabilities. In physiological terms, the reactions to these physical stimuli are protective reactions used by physiatry to provoke one's own reactions of the body. The effect of physiatric stimuli depends on the reactivity of the body, and also on the kind, form, intensity and duration of the physical stimulus.

Physiotherapy – forms Physiotherapy can be
• *natural* For example solar radiation, atmospheric pressure, atmospheric electricity, effects of gravity, thermal climatic effects, natural radioactive radiation, magnetic radiation.
• *artificially prepared* The sources of various energies: mechanic, acoustic, electric, thermal; sources of magnetic and electromagnetic radiation. Also included are certain manual activities such as classical and reflex massages, passive movements, positioning, manipulation, mobilisation, acupuncture, acupressure and active motion exercises – therapeutic physical training.

PICP (procollagen I carboxyterminal propeptide) → see Procollagen peptides

Pigmented villonodular synovitis A rare benign, slowly progressive disease of unknown aetiology caused by proliferation of synovial cells and mesenchymal connective tissue of affected joints, tendon sheaths and bursae. It is characterized by villous and nodular growth of synovia. It mainly affects young to middle-aged adults. Most frequently it affects the knee, hip, less frequently wrist,

elbow, temporomandibular joint and hands. The affected joint is swollen; roughened synovia resembles a foam structure. Synovial fluid is xanthochromic or sanguinous, with cell counts around $3,000/mm^3$, mainly mononuclear cells.

Biopsy of synovial membrane is diffusely brown with deposits of haemosiderin and the presence of multi-nuclear large cells. Opinions about malignant transformation are still not consistent. Treatment consists mainly of rheumatologic and orthopaedic interventions with subtotal synovectomy.

Pilates technique → see Exercise techniques

PINP (procollagen I N-terminal propeptide) → see Procollagen peptides

Piper fatigue scale (PFS) → see Instruments of assessing (health status measurements, outcome measurement)

Plantar fasciitis → see Calcaneal Spur

Plantogram An area print of the foot. It is obtained by tracing the contour of the foot of a standing patient with a pen pointing vertically on the paper. A plantogram is used to obtain prints of the foot, where the patient stands on the paper fixed above the base saturated with paint. The plantogram shows the distribution of pressures on the sole of the foot in the standing position.

Plasmocytoma and its musculoskeletal symptoms (MM; multiple myeloma) One of the most frequent malignant haematologic diseases characterised by malignant transformation of mature plasma cells and their precursors (B lymphocytes, lymphoplasmacytoid cells).

Clinical symptoms: Systemic symptoms (fatigue, bone pain, weight loss and frequent infections) are prevalent in advanced disease. Depending on the grade of infiltration of bone marrow with myeloma cells and their metastatic and secretory activity, the following symptoms occur:

- haematologic symptoms (anaemia, thrombocytopenia or pancytopenia due to increased numbers of atypical plasma cells in bone marrow with subsequent reduction of normal haematopoesis),
- symptoms arising from paraproteinemia and a general increase in plasma protein concentration markedly increased erythrocyte sedimentation rate, hyperproteinemia, proteinuria, increased serum viscosity, increased concentration of monoclonal Ig-paraprotein IgG, IgA, rarely IgM, IgE, IgD and more frequently kappa,
- bone changes on X-ray with osteolytic lesions (approximately in 2/3 patients), pathological fractures or diffuse osteoporosis; increased osteoclastic remodelling and subsequent bone resorption lead to hypercalcaemia and increased levels of collagen degradation products.

Platelet-derived growth factor (PDGF)
A polypeptide acting as a systemic and local regulator of tissue growth. Its function is similar to FGF. It stimulates the replication of osseous cells and collagen synthesis. The synthesis of locally produced PDGF is regulated by growth factors.

Plyometric exercises
The principle of the exercise is the stretch-shortening cycle of muscle movement. Before the prime movement, e.g. flexion, the individual performs a short quick movement in the opposite direction, i.e. extension. It is applied mainly in sports medicine when rehearsing extreme exertion, e.g. jumps.

Podiatry
The field of health care involved in the study and treatment of disorders and deformities of the feet, ankle and lower leg.

Podogram
Examination of the footprint of the bare planta pedis (sole) in the normal standing position. A podogram provides information on the patient's skeletal and muscular system. A podogram has geometric (informing mainly about body height) and dynamic signs (informing about body weight).

POEMS syndrome
An acronym for this multisystem multiorgan disease, which includes polyneuropathy (P), organomegaly (O), endocrinopathy (E), monoclonal gammopathy (M) and skin abnormalities (S). Described for the first time in 1956 by Crow, in 1968 by Fukase and in 1983 by Takatsuki, it is also known as Crow-Fukase-Takatsuki syndrome. The major criteria consist of polyneuropathy and monoclonal gammopathy (paraproteinaemia), with minor criteria consisting of sclerotic bone lesions, organomegaly, oedema, endocrinopathy, skin changes, and papilloedema. The complete form of POEMS syndrome requires the presence of at least the two major criteria, otherwise it is referred to as the incomplete form.

The neuropathy is of a distal, symmetric sensomotor type, with proximal progression. Electromyography reveals denervation, demyelination and axonal degeneration. Hepatosplenomegaly and lymphadenopathy occur. Symptoms and signs of endocrinopathy include impotence, testicular atrophy, gynaecomastia, amenorrhea, hyperprolactinaemia and hyperoestrogenaemia. Hypothyroidism and diabetes mellitus are usually present. The paraproteinaemia involves immunoglobulin IgA and free chains of the lambda type in 90% of patients. Markers of increased osteoclastic resorption may be present. Skin changes include hyperpigmentation, hyperkeratosis, hypertrichosis, and Raynaud's phenomenon.

Polarised light
→ see Birefringence (Double refraction)

Polyarteritis nodosa (PAN)
A disease of small and medium-sized arteries characterised by the involvement of all three layers of the vessel wall, leading to the formation of multiple aneurysms, thrombi and infarctions. Its aetiology is unknown but deposition of immune complexes in arterial walls is considered to be an important pathophysiological mechanism. This inflammatory reaction activates complement and neutrophils (immunopathology). It may be associated with certain viral infections such as hepatitis B. At present, two types of PAN are known:

1. *typical PAN* is defined as necrotising inflammation of medium and small sized arteries without vasculitis affecting arterioles, capillaries or venules, and without glomerulonephritis,
2. *microscopic polyarteritis* or more precisely *polyangiitis* is a necrotising vasculitis with minimal or total absence of immune complex deposits; affects small vessels (capillaries), venules or arterioles; concurrently, necrotising arteritis of small and medium-sized arteries can be present. This second form occurs considerably more frequently.

Clinical symptoms: Apart from systemic symptoms, various polymorphic exanthemas with typical livedo reticularis, non-specific arthralgias and even arthritis, involvement of peripheral nerves (asymmetric polyneuropathy), kidneys (renal impairment and hypertension) and gastrointestinal tract (bowel infarction) can occur.

Polyarthralgias Concurrent, mainly symmetric, pain in several joints is referred to as polyarthralgias, as long as symptoms of the inflammation process are absent.

Most frequent causes include:
- viral diseases, particularly their prodromal period (e.g. hepatitis, rubella, influenza, AIDS),
- diffuse connective tissue diseases, polyarthritis, particularly in prodromal period, Sjögren's syndrome, systemic lupus erythematosus, polymyositis, rheumatoid arthritis,
- polyarthralgias associated with internal diseases (ulcerative colitis, Crohn's disease, multiple myeloma, hypertrophic pulmonary osteoarthropathy = HPOA, chronic pancreatitis, myxoma of the heart, etc.),
- metabolic diseases (hyperlipidaemia, haemochromatosis),
- endocrine disorders, menopause, hyperthyroidism, hypothyroidism, hyperparathyroidism, Cushing's disease, acromegaly,
- bacterial infections, sepsis, chronic infections, infectious foci (teeth, tonsils), bacterial endocarditis,
- drugs (retinoids, cimetidine, fluorides, quinolones, hydralazine, β-blockers, pyrazinamide, gold, thiazides and also termination of steroid therapy),
- para-neoplastic syndrome,
- changes of atmospheric pressure (weather, caisson disease),
- joint hyperlaxity,
- incipient generalised osteoarthrosis.

Psychogenic rheumatism is a psychosomatic disease with arthrodynia as a major symptom. Inflammatory symptoms are absent and organic disease can be ruled out. The patient must be assured that he/she does not suffer from inflammatory joint disease. Depending on need, psychiatric referral and treatment should be considered.

Polyarticular juvenile idiopathic arthritis → see Juvenile idiopathic arthritis (JIA)

Polychondritis → see Relapsing polychondritis

Polymerase chain reaction → see PCR (polymerase chain reaction)

Polymorphism A phenomenon in biology which occurs when several morphological forms exist within a single population of the same species of organism. It also occurs at the level of protein molecules, when it is referred to as genetic polymorphism. A locus of a particular gene in individuals of a particular population may contain one of several variants (alleles). They therefore encode different variants of a corresponding protein product. The major histocompatibility complex (MHC) is considered to be the most polymorphic system.

Polymorphonuclear leukocytes Not an entirely clearly used term by which the majority of authors indicate neutrophils, whereas others indicate granulocytes.

Polymyalgia rheumatica A clinical syndrome, affecting individuals over the age of 50, characterised by myalgias and stiffness of the shoulder and/or pelvic muscles and is often accompanied by non-specific systemic symptoms. The rapid response of clinical symptoms to low doses of glucocorticoids is characteristic of this disease.

Myalgias and muscle stiffness are usually symmetrical, most often worse after rest and in the morning. Muscle strength is unaffected but may be limited by myalgias when examining the patient. Musculoskeletal symptoms are frequently accompanied by systemic symptoms like fatigue, tiredness, loss of appetite, loss of weight, and fever. Raised erythrocyte sedimentation rate (ESR) is the most dominant laboratory test, other acute phase reactants (plasma viscosity, CRP) may be elevated. Glucocorticoid treatment is necessary for several months sometimes up to two years, though lifelong treatment may be needed in some patients.

Polymyositis → see Idiopathic inflammatory myopathies (IIM), Non-inflammatory myopathies

Polyostotic fibrous dysplasia → see McCune-Albright syndrome (polyostotic fibrous dysplasia)

Poncet's disease A reactive arthritis associated with acute tuberculosis. The presence of mycobacterium in the joint has not been proved. Synovial biopsy does not reveal myobacterial involvement, but shows non-specific inflammation.

Treatment: Non-steroidal anti-inflammatory drugs are administered in addition to treating the primary disease.

Popliteal cyst → see Baker's cyst

Positioning Two basic positions are used in rheumatic diseases:
1. General standstill regime in bed when patient is lying on his back, his upper extremities are at an abduction of 30°, forearms in a middle position between pronation and supination, with mild extension of the wrists; lower extremities at an abduction of 15°, knees straight and dorsiflexion of 90° at ankles. The head rests on a small pillow; shoulders are off the pillow.

The position of the back is alternated with the prone position.
2. Either preventive splints fix the local standstill positioning of a joint affected by inflammation or if there are existing contractures must be positioned in a set of corrective splints. The period of corrective splinting is 5 to 30 minutes. The positioning of affected joints can also be secured by traction, which at the same time enables performance of movement therapy without gravity.

Positron emission tomography (PET)
A method of nuclear medicine imaging based on the detection of photons of gamma-radiation, which are emitted during transformation of positron-emitting radioisotope that are administered into the body for diagnostic purposes. These radioisotopes can be incorporated into molecules of many biologically active substances and thus enable monitoring of their metabolism and distribution in various parts of the body.

A detection scanner measures the distribution of specific activity of the radio indicator in the body. A final tomographic picture can be achieved from this data using computer analysis to create numeric reconstruction algorithms resulting in a three-dimensional picture or a map of functional processes within the body.

Post-dysenteric arthritis A sterile reactive oligoarthritis may occur 1 to 3 weeks after dysentery induced *Shigella flexneri* infection, and usually settles within a few weeks.

Post-isometric relaxation This belongs to neuromuscular techniques. Apart from isometric muscle activation, it utilises mainly inspiration and looking in a certain direction as a facilitating manoeuvre and expiration while looking in the opposite direction as an inhibitory manoeuvre. The initial position of particular segments of the locomotion system lets us target the facilitation and inhibition into particular muscles or muscle groups.

Postmenopausal Osteoporosis (type I)
Oestrogen deficiency is regarded as the main pathophysiological mechanism for the development of postmenopausal osteoporosis. Its onset is typically 15–20 years after the menopause with trabecular bone being mainly affected. The main clinical manifestations are fractures of bones with a higher trabecular bone fraction (distal forearm, vertebrae), but also involves cortical bone in the elderly, predisposing to hip fractures.

Postmenopausal Osteoporosis – treatment guidelines
- general treatment and recommendations: a healthy lifestyle with adequate physical activity, sufficient dietary supply of calcium and vitamin D, and prevention of falls. Minimising risks by avoidance of drugs with adverse effects on balance and calcium metabolism (hypnotics, long-term anticonvulsants, anticoagulants, phosphate-binding antacids, glucocorticoids, and others) are also important.
- basic treatment: calcium and vitamin D supplementation,
- specific treatment with antiresorptive agents and stimulators of osteoformation. This type of treatment must be optimised to the age, health status and contraindications for the individual patient.

Post-Salmonella reactive arthritis
This reactive arthritis occurs 1 to 2 weeks after infection (diarrhoea) and is similar to post-Yersinia arthritis. In most cases the inflammatory process affects the knee and/or ankle joints, and fever may occur. The diagnosis is confirmed by a rising titre of antibodies against salmonella. The infectious agent can be cultured in the stools.

Post-vaccination arthritis
In isolated cases, arthritis with a clinical picture of reactive arthritis with a tendency to gradual regression occurs after administration of certain vaccines (rubella, BCG, hepatitis B).

Post-Yersinia reactive arthritis
Yersinia enterocolitica or *Yersinia pseudotuberculosis* is the agent causing transitory diarrhoea with mesenteric lymphadenitis, and after 1 to 3 weeks oligo- or polyarthritis develops, often accompanied by myalgia, endocarditis, erythema nodosum, conjunctivitis, lymphadenopathy and splenomegaly. Arthritis of the knee and/or ankle joints is characteristic. The joint is swollen and warm, and often associated with a fever.

Laboratory diagnostics: Besides evidence of inflammatory activity, the dynamics of the rise of anti-Yersinia antibody titre is crucial. Unilateral sacroiliitis can be observed.

Prednisolone → see Glucocorticoids

Priessnitz compress
A cold compress attached to the surface of the body in order to achieve better local blood perfusion. The first layer consists of a wet compress, the second consists of waterproof material and the third one consists of a dry warm compress. The steam effect is thus achieved. Local vasodilatation develops within one hour (local hyperaemia). In rheumatology, the Priessnitz compress is used particularly in degenerative disease of joints. Cold herbal infusion may be used instead of cold water; thereby the steam effect is amplified (so-called Tripes compress). Vincenz Priessnitz, also written Prießnitz, (1799–1851) lived in Austrian Silesia (now Czech Republic) and is considered as the founder of hydrotherapy.

Primary immunodeficiency
Immunodeficiency is defined as a defect of the immune system due to the absence, decrease or functional alteration of one of its components. It is classified as primary or secondary immunodeficiency. Primary immunodeficiencies are usually genetic disorders due to a defect in embryonic development, an enzyme defect, or of unknown cause. Secondary immunodeficiencies develop due to impairment of the existing evolved immune system as a consequence of various pathological conditions including malignancies, metabolic diseases, malnutrition, and drugs. Primary antibody immunodeficiency comprises 50–70% of all primary immunodeficiencies.

Clinical symptoms: Both primary and secondary immunodeficiencies have basically the same symptoms with recurrent and chronic infections and frequently are associated with autoimmune diseases, e.g. pernicious anaemia, autoimmune haemolytic anaemia, idiopathic thrombocytopenic purpura, thyroiditis, chronic active hepatitis, systemic lupus erythematosus, Sjögren's syndrome, juvenile idiopathic arthritis or dermatomyositis. Aseptic non-erosive polyarticular arthritis, suggestive of rheumatoid arthritis, occurs in 10–30% of patients with hypogammaglobulinaemia. Arthritis can be the first clinical symptom of primary hypogammaglobulinaemia.

Primary hyperparathyroidism An autonomous overproduction of parathormone. The most frequent causes comprise adenoma, hyperplasia and rarely carcinoma of the parathyroid glands. Clinically typical changes of bones, nephrolithiasis, nephrocalcinosis, gastroduodenal ulcer disease, acute pancreatitis, arterial hypertension and arrhythmias may be present. Typically, the serum and urinary calcium levels are elevated in the presence of an elevated parathormone level. The concentration of phosphate is decreased in the serum and increased in the urine. Surgical removal of affected parathyroid glands is the treatment of choice.

Prion Currently, it is the smallest known infectious particle consisting only of protein causing universally fatal diseases affecting brain and neural tissues. Prion invokes both human diseases (Kuru disease, Creutzfeldt-Jakob disease, Gerstmann-Sträussler syndrome) and animal diseases (sheep scrapie, bovine spongiform encephalopathy or BSE, infectious mink encephalopathy). Prions are usually species specific, but BSE most probably originated when beef-cattle were fed with meat-bone powder prepared from animals that perished from scrapie and so the species barrier was broken and BSE prion developed. Similarly, new variant Creutzfeldt-Jakob disease developed when BSE prion was transformed into human prion, invoking such a disease.

Procollagen peptides Procollagen is a precursor of collagen and the terminal peptides are released via proteolytic cleavage into the circulation prior to the formation of collagen fibrils. Procollagen has accessory peptides on the C- and T-terminal ends, which are referred to as the procollagen I N-terminal propeptide (PINP) and procollagen I carboxyterminal propeptide (PICP). The serum procollagen I carboxyterminal propeptide (PICP) has been monitored as a marker of osteoformation. Its value falls in postmenopausal women. Antiresorptive treatment, as well as glucocorticoids, lowers the PICP concentration. Determination of these peptides is utilised in the monitoring of disturbances of collagen synthesis (decreased levels in osteogenesis imperfecta and hypercorticism).

Progressive osseous heteroplasia A very rare condition of children in which progressive ossification occurs in subcutaneous and deeper connective tissue. In contrast to fibrodysplasia ossificans progressiva, the hereditary skeletal malformation is absent (see myositis ossificans progressive) and heterotopic ossification is of an intramembranous than an enchondral feature. Ankylosis and local defect in growth of the affected extremity develop when a joint is involved. The disease is autosomal dominant with variable expressivity.

Progressive type of myositis ossificans (myositis ossificans progressiva) A rare disease manifesting itself by the ossification of skeletal muscles, muscle fascia and aponeurosis. The onset of the disease frequently occurs in childhood and is often associated with typical inherited skeletal abnormalities (microdactyly or absence of digits affecting either the hands or feet). A familial occurrence has been observed with an autosomal dominant type of heredity with variable expressivity.

Clinical picture: Initially localised oedema, erythema and warm sensation, particularly in the neck and paravertebral area, occur. At this stage patients suffer from severe pain. The inflammation subsides slowly within a few days and subsequently fibrous changes with consequent ossification develop in the next few weeks. Replacement of muscle tissues and tendons by osseous tissue leads to contracture and deformity. After the development of osseous tissue, the subsequent changes are minimal. Restrictive lung disease may develop due to involvement of thoracic muscles. Subsequently, respiratory impairment develops, and associated pneumonias are the major cause of death in patients with the progressive type of myositis ossificans.

Prolapsed lumbar intervertebral disc

Prolapse of the intervertebral disc often develops as a consequence of its chronic degeneration. The fibrous ring surrounding the intervertebral disc becomes diseased and the inner softer part of the disc bulges out. It most frequently involves the L_4-L_5 and L_5-S_1 segments. Compression of the nerve root of L_5 or S_1 respectively, is caused by dorsolateral prolapse of the disc. Multiple root impairments develop in the case of medial prolapse of the disc (cauda equina syndrome). Urgent surgical intervention may be necessary.

Clinical symptoms: Long-term compression of the cauda equina invokes permanent paralysis of the pelvic muscles with subsequent urinary and faecal incontinence. The clinical picture of intervertebral disc protrusion with spinal root compression is characterised by pain in the corresponding lumbar area and root zone of the lower extremity. Spasm of paravertebral muscles on the side of disc protrusion occurs. The root palsy is manifested by sensory impairment in the corresponding dermatome, and by muscle weakness and decreased, eventually absent reflexes in the corresponding myotome.

Proliferating cell nuclear antigen → see

Anti-PCNA/cyclin antibodies (proliferating cell nuclear antigen)

Properdin Also referred to as factor P. It comprises the regulatory function in the course of activation of complement via the alternative pathway. This pathway was previously known as the properdin system. Indi-

viduals with properdin deficiency (less than 2% of normal serum level) are more suspectible to infections due to Neisseria.

Prostacyclin A metabolite of arachidonic acid (PGI_2) with inhibitory effects on platelet aggregation. PGI_2 is an effective vasodilatator and increases vascular permeability. It has opposite properties to those of thromboxane.

Prostaglandins A family of biologically active lipids, which originate from arachidonic acid by the influence of the enzyme cyclooxygenase. They belong to the group of local hormones and are present in virtually all human and mammalian tissues. They are involved in regulation of inflammatory reactions, particularly prostaglandin E_2 (PGE_2), which is an endogenous pyrogen, causing vasodilatation, a drop in blood pressure and increased vascular permeability. PGD_2 with similar properties, except the pyrogenic property, is released in the anaphylactic reaction mediated by IgE. Both PGE_2 and PGD_2 inhibit platelet aggregation, and in addition, PGD_2 inhibits the expression of MHC (major histocompatibility complex) class II molecules on the surface of T lymphocytes and macrophages. The involvement of prostaglandins in the regulation of the inflammatory response is based on the fact that a typical anti-inflammatory drug, such as acetylsalicylic acid, acts through the inhibition of cyclooxygenase which is the enzyme responsible for the biosynthesis of prostaglandins.

Prosthesis An artificial extension that replaces a missing part of the body. Prosthesis can be classified as epiprosthesis, whose function is cosmetic replacement such as dental or eye prosthesis, or endoprosthesis with replacement of parts of the body such as heart valves, blood vessels and partial or total joint replacements.

Proteases Proteolytic enzymes that are capable of degrading protein chains into minor fragments, even into amino acids. Depending on the localisation of the peptide bond within the polypeptide chain, proteases are divided into two main groups; endopeptidases which break the peptide bond inside the protein chain thereby forming polypeptide fragments and exopeptidases which break only terminal amino acids or hydrolyse small oligopeptides. Peptidases are further divided into carboxypeptidases (split terminal amino acids from C-ending of polypeptide chain) and aminopeptidases (split N-terminal amino acids). Usually a number of proteinases are involved in the degradation of one particular protein.

Proteasome A cellular organelle located in the cytoplasm which plays a significant role in antigen presentation in which HLA class I molecules are involved. It is of spherical shape and consists of 12 to 14 circularly arranged units. Proteasome contains proteolytic enzymes, which are able to break antigens into peptide fragments. The most favourable fragments are those consisting of 8 or 9 amino acid subunits as these can optimally bind to binding channels of HLA class I antigens (antigen presentation).

Protein A A protein located in the cellular wall of Staphylococcus aureus. It is able to bind onto the Fc domains of IgG molecules (in humans except for IgG3 subclass). It is suggested that the protein protects Staphylococcus against IgG antibodies by disabling their interaction with complement and Fc-receptors on the surface of professional phagocytes. Protein A is utilised in IgG antibody purification, in the detection of these antibodies using ELISA techniques, and also as a polyclonal mitogen of B lymphocytes.

Protrusion of intervertebral disc Protrusion of intervertebral disc reveals similar symptoms as prolapse but the pathological picture is different. In disc protrusion, the fibrous ring surrounding the intervertebral disc remains intact but deformation causes it to bulge out.

Pseudo-Felty's syndrome A variant of Felty's syndrome characterised by the presence of neutropenia and an increased number of large granular lymphocytes in the patient's blood and bone marrow. Most patients also suffer from thrombocytopenia, anaemia and splenomegaly. The syndrome usually affects elderly patients, and recurrent infections are prominent and the major cause of death. It can occur relatively early in the course of arthritis. Treatment is difficult, but consists of a combination of immunosuppressive drugs (including methotrexate and cyclosporin) or glucocorticoids, either alone or in combination with an immunosuppressive agent. Splenectomy is contraindicated.

Pseudogout → see Chondrocalcinosis, Crystalline-induced arthropathy

Pseudohypoparathyroidism A group of inherited diseases characterised by laboratory findings typical for hypoparathyroidism (hypocalcaemia, hyperphosphataemia but with an increased concentration of parathormone (PTH)). Fuller Albright (American physician, 1900–1969) first described the condition in 1942. The condition is due to a lack of effect of PTH on the target organs (bone and kidney). Under normal circumstances, PTH binds to a specific receptor on the plasma membrane of target cells. This receptor is connected with the signal effector molecule on the inner surface of the membrane by regulating nucleotide guanine (G), which is attached to protein (Gs protein). The synthesis of many 'secondary messengers', including cyclic adenosine monophosphate (cAMP), initiates rapidly after the hormone binds to the receptor with subsequent activation of adenylyl cyclase and other enzymes. Cyclic adenosine monophosphate activates protein kinase A, as well as stimulating other enzymes, ion channels and proteins. Administration of PTH in a healthy individual leads to a significant increase in nephrogenic cAMP excretion into the urine. Neither the concentration of cAMP nor phosphaturia increases in the group of diseases referred to as pseudohypoparathyroidism type I, due to mutations of the Gs alpha gene (GNAS1). The excretion of cAMP into the urine increases but the phosphaturic response is miss-ing after oral administration of PTH in the case of pseudohypoparathyroidism type II.

Psoriatic arthritis (PsA) Arthritis associ-ated with psoriasis, usually seronegative and without rheumatoid nodules.

Clinical symptoms:
- Arthritis, frequently asymmetric, affecting DIP (distal interphalangeal) joints and joints of the anterior chest wall
- Dactylitis
- Enthesitis
- X-ray signs of new bone formation and erosions of terminal phalanges
- Typical extra-articular manifestations (ophthalmic).

Psychogenic pain → see Types of pain

Purine analogues Azathioprine and 6-mercaptopurine belong to purine ana-logues. Currently, neither azathioprine nor 6-mercaptopurine is the drug of first choice in the treatment of rheumatoid arthritis (RA) but they both remain a valuable therapeutic option for RA when complicated by vasculitis, glomerulonephritis or when other DMARDs are not tolerated.

Dosage: Azathioprine in RA is adminis-tered orally in a daily dose from 1.5 to 2.5 mg/kg (75 to 200 mg daily). Its full effects take a couple of months. It is necessary to monitor the blood count and liver function tests dur-ing treatment: every 14 days for the first two months, and subsequently every 6–8 weeks. The occurrence of leukopenia is an indica-tion for withdrawal of treatment.

Clinical efficiency: Several clinical trials show comparable clinical efficiency of azathi-oprine with antimalarials, penicillamine, par-enteral gold, cyclophosphamide and cy-closporin, but less when compared to metho-trexate in RA.

The therapeutic efficiency and toxicity of azathioprine are dose dependent and increase proportionally to the administered dose. How-ever, patients with a genetic deficiency of thio-purine methyltransferase (TPMT) are at in-creased risk of severe myelosuppression and liver toxicity, so studies are looking at the ef-ficacy of measuring the TMPT genotype and/or enzyme activity in patients prior to treat-ment (Pavelka 2000). Azathioprine is well tolerated in pregnancy and is not associated with congenital malformations in humans. In spite of data showing that only very small amounts transfer into breast milk, its admin-istration during breast-feeding is not recom-mended.

Adverse effects: Gastrointestinal symp-toms such as nausea and vomiting, leukope-nia and increased liver transaminases. Clinical symptoms resolve after withdrawal of treat-ment. Long-term treatment with azathioprine is associated with a higher risk of malignan-cies, particularly haematopoietic and lym-phoreticular malignancies.

Pyoderma gangrenosum A rare derma-tological ulcerative disease of unknown ori-gin which belongs to the group of non-infec-tious neutrophilic dermatoses.

Clinical symptoms:
- Typical lesions sometimes develop after minor injuries, have a dark red to purple colour, most commonly involving the legs and their margin often overreaches the ul-ceration (referred to as 'undermined mar-gin')
- Ulceration is usually very painful
- Systemic diseases (inflammatory bowel dis-ease, arthritis or lymphoproliferative disor-ders) are often associated with the pyoder-ma gangrenosum
- The diagnosis of pyoderma gangrenosum is confirmed when other conditions caus-ing skin ulcerations are excluded

Quantitative Computerised Tomography (QCT) In contrast to DEXA, QCT measures the volumetric bone density (mg/cm^3). It can separately measure trabecular bone. QCT scans the whole region of interest using a multi-slice or spiral CT and specific software is needed. Its use is not recommended in the diagnosis of osteoporosis. A greater error of measurement occurs than with DEXA, a relatively high radiation dose for the patient, the high cost of the investigation and a lower accessibility for diagnosing of osteoporosis are all disadvantages of this method. Therefore, CT is used mainly in the differential diagnosis of bone changes.

Quantitative Ultrasound (QUS) This has a relatively good predictive value for the risk of fracture, and is therefore a suitable method for selecting patients with high risk of fracture. However, it is not suitable for confirming the diagnosis of osteoporosis based on the WHO criteria. Low costs, portability and safety are all advantages of this method. The measurement has lower reproducibility and it is therefore not suitable for monitoring the effectiveness of treatment. Measurement only in peripherally localised bones (heel, tibia) is a disadvantage of this method. In contrast to radiological methods, the measured value is influenced not only by the bone mineral density, but also by the structure of the measured bone. Changes in bone architecture also influence the mechanical firmness of bone, but at present we are unable to interpret them unambiguously.

Radiography The radiograph (X-ray) is still "a golden standard" of musculoskeletal system examination even in the era of novel diagnostic imaging methods such as USS, CT and MRI. It enables evaluation and assessment of changes to the skeleton in arthritic and orthopaedic disorders, monitoring the potential progression of the disease over time and assessment of their changes with respect to treatment. Projectional radiography is commonly used in examining the joints and the spine and involves taking two X-rays, usually at right-angles to each other, to produce 2D X-ray images. Image intensification may be used for targeted joint injections (e.g. hip joint or spinal injections) or in internal fixation of fractures. Radiographic examination with contrast medium is used in rheumatology for diagnosing oesophageal dysmotility in systemic sclerosis.

Radiographic examination after an intra-articular application of contrast medium (arthrography) is utilised less in the era of CT, MRI and arthroscopy. Radiographic examination of the vascular system after intravenous injection of a contrast medium (classical angiography, digital subtraction angiography – DSA) is utilised, for example, in the diagnosis and assessment of vasculitis.

Radioimmunoassay An analytical method used to assess the concentration of soluble antigens or haptens. In this method, the antigen or hapten is labelled with a radioactive isotope which competitively inhibits the binding of unmarked antigen with specific antibody. The relation between the inhibition and concentration of the analysed antigen is assessed by a set of standard solutions of unmarked antigen of known concentration. It was the first method to enable quantification of various proteohormones, neuropeptides and other substances in complex biological fluids.

Radioimmunoelectrophoresis An electrophoretic analysis with radioactive labelled antigen or antibody to identify the precipitation line.

Radioimmunoscintigraphy Monoclonal antibodies directed against antigens associated with malignancies is used in this in vivo diagnostic method. After the conjugation of antibodies with radioactive nuclides and their administration to a patient affected by a malignancy, these conjugates bind exclusively to the malignant cells and identify them. Contemporary radioimmunoscintigraphy is a sensitive method able to identify a tumour weighing as low as 0.1–1.0 gram, including possible metastases.

RANK (receptor-activator of nuclear factor κ-B) A transmembrane protein consisting of 616 amino acids that is localised on precursors of osteoblasts. Binding OPG-L (RANKL) to ODAR (RANK) leads to the differentiation and activation of osteoblasts.

RANKL (receptor-activator of nuclear factor κ-B ligand) Produced by osteoblasts. It belongs to the TNR-receptor family. Initially it was called osteoclast differentiation factor, which represents its main role in the body. It is produced by osteoblasts in soluble and membrane-binding forms. Binding to its receptor (RANK) on the surface of osteoclasts and their precursors leads to the activation of differentiation, maturation and production of new osteoclasts and stimulation of their osteolytic activity.

Rapamycin A relatively new immunosuppressive agent, originally developed as an antifungal agent, with a structure similar to tacrolimus but with a different mode of action. It inhibits the response to IL-2 and thereby blocks the proliferation of B and T lymphocytes, the synthesis of lymphokines and responsiveness of T cells. Its immunosuppressive concentrations are significantly lower than those of tacrolimus and cyclosporin.

Rapid assessment of disease activity in rheumatology (RADAR) → see Instruments of assessing (health status measurements, outcome measurement)

Raynaud's phenomenon (RP) A symmetrical non-progressive vasospastic disorder affecting the fingers and toes, which manifests as paleness and/or cyanosis. Such a symptom is due to cold exposition or emotional stress. Maurice Raynaud (1834–1881, French physician) first described the phenomenon in 1862.

Clinical symptoms: The typical clinical picture consists of three phases. In the first phase, the fingers become pale due to vasospasm of the digital arteries. In the second phase, dilatation of the capillaries and venules occurs, leading to cyanosis due to blood stasis and its subsequent deoxygenation. The patient usually complains of cold sensations and paraesthesia during these phases of RP. When heating the limb, vasospasm retreats and blood perfusion dramatically increases. This phase of reactive hyperaemia is characterised by a bright red colour of the fingers and is often associated with unpleasant pulsating sensations. The changes to the fingers extend from distal parts towards proximal areas and never proximal of the metacarpophalangeal joints. The fingers and toes are most often affected, particularly the 2nd, 3rd and 4th fingers of the hand, less frequently the toes. The acral part of the nose, the tongue and ear can be affected. Infrared thermography can be used in the detection and quantification of RP.

Reactive arthritis (ReA) Aseptic immunologically mediated joint inflammation, which develops in association with distant infection in the body. The disease has a systemic character and usually develops after upper airway infections, urogenital or gastrointestinal infections. However, ReA may de-

velop after infection localised anywhere in the body and often the association between clinically and microbiologically defined previous infection and ReA may not be found.

Main features of ReA:
- Arthritis, eventually other musculoskeletal symptoms (myalgia, tendinitis, osteitis, enthesopathy),
- Skin and mucosal lesions,
- Ophthalmic lesions (uveitis, conjunctivitis),
- Organ lesions are rare (nephritis, carditis),
- The prognosis is usually favourable with spontaneous remission,
- Chronic course of the disease with functional impairment is rare,
- Significant association with the HLA-B27 antigen.

Reactive nitrogen intermediates (RNI) Nitric oxide, for which NO synthase is involved in its synthesis, is the main representative RNI. NO is involved in a number of protective, regulatory and also harmful reactions in the immune, nervous and cardiovascular systems. Other oxides of nitrogen, anions of peroxynitrous and nitrous acid and finally anions of nitric acid can originate from nitric oxide.

Reactive oxygen intermediates (ROI) Unstable molecules that possess an uncoupled electron (free radicals) or excited-state electrons (singleton oxygen). The basic free radical derived from molecular oxygen is superoxide from which hydrogen peroxide and subsequently hydroxyl radicals are formed. ROI are formed in higher concentrations, particularly in professional phagocytes (neutrophils, macrophages), where they are involved in the destruction of phagocytosed micro-organisms. They are also very effective cytolytic substances and may damage the cells and tissues of the hosting organism during immunopathological reactions.

Receptor A complex of atoms or molecules that form a site with stereochemically specific affinity for a particular substance known as ligand (agonist in pharmacology). The recep-

R

tors are usually present on the surface of cells but may also be located on the inner part of the cytoplasmic membrane or in the cytoplasm. The binding of ligand (agonist) to the receptor is the signal for the cell to perform certain physiological (in some cases pathological) responses. The binding of an inhibitor (antagonist) to this receptor leads to inhibition of the receptor's function. Neurotransmitters, hormones, antigens, cytokines, or other mediators transmit their signal through receptors and thereby information is transmitted between cells. One cell can transfer the information to another cell directly without the need for any chemical messenger. In such a case, the receptor of one cell reacts with the receptor (effector) of the other cell.

Receptor-activator of nuclear factor κ-B → see RANK (receptor-activator of nuclear factor κ-B)

Receptor-activator of nuclear factor κ-B ligand → see RANKL (receptor-activator of nuclear factor κ-B ligand)

Referred pain The pain felt in an area that is distinct from the affected area. It is common in lesions of visceral organs. It is usually felt in the area that is innervated from the same spinal segment as the involved viscus.

Reflex A basic functional unit of the nervous system function. It can be defined as an involuntary, rapid and stereotypic response to a peripheral stimulus.

Reflex sympathetic dystrophy → see Algodystrophic syndrome (ADS)

Reflexive massage The fundamental of this massage is the knowledge that functional connections exist between skin and muscle areas, bones, vessels, nerves and subcutaneous tissue and inner organs, which are supplied from the same spinal segments. Reflexive massage can be used in both organic and functional disorders, particularly in the chronic stage. The main indications are spinal pain syndrome and extra-articular rheumatism.

Reflex arc The set of structures involved in the reflex pathway. It consists of 5 components: receptor, afferent nerve pathway, integration centre, efferent nerve pathway and effector. The connection with the central nervous system runs through the integration centre.

Rehabilitation methods Rehabilitation methods in rheumatoid arthritis are focused on maintaining the scope of movement and muscle strength. The patient must be taught the knowledge of how to protect affected joints by improving muscle power and how to improve their daily routine. The use of orthoses and various auxiliary instruments in performing daily routines is, apart from rehabilitation, one of the basic components of joint protection. The resources of physical therapy (PT) need to be used to minimise the symptoms and signs of RA, such as pain, atrophy, decreases in local metabolism, spasms etc. Balneotherapy, both local and systemic, is also important in the management of RA.

Relapsing polychondritis A very rare disease affecting a number of organs. The disease is episodic, but occasionally progressive. It is an inflammatory process affecting structures of the cartilage and tissues with a high content of glycosaminoglycans. Clinical symptoms appear in the areas of the pinna of the ear, nose, larynx, upper airways, joints, heart, blood vessels, inner ear, cornea and sclera.
Clinical symptoms:
- Chondritis of ear, nasal, laryngotracheal, costal and joint cartilages,
- Inflammation of eye and inner ear,
- Collapse of laryngotracheal structures, subglottic area leading to increased upper airways infections and stridor,
- Concurrent presence of vasculitis or glomerulonephritis may contribute to increased morbidity and mortality,
- Clinical symptoms, the course of disease and response to treatment vary.

Relaxation An essential component of rehabilitation when both muscle and psychological relaxation occurs. Relaxation in the rhythm of breathing, autogenic training (Schultz' autogenic training psychomotor relaxation therapy; Johannes Heinrich Schultz, German physician, 1884–1970), Jacobsons' relaxation method (Edmund Jacobson, American physician, 1888–1983) and yoga elements are among such techniques.

Remitting seronegative symmetrical synovitis with pitting oedema) → see Syndrome RS3PE (remitting seronegative symmetrical synovitis with pitting oedema)

Reverse transcriptase An RNA dependent DNA polymerase, which is the enzyme that synthesises DNA on the RNA chain matrix and transfers the genetic information from RNA into DNA. RNA viruses contain this enzyme.

Rhesus blood group system The set of antigens present on the surface of erythrocytes in humans and *Rhesus* apes (that is why Rh). They are encoded by gene loci on chromosome 1 which possesses at least three allele pairs Dd, Cc and Ee. The most clinically significant is antigen D, so individuals are either Rhesus factor positive (RhD⁺) or Rhesus factor negative (RhD⁻) depending on whether they do or do not possess Rhesus factor on the surface of their erythrocytes. Individuals who do not possess this antigen (RhD⁻) and receive erythrocyte RhD⁺ transfusion will develop alloantibodies directed against the antigen. Anti-RhD antibodies will evoke severe post transfusion reactions during another transfusion of RhD⁺ blood. In pregnant women who are RhD⁻ and who have a foetus with RhD⁺ erythrocytes (antigen RhD inherited from father), the transfer of foetal erythrocytes into the maternal circulation (e.g. during labour or amniocentesis) may evoke the formation of anti-RhD antibodies. Such alloantibodies will cause haemolytic disease in newborns in subsequent pregnancies. Contrary to alloantibodies against ABO blood groups antigens, anti-Rh antibodies do not cause agglutination of Rh-positive erythrocytes and that is why they must be detected by a different method (Coomb's test).

Rheumatic fever Systemic inflammatory disease which develops 2 to 5 weeks after infection with group A beta-haemolytic streptococcus. It is characterised by a number of pathological reactions in which the immune system is involved and which affect mainly the heart and joints.

Clinical symptoms: The disease is characterised by fever, migratory arthritis and symptoms of rheumatic heart inflammation (carditis). The inflammation may affect endocardium, myocardium or pericardium – either selectively or completely (pancarditis). In certain cases, permanent heart damage may develop, primarily rheumatic valve disease. Central nervous system involvement can result in chorea, pneumonitis when the lungs are affected, and erythema marginatum when the skin is affected. Laboratory findings include increased titre of streptococcal antibodies and the presence of elevated acute phase reactants.

Jones criteria JONES is an abbreviation summary often used to recall the major criteria (joints, o-shaped heart on imaging, nodules, erythema marginatum, Sydenham's chorea). The presence of two major symptoms or 1 major + 2 minor symptoms are necessary to make a diagnosis of rheumatic fever:
- Major symptoms: migratory polyarthritis, carditis, chorea, erythema marginatum, rheumatic nodules,
- Minor symptoms: fever, arthralgias, increased erythrocyte sedimentation rate, elevated C-reactive protein, leukocytosis, the confirmation of beta-haemolytic streptococcus infection, prolonged P-R interval on ECG (first degree heart block), a history of rheumatic fever.

Rheumatoid arthritis (RA) A common inflammatory joint disease that affects individuals of all ages, with maximal onset in women around the menopause. The disease is multifactorial in origin with certain genetic predispositions and unknown trigger factors. It is characterised by chronic inflammation, which is initiated and maintained by immunopathological mechanisms. The course of RA is very variable in pattern, but generally is progressive and can lead to significant disability.

General features:

- RA is not a benign disease as it shortens the life of affected individuals by 5–10 years
- Joint erosion develops early – usually during the first two years
- Early RA affects mainly joints, later systemic symptoms may develop
- Therapeutic management is effective particularly in the early stages of RA,
- RA is a very variable disease; most forms progress slowly, have long periods of clinical remission and a low tendency towards destruction; approximately 10% develop severe disease with joint destruction and deformities, leading to severe disabilities,
- The course of RA is unpredictable but risk factors associated with unfavourable prognosis have been defined based on large studies of patients (Rovenský et al. 2000, Scott 2000, Plant et al. 1994).

Rheumatoid arthritis (RA) – aetio-pathogenesis

The cause of RA is currently unknown. It is hypothesised that RA is a disease that develops in individuals with a genetic predisposition after induction by an unknown microorganism. A genetic element is well established, particularly in the studies of concordance in monozygotic twins, which is 12–15%, compared to 2–4% in dizygotic twins (Silman 1997, Seldin et al. 1999, Wiles et al. 1999). RA is a polygene-determined disease with major involvement of the HLA complex, which is thought to account for up to 40–50%. RA is associated with the HLA-DR4 antigen. This antigen can be divided into 5 subtypes: HLA-Dw4, HLA-Dw10, HLA-Dw13, HLA-Dw14, and HLA-Dw15. The association of RA with antigens HLA-DR4, HLA-Dw4 and antigens HLA-DR4, HLA-Dw14 is typical for the Caucasian population. However, only 70% of RA patients possess the antigens HLA-DR4, HLA-Dw4 or HLA-DR4, HLA-Dw14 in the Caucasian population; other patients possess other antigens, particularly HLA-DR1.

The major biological function of HLA molecules is to present peptides originating from protein antigens of endogenous or exogenous origin. These antigens are consequently recognised by T lymphocytes, which, by a number of interactions with other immune cells, initiate the immune response. It is unknown from which antigen the "arthritogenic" peptide originates in RA. It is hypothesised that the whole autoimmune process is initiated by infection.

Pathogenesis: RA is definitely associated with immune mechanisms and direct damage of target structures in the initial stages of the disease. Initially, T lymphocytes play a major role. Lymphocytes (especially $CD4^+$) represent 50% of all cells present in the inflammatory infiltrate and accumulate in the synovial membrane. The profile of cytokines suggests that these cells belong to the T_H1 subpopulation. Insufficient synthesis of T_H2 cytokines, particularly IL-4, IL-3 and IL-10 may contribute to an uncontrolled inflammatory process, as these cytokines belong to the anti-inflammatory group of cytokines and so they may antagonise the unfavourable pro-inflammatory cytokines IL-1, IL-6 and TNF-α. TNF-α is a cytokine, which alone is responsible for the development of local and systemic inflammatory reactions, and is also the key regulating mediator of other cytokines production. Another important cytokine, IL-7 increases the production of other cytokines by acting on macrophages and synoviocytes. Activated T lymphocytes are present particularly in the perivascular space, contrary to $CD8^+$ T-lymphocytes, which are dispersed in synovial membrane. Macrophages are also present. With these features, the conditions for initiation and maintenance of the immune response are assured, as particularly macrophages, through their class II HLA antigens, present the pathogenic antigen to T lymphocytes. Macrophages are important producers of pro-inflammatory cytokines and chemokines. Germinal centres typical for B lymphocyte areas of the lymph nodes are also present in the synovial membrane. A number of autoantibodies that after binding to their autoantigens form immune complexes are produced in the germinal centres. The immune complexes subsequently induce an inflammatory process in which polymorpho-nuclear leukocytes are particularly involved. Neutrophils through the medium of prote-olytic enzymes and reactive oxygen and ni-trogen radicals damage the extracellular ma-trix and cartilage. The invasion of neutrophils into synovial fluid contributes to other typi-cal changes for RA, especially involving neo-vascularisation. Neovascularisation and pro-liferation of synoviocytes are among the ma-jor changes that contribute to development of the pathological process.

Chronic inflammation of synovial mem-brane leads to pannus formation. Such gran-ulation tissue consists of a number of cells of different types, such as lymphocytes, mac-rophages, fibroblasts, synoviocytes and mast cells. The invasion of pannus and the synthe-sis of proteolytic enzymes are directly respon-sible for cartilage destruction, erosion of sub-chondral bone and damage to periarticular structures. Metalloproteinases (collagenase, stromelysin) and other proteolytic enzymes (elastase, cathepsin B and G, gelatinase) re-leased from activated macrophages, fibro-blasts, synoviocytes and chondrocytes in re-sponse to pro-inflammatory cytokines, par-ticularly IL-1 and TNF-α, are involved in damaging the tissues. Periarticular osteope-nia is caused by increased activity of osteo-clasts, which are stimulated by IL-1 and IL-6.

Rheumatoid arthritis (RA) – classification criteria

Criteria suggested by Arnett et al. in 1987 are used for the purposes of the ACR (American College of Rheumatology; table 11). A patient suffers from RA if at least 4 criteria are present, 1–4 criteria must last at least 6 weeks.

Rheumatoid arthritis (RA) – clinical symptoms

The initial symptoms of RA can involve the joints alone or be more systemic. Joint symptoms include pain of various in-tensities with more intense pain occurring in the morning. Another prominent symptom is morning stiffness, usually lasting more than one hour, which distinguishes the pain from that occurring in osteoarthrosis. Systemic symptoms include general malaise, tiredness, fatigue, subfebrile temperatures, weight loss and sleep disturbance. Metacarpophalangeal (MCP), proximal interphalangeal (PIP) joints and wrist (RC) are the most frequently af-fected in early RA.

Symmetric joint involvement is typical. The basic clinical signs of joint inflammation are soft tissue swelling and tenderness on pal-pation. The joint is considered to be active from an inflammatory point of view when it is swollen and sore during palpation. The joint swelling can be intra-articular or peri-articular. Fluid can be found with intra-artic-ular swelling. Joint destruction can be detect-

Table 11. ACR classification criteria for diagnosis of rheumatoid arthritis 1987

Criteria	Definition
• morning stiffness • arthritis of three or more joint groups	• morning joint stiffness that lasts at least 1 hour • soft tissue swelling or fluid observed by a physician is present at least in 3 of 14 joint areas (right or left PIP, MCP, RC, elbow, knee, ankle, MTP joints)
• arthritis of hand joints • symmetric arthritis	• swelling of at least one area – RC, MCP or PIP • concurrent involvement of the same joints on both sides of the body
• rheumatoid nodules	• subcutaneous nodules over the bone eminences or extensor areas around joints observed by a physician
• serum rheumatoid factor	• verification by any method where outcomes are not positive in more than 5% of the normal population
• X-ray changes	• X-ray changes typical for RA that are visible on an X-ray picture taken in PA projection of the hand and wrist with the discovery of erosions or decalcification of affected joints or in their proximity

R

ed clinically or radiologically. The course of the disease is very variable. RA is not a benign disease; it shortens the life of affected individuals by 5 to 10 years. The diagnosis of RA is confirmed by the presence of ACR classification criteria, though early disease may not fulfil four of these criteria.

Rheumatoid arthritis disease activity index (RADAI) → see Instruments of assessing (health status measurements, outcome measurement)

Rheumatoid arthritis (RA) – extra-articular symptoms
Ophthalmic complications in RA:
- Keratoconjunctivitis sicca (dry eyes),
- Episcleritis,
- Scleritis,
- Uveitis,
- Episcleral nodules,
- Peripheral ulcerative keratitis,
- Secondary cataract,
- Glaucoma,
- Keratopathy,
- Retinopathy.

Cardiac complications in RA:
- Pericarditis,
- Myocarditis,
- Disease of endocardium,
- Coronary arteritis,
- Cardiac amyloidosis,
- Vasculitis.

Haematological abnormalities:
- Anaemia accompanying chronic disease,
- Anaemia due to iron deficiency,
- Thrombocytosis,
- Thrombocytopenia,
- Felty's syndrome (neutropenia)
- Large granular lymphocyte syndrome,
- Lymphadenopathy,
- Lymphoproliferative disease.

Pulmonary complications in RA:
- Pleuritis,
- Rheumatoid nodules in the lung,
- Caplan's syndrome,
- Diffuse interstitial pulmonary fibrosis,
- Bronchiolitis obliterans,
- Constrictive bronchiolitis,
- Drug toxicity symptoms.

Renal complications:
- Glomerulonephritis,
- Secondary amyloidosis,
- Pyelonephritis,
- Interstitial nephritis.

Neurological complications:
- Compressive syndromes (carpal tunnel syndrome, ulnar nerve compression, tarsal tunnel syndrome),
- Distal sensory neuropathy,
- Sensory-motor neuropathy.

Soft tissue complications:
- Tendinitis,
- Tenosynovitis,
- Bursitis,
- Myositis (non-specific).

Rheumatoid arthritis pain scale (RASP)
→ see Instruments of assessing (health status measurements, outcome measurement)

Rheumatoid arthritis (RA) – pathological anatomy
In RA, the inflammatory process is located in the synovial membrane, which normally plays a significant role in the nutrition of avascular hyaline cartilage in synovial joints. The synovia of tendon sheaths and bursae are also affected by the inflammation. The joint cartilage is gradually damaged as its nutrition and drainage of the articular cavity is affected by the inflammation. Pannus tissue is formed in the area of the synoviochondral junction. The pannus expands into articular cartilage and gradually replaces the cartilage – initially at the margin. Tendon sheaths, ligaments and discs are affected secondarily.

Macroscopic changes of synovial membrane

In the early stage of RA, the synovial membrane is oedematous, hyperaemic and opalescent and straw-coloured synovial fluid leaks from the membrane. Villi and fibrin are present on the surface of synovia; 'rice shaped' particles may be present in the synovial fluid. The articular cavity may be obliterated (fibrosed ankylosis), but the presence of synovial fluid frequently prevents the formation of adhesions. Synovial villi may atrophy over time and the synovial membrane affected by inflammation transforms into thin tissue membrane.

Microscopic changes of synovial membrane

A distinct hyperplastic layer of synovial cells is typical. Blood plasma gradually leaks from dilated capillaries and venules into the articular cavity and along with infiltrating cells forms an inflammatory exudate. Polymorphonuclear leukocytes and later also mononuclear inflammatory cells migrate from vessels into the interstitium of the synovial membrane and to synovial fluid. Fibrinogen, which leaked from blood vessels, forms polymerised aggregates of fibrin on the synovial membrane. Deposits of fibrin, necrosis, poorly differentiated mesenchymal cells and decomposition of collagen fibrils are found in the synovial membrane.

Rheumatoid arthritis (RA) – remission criteria (according to American College of Rheumatology; ACR)

- Morning stiffness lasting less than 15 minutes,
- No tiredness,
- No joint pain,
- No joint tenderness or pain during passive movement,
- No soft tissue swelling of joints or tendon sheaths,
- Erythrocyte Sedimentation Rate does not exceed 30 mm/hour in women and 20 mm/hour in men.

Exceptions that exclude clinical remission include the clinical manifestation of active vasculitis, pericarditis, pleuritis, myositis, weight loss or fever which cannot be explained other than in association with RA.

Rheumatoid factors (RF) Autoantibodies
that react with antigenic determinants on the Fc-component of the IgG molecule. The presence of IgM RF is a serological diagnostic criteria for rheumatoid arthritis (RA); it is present in 75 to 90% of cases. RF can be detected either in serum or in various body fluids, including synovial fluid. Synthesis takes place mainly in the lymphatic tissue of the joint affected by inflammation, but also in bone marrow, lymph nodes, spleen and subcutaneous rheumatoid nodules. RF's can be of various immunoglobulin isotypes, i.e. besides IgM RF, there are also IgG RF, IgA RF and IgE RF.

Agglutination tests are still the most popular methods for RF assessment. In routine use, sheep erythrocytes bond with rabbit IgG (Waaler-Rose haemaglutination test) are often replaced by inert latex particles, which are coated with human IgG. A latex fixation test has a higher sensitivity for detecting RF but has a slightly lower specificity for diagnosing RA. A greater frequency of positivity of the latex test is probably based on the fact that human IgG react also with anti-allotypic antibodies and anti-Fab antibodies. The test particularly detects pentameric IgM RF that, in view of the higher number of bonds, produces macroscopically visible agglutination. The contribution of IgG RF and IgA RF to the positivity of the agglutination test is minimal. The result is taken as the highest titre of serum dilution when agglutination is apparent. A titre higher than 1:80 is considered positive.

IgG present in the serum may during the agglutination test compete with IgG coating the particles. In certain RF's, the binding sites of RF are already bound by normal serum IgG and so the agglutination is negative. Such RF's are referred to as hidden rheumatoid factors and can be detected by the latex fixation test only when the IgM fraction of serum is separated from IgG fraction. Hidden RF's are found more commonly in juvenile idiopathic arthritis.

Recently, the ELISA method, which has a number of advantages, has been used more frequently for detecting RF. In particular, ELISA allows the detection of immunoglobulin isotypes of rheumatoid factors depending on the specificity of the secondary antibody which is marked by enzyme; ELISA is also more sensitive in detecting IgM RF than the agglutination test.

The presence of RF is not associated only with RA. Increased levels are found in certain other acute and chronic inflammatory diseases. The frequency and level of rheumatoid factors is increased in individuals over the age of 60, and so it is recommended to reconsider the titre of a positive test, e.g. a positive titre in the latex fixation test is 1:1280. Such an increase in the frequency and levels of RF is reduced again in individuals over the age of 80, probably due to the higher mortality of individuals with autoantibodies.

Permanently increased levels of RF are more frequently present in chronic bacterial infections, such as subacute bacterial endocarditis, tuberculosis, syphilis or leprosy. They are usually temporarily increased in viral infections (e.g. infectious mononucleosis, hepatitis, influenza, AIDS) or after vaccination. RF positivity can be also found in other systemic or rheumatic diseases (systemic lupus erythematosus, scleroderma, Sharp's syndrome, Sjögren's syndrome, myositis), parasitic infections, pulmonary and liver diseases, sarcoidosis, mixed cryoglobulinaemia, hypergammaglobulinaemic purpura, Waldenström's macroglobulinaemia, chronic lymphocytic leukaemia and finally, in some patients with malignancy. Low levels of RF can occur in all healthy individuals. B lymphocytes with membrane-bound receptor with RF activity are a normal physiological finding and are presumably involved in normal immune system function.

Rheumatoid nodules Occur in 20 to 35% of patients with positive rheumatoid factors. They usually accompany more active forms of the disease. The nodules develop in areas exposed to pressure, such as the olecranon process, hand joints, sacral eminence or Achilles tendon. Rheumatoid nodules often bind tightly to the periosteum. Histologically, they consist of central necrosis surrounded by fibroblasts. The nodules are most likely the consequence of vasculitis of a small vessel with fibrous necrosis, which forms the central part of the nodule, surrounded by the proliferation of fibroblasts. Rheumatoid nodules are benign and mainly represent a cosmetic problem but if they develop in a problematic location (e.g. the sole of the foot), they may be surgically removed.

Rheumatoid pneumoconiosis (Caplan's syndrome) Is characterised by pulmonary rheumatoid nodules and pneumoconiosis in patients with rheumatoid arthritis (RA). The nodules are multiple and usually occupy the subpleural areas of pulmonary tissue. The X-ray picture suggests massive pulmonary fibrosis. The nodules are visible as concentric light and dark strips and consist of a central necrosis, an inflammatory zone with macrophages containing dust particles, a zone of fibroblasts and a surrounding layer of fibrous tissue. Caplan's syndrome (Anthony Caplan, English physician, 1907–1976) develops in individuals with RA who have had considerable exposure to coal-dust. However, a similar condition develops after silica and asbestos exposure.

Rheumatoid-surgical treatment Synovectomy, implantation of total joint prosthesis and joint arthrodesis belong to conventional corrective rheumatoid-surgical treatments. They are indicated in patients with rheumatoid arthritis (RA) in order to reduce tissues affected by inflammation (synovectomy), to provide pain relief and improve joint function. Synovectomy is indicated after failure of courses of DMARD treatment and only short term benefit from intra-articular glucocorticosteroids if only a few joints are affected. However, surgical synovectomy is often of limited success as it is impossible to remove all inflamed synovium. Prophylactic synovectomy of the wrist with excision of the head of the ulna should be considered in patients with severe wrist disease in order to prevent the rupture of extensor tendons. Other suitable rheumatoid-surgical interventions include total hip, knee and shoulder replacements, replacement of metacarpal or proximal interphalangeal joints and resection of metatarsal heads in patients with subluxation of metatarsal joints, and finally operation of hallux valgum with bursitis affecting the first metatarsal bone. In selected patients, reconstructive hand surgery on joints and tendons may be very beneficial. In arthrodesis, the joint pain is abolished but at the detriment of complete loss of joint mobility. Fusion of C1 and C2 vertebrae is indicated in atlanto-axial subluxation (>4 mms) with associated neurological symptoms and signs. The rheumatologist in liaison with an orthopaedic specialist can recommend rheumatoid-surgical interventions.

Rheumatological rehabilitation Has three functions:

1. *Preventive* – focusing on educating the patient to learn all the elements of rehabilitation treatment before the development of functional deficits,
2. *Corrective* – the aim is to influence reversible functional deficits,
3. *Maintaining* – to maintain existing functional levels.

Rhizarthrosis → see Osteoarthritis (OA) of the first carpometacarpal (CMC) joint (Rhizarthrosis)

Rickets A generalised skeletal disorder occurring in children characterised by inadequate mineralisation of bone matrix (osteoid). Newly formed trabecular and cortical bone and the growth plate (in contrast to osteomalacia, which does not interfere with the growth plate) are all affected. Clinically, its presentation varies with age. Rickets within the first year of life may present with craniotabes (thin deformed skull), and later with widened epiphyses at the wrists and beading of the costochondral junction (rickety rosary). In older children, typical bow-leg deformities occur. A number of acquired and genetically conditioned causes for rickets have been identified (table 12). From a biochemical perspective, rickets can be divided into those arising due to a calcium deficiency (hypocalcaemic rickets) or phosphate depletion (hypophosphataemic

Table 12. Classification of rickets (modified according to a review of Kutilek et al., 1998)

Genetically conditioned	hypocalcaemic:
	vitamin D-dependent (type I; an enzymatic defect in synthesis of the active form of vitamin D)
	vitamin D-dependent (Type II; pseudovitamin D deficiency caused by mutation in the gene encoding the vitamin D receptor)
	25-hydroxylase deficiency
	magnesium-dependent
	vitamin D-resistant
	hypophosphataemic:
	vitamin D-resistant (X-linked or autosomal dominant types)
	hereditary hypophosphataemic with a hypercalciuria
	renal Fanconi syndrome
	renal tubular acidosis (RTA type I; distal RTA)
	renal tubular acidosis (RTA type II; proximal RTA)
	Dent disease
	Lowe's (oculocerebrorenal) syndrome
	Inborn errors of metabolism (cystinosis, glycogenosis I, hypertyrosinaemia (tyrosinaemia type I),
	Wilson's disease)
Genetically unconditioned	hypocalcaemic:
	vitamin D-deficiency
	calcium-deficiency
	magnesium-dependent vitamin D-resistant
	hepatopathy
	renal osteodystrophy
	anticonvulsant therapy
	hypophosphataemic:
	phosphate deficiency (metabolic osteopathy of the prematurely born, other acquired hypophosphataemias)
	oncogenic
	acquired Fanconi syndrome, acquired renal tubular acidosis (intoxications, interstitial nephritis)

R

rickets). Conventionally, blood tests show a low serum calcium, phosphate and vitamin D with an elevated alkaline phosphatase.

The most frequent cause of rickets is acquired deficiency rickets due to lack of vitamin D. The disease occurs sporadically, particularly in older breastfed children and toddlers. In most cases the cause is a combination of a lack of calcium intake and borderline levels of vitamin D. Treatment is dependent on the cause, but many acquired rickets respond to calcium and vitamin D replacement. Other types of rickets are relatively rare. Hypophosphataemic vitamin D resistant rickets linked to the X chromosome has an incidence of 1:20,000 and is the most frequent congenital type of rickets.

Risedronate A bisphosphonate licensed for the treatment of postmenopausal osteoporosis to reduce the incidence of vertebral and hip fractures. It is also licensed for the prevention of glucocorticoid-induced osteoporosis and is used in men with osteoporosis. The drug should be taken on an empty stomach and washed down with a cup of water in an upright posture. The patient should not sit, lie down or eat for thirty minutes after drug ingestion. The normal drug regime is 35 mg once weekly or (rarely nowadays) 5 mg daily.

Rolf technique → see Exercise techniques

Rubella-associated arthritis Occurs in 15 to 20% of all rubella infections affecting adults. The arthritis can be divided into mono-, oligo-, or polyarthritis.

Clinical symptoms: Myalgias, suboccipital lymphadenopathy. Exanthema does not always occur.

Laboratory diagnostic criteria: Prevalence of mononuclear cells is typical in differential blood account. Mononuclear cells are also found in synovial fluid. Serologic screening reveals antibodies against the rubella virus.

Treatment: The disease recovers spontaneously, though symptomatic treatment may be needed.

R

Sacroiliac block (SI block) Sacroiliac pain is a frequent reason for vertebrogenic pain syndrome. SI block is blockade of one or both SI joints. Symptoms can be confirmed as arising from the sacroiliac joint by various methods, e.g. hyperabduction phenomenon according to Patrick, by springing the SI joints in the prone and supine positions, by tenderness over the affected SI joint in the standing position

Sanfilippo's disease → see Mucopolysaccharidosis (MPS)

SAPHO syndrome It is characterised by a unique arthropathy predominantly affecting the sternocostoclavicular area and accompanied by skin lesions of acne or pustulosis type and chronic recurrent multifocal osteomyelitis. The syndrome affects particularly the European and Japanese populations. The nomenclature SAPHO reflects **s**ynovitis, **a**cne **p**ustules, **h**yperostosis and **o**steomyelitis. Clinical symptoms include pain in the area of the sternum and the costoclavicular area. Ossification of the costoclavicular ligaments may be visible on X-ray. The triad of sacroiliitis, syndesmophytes and discitis is present when the vertebral column is affected. The skin lesions include palmoplantar pustulosis, acne conglobata or acne fulminans. Pathologically, the skin lesions are referred to as neutrophilic pseudoabscesses. Joint impairment is peripheral and symmetric. The symptoms on the axial skeleton are similar to those of seronegative spondyloarthropathy. There's no direct association with the HLA-B27 antigen.

The clinical picture is characterised by pain and oedema in the sternal area. The disease leads to limited movement of the arms and shoulders. Pain localised to the acromioclavicular joints may also be present. Osteolytic lesions in the sternum and rarely in the mandible may develop later on in the course of the disease. Less frequently, ossification of the ribs, sternum and sternoclavicular joint occurs. Focuses of sterile osteomyelitis are present in the histopathological picture. The aetiology of the disease is unknown, though in a few cases disseminated infections due to *Propionibacterium acne* were reported. Treatment is non-specific; antibiotics are not effective. Non-steroidal anti-inflammatory drugs, sulphasalazine and methotrexate have benefited certain patients. Recent studies have shown significant improvement after intramuscular administration of calcitonin or intravenous pamidronate. The differential diagnosis includes ankylosing spondylitis, psoriatic arthritis, fibromyalgia, bacterial infections and relapsing polychondritis (Schilling et al. 2000, Olivieri et al. 2006).

SARA → see Sexually acquired reactive arthritis (SARA)

Sarcoidosis → see Musculoskeletal manifestations of sarcoidosis

Sausage toe → see Toe swelling/deformity and associated diseases

Scheie's disease → see Mucopolysaccharidosis (MPS)

Scheuermann's disease Juvenile kyphosis and idiopathic scoliosis are severe disorders of a growing vertebral column. Hereditary, hormonal, nutritional factors, blood supply impairment and mechanical overloading cause osteochondrosis of vertebral end plates and herniation of the nucleus pulposus into vertebral bodies called Schmorl's nodes (Christian Georg Schmorl, German pathologist, 1961–1932). The condition leads to wedging deformities of vertebrae, narrowing of inter-vertebral discs and kyphosis of the thoracic spine compensated by significant cervical and lumbar lordosis.

Schmid's dysplasia An autosomal dominant hereditary metaphyseal dysplasia associated with mild short-limbed dwarfism without shortening of the vertebral column. Epiphyses of long bones are denticulate; metaphyses are deformed in caliculus shape. Affected individuals suffer from genu varum and coxa vara. Schmid's dysplasia becomes obvious after the third year of life; initially the dysplasia may suggest rickets but serum levels of calcium, phosphate and alkaline phosphatase are within the normal childhood range.

Schmorl's nodes → see Scheuermann's disease

Schober's test → see Metric measurement of vertebral column in spondyloarthritis (SpA)

Schober's test modified → see Metric measurement of vertebral column in spondyloarthritis (SpA)

SCID → see Severe combined immunodeficiency (SCID)

SCID mice (Severe Combined Immunodeficiency mice) A species of mice with serious genetic combined immunodeficiency (SCID) which causes them not to develop antibody or T-cell immunity and so allow them to serve as "live test-tubes" for implanting lymphocytes from other animal species. When, for example, human lymphocytes are injected, they can produce antibodies of human isotypes after antigen stimulation. The nature of the primary disorder is a mutation on chromosome 16 causing deficient activity of an enzyme involved in DNA repair, leading to failure of haematopoietic stem cells of the lymphoid line to mature.

Sclerosteosis A progressive autosomal recessive disorder characterised by an excess of bone stock due to insufficient expression of the SOST gene. It shows radiologically as a generalised hyperostosis and sclerosis leading to a markedly thickened and sclerotic skull, mandible, ribs, clavicles and all long bones. Sclerostin is a protein product of the SOST gene competing with bone morphogenic products (BMPs) for receptor types I and II of these proteins on osteoblasts. Sclerostin decreases the signalling induced by BMPs and suppresses the osteoblast-induced mineralisation. The expression of SOST has been detected in osteoblast cultures and in sites of mineralisation of the skeleton. A strong expression in osteocytes indicates that through these cells sclerostin modulates bone homeostasis. Transgenic mice with increased expression of SOST have low bone stock and decreased firmness of the bones.

Sclerostin (SOST) A glycoprotein that is homologous with other BMP (bone morphogenic products) antagonists from the DAN (differential screening-selected gene aberrant in neuroblastoma) family, such as noggin, gremlin and dan. It plays an important role in bone homeostasis and a specific role in the differentiation of osteoblasts and osteoformation induced by these cells. It acts as an integration link for osteocyte-mediated regulation of osteoformation. Sclerostin released from osteocytes may control the proliferation and differentiation of osteoprogenitor/preosteoblastic cells as well as the activity of mature osteoblasts via inhibition of activity of BMP proteins.

Scoliosis The curvature of the vertebral column in the frontal plain. Scoliosis is considered to be the lateral curvature of the vertebral column in a range greater than 11°. Scoliosis can be functional (the curves are not fixed and can be corrected actively or passively) or structural (the curves are fixed).

Scurvy → see Musculoskeletal symptoms in scurvy

Secondary gout A condition in which gout is caused by hyperuricaemia secondary to overproduction of uric acid from increased cellular turnover or decreased excretion of uric acid by renal disease or effects of drugs. Lymphoproliferative and myeloproliferative diseases, certain malignancies (usually carcinomas in disseminated malignancies and more frequently in anaplastic malignancies) and haemolytic anaemia belong to those conditions that are associated with overproduction of uric acid. Chronic renal insufficiency, chronic lead poisoning, drugs (diuretics, low dose salicylates, pyrazinamide, nicotinic acid and ethambutol) and also endocrinopathies (hyperparathyroidism, hypothyroidism) are among conditions associated with decreased renal elimination of uric acid.

Secondary hyperparathyroidism The increased concentration of parathormone is in response to calcium deficiency with the most frequent cause being a vitamin D deficiency. Treatment of the underlying cause is the treatment of choice.

Secondary Osteoporosis Develops as a result of another primary disorder or as a consequence of treatment. In spite of its low prevalence, approximately 10%, it is important to rule it out as a cause of osteoporosis. Exclusion of secondary osteoporosis is often demanding especially in patients in whom it is suspected on the basis of the medical history, clinical examination and laboratory findings, as well as in patients in whom the bone mineral density measured for age is low or the elapsed time since the menopause. In men, a thorough differential diagnosis is imperative as several authors report its occurrence in more than 70% of cases. The importance of distinguishing secondary osteoporosis often lies in a diametrically different therapeutic approach. The most frequent causes of secondary osteoporosis include: disorders of the gastrointestinal tract, pancreas, liver and kidneys, endocrine and rheumatic diseases and drug-induced osteoporosis.

Secondary Osteoporosis – classification
- Osteoporosis due to hormone deficiency – deficiency of sex hormones (several authors include postmenopausal osteoporo-

sis as a consequence of oestrogen deficiency in this group) and growth hormone.
- Osteoporosis due to excess of hormones – hypercorticism, hyperthyroidism, hyperprolactinaemia, and hyperparathyroidism.
- Osteoporosis caused by dietary deficiencies – insufficient calcium and vitamin D intake, disturbances of digestion and malabsorption syndromes.
- Renal osteopathy.
- Inactivity-induced osteoporosis.
- Osteoporosis due to chronic inflammatory disorders.
- Osteoporosis due to neoplastic disease.
- Drug-induced osteoporosis – corticosteroids, excess thyroid hormones, anti-convulsants, heparin, cyclosporin A, and methotrexate.

Selectins A family of glycoprotein leuko-adhesive molecules which consist of three members: L-selectin (CD62L, previously referred to as MEL-14), P-selectin (CD62P, previously referred to as PADGEM) and E-selectin (CD62E, previously referred to as ELAM-1). The nomenclature is derived from the cell types, which possess particular selectins on their surface: L-selectin on leukocytes, P-selectin on platelets and after induction by cytokines on endothelial cells, and E-selectin on endothelial cells. The molecules of selectin have the lectin domain on the N-terminal of the molecule through which they can bind to the specific ligand. These are saccharides in adhesive molecules similar to mucin. This is the fundamental of their biological function as such lectin-saccharide interactions (lectins) are particularly involved in the binding of leukocytes to the vascular endothelium and subsequently in their migration from postcapillary venules to the tissue affected by inflammation.

Selective Oestrogen Receptor Modulators (SERM) At present, raloxifene is the only member on the market licensed for the treatment of osteoporosis. It acts on bone as an oestradiol agonist, producing a decrease in bone resorption and an increased proliferation of osteoblasts. As an oestradiol agonist, it influences the cardiovascular system (even though

S

in contrast to oestradiol, it does not increase the total HDL and CRP). Raloxifene is an oestrogen antagonist of receptors in the endometrium and breasts. It significantly reduces the risk of vertebral and nonvertebral fractures in women with severe osteoporosis, and a reduced risk of invasive breast cancer (84%) is considered an additive and very important effect. A possible positive influence on cardiovascular events is promising. Raloxifene is also effective in the prevention of osteoporosis. An increased risk of venous thromboembolism with raloxifene is comparable to oestrogens and hot flushes may also be accentuated. Therefore, it is not suitable for patients with a history (or family history) venous thrombembolism and for women with climacteric problems.

Semiquantitative assessment of vertebral deformities
The assessment of changes in the height of vertebral bodies in the lateral projection has a great significance, especially in predicting further fractures, in patients with osteoporosis. A semiquantitative assessment, according to Genant, is the most frequently used method in clinical practice. A decrease of anterior height of a vertebra by 20 to 25% is assessed as 1st degree or mild fracture, with a decreased height by 25 to 40% as 2nd degree or moderate vertebral fracture and a decrease by 40% and more as 3rd degree or severe fracture.

Senile shoulder
Chronic shoulder pain with polytopic symptomatology. The pain is caused by degenerative changes of periarticular soft tissue in old age. Tendon ruptures and atrophy of the rotator cuff are often present.

Senile Osteoporosis (type II)
A mild degree of atrophy of the bones is a physiological phenomenon and belongs to the normal involution of ageing. A pathological state occurs when bone loss is excessively enhanced and the bone mineral density level decreases below the osteoporosis limit defined in the individual age groups of men and women on the basis of WHO criteria – see the entry diagnostics of osteoporosis.

Senile osteoporosis usually occurs in people older than 70 years. It affects women just a little more often than men. The most important pathogenic factors of senile osteoporosis include age-related decrease of osteoformation (decreased vitality and activity of both the osteoblasts and osteoclasts), circulation and neurotrophic disturbances of bone, age-related structural changes in bone collagen and secondary hyperparathyroidism consequent on decreased absorption of calcium due to decreased production of calcitriol. It is characterised by fractures, both in the cortical and trabecular bones (hip, vertebrae, proximal humerus, tibia and other long bones).

Septic arthritis
Is caused by a group of bacteria: *Staphylococcus aureus* (more than 50%), *Staphylococcus epidermidis*, *Streptococcus pyogenes* (15 to 20%), *Enterococcus faecium*, *Enterococcus faecalis*, *Haemophilus influenzae*, *Escherichia coli*, *Klebsiella pneumoniae*, *and Salmonella species*. Bacterial arthritis is most frequently caused by *Staphylococcus aureus*, *Streptococcus haemolyticus*, *Pseudomonas*, and by *Haemophilus influenzae* and *Escherichia coli* in children. The risk factors are listed in table 13.

Table 13. Risk factors of septic arthritis

- elderly
- underlying disease: RA, SLE, diabetes mellitus, liver cirrhosis, chronic nephropathy, malignancies, haemophilia, hypogammaglobulinemia
- orthopaedic interventions
- joint replacements
- extraarticular infections: skin, pneumonia, pyelonephritis
- long-term therapy using corticosteroids and immunosuppressive drugs
- haemodialysis
- IV drug abuse
- acquired immunodeficiency syndrome
- organ transplantations

The onset of disease is acute with systemic symptoms such as shivering, fever, lethargy, and fatigue. Pain, oedema with erythema, local hyperaemia and reduction of active and passive locomotion in the affected joint are dominant symptoms and signs of the disease. Antalgic posture is frequent. Increased synovial fluid is present in the joint (more than 90% of all cases). Clinical symptoms in the hip or sacroiliac joint may be atypical or modified. Atypical symptoms occur in the newborn, drug abusers and individuals with immunodeficiencies. The pain and oedema localised in the pubic symphysis, sacroiliac and the sternoclavicular joint in children and IV drug abusers may suggest Gram-negative infection. Micro-organisms of low virulence may cause chronic synovitis.

Early diagnosis is very important, as joint sepsis may lead to destruction of the affected joint, or even fatal septicaemia.

Laboratory findings: The laboratory picture includes a high erythrocyte sedimentation rate, C-reactive protein and leukocytosis referred to as left shift. Aspiration of synovial fluid is diagnostically very important. The fluid is usually opaque, and often purulent. The cell count is usually more than 3,000 and up to 50,000 WBC/mm^3 with a majority of polymorphonuclear cells. The X-ray picture initially only shows soft tissue swelling and an apparent increase in joint space where there is significant synovial fluid. Later osteoporosis, erosion and cartilage destruction develop, the articular cavity gradually narrows, or even disappears. Isotope scintigraphy (using ^{67}Ga or marked leukocytes) helps to confirm the diagnosis in cases where affected joints are located in areas of difficult access (sacroiliac and hip joint).

Treatment: Hospital admission to an orthopaedic or rheumatology ward is necessary, as apart from confirmation of diagnosis and assessment of antibiotic sensitivity, bed rest, parenteral administration of antibiotics, pain management and monitoring of the clinical response must be ensured. Treatment with broad-spectrum antibiotics, which can be later modified according to the results of cultures and sensitivity, must be started immediately after taking the sample of synovial fluid. Intravenous administration of antibiotics is necessary to ensure effective concentrations of the antibiotics in the serum and synovial fluid. Oral, intra-articular or intramuscular antibiotics are not suitable for the initial treatment of septic arthritis.

SERM → see Selective Oestrogen Receptor Modulators (SERM)

Seronegative spondyloarthritis A relatively heterogeneous group of inflammatory rheumatic diseases in the course of which rheumatoid factors remain negative (seronegative) by the use of standard tests. Involvement of the axial skeleton and major peripheral joints along with skin, mucosal, gastrointestinal and urogenital symptoms are common clinical signs in this disease.

Clinical symptoms:
- Absence of subcutaneous nodules,
- Inflammatory arthritis of peripheral joints,
- Sacroiliitis, spondylitis (sometimes localised),
- Skin, mucosal, ophthalmic, gastrointestinal and urogenital symptoms,
- Familial incidence
- Frequent association with HLA-B27,
- Ossification in areas of inflammatory enthesopathies (pelvis, os calcis etc.).

Serum amyloid A (SAA) A family of polymorphous proteins encoded by various genes on chromosome 11 in a number of mammalian species. There are two human acute-phase SAA proteins (SAA1 and SAA2), with 5 isoforms of SAA1 and 2 isoforms of SAA2. The physiological concentration of SAA in serum is approximately 2 to 3 mg/L, but can increase by one thousand times in acute inflammation (similarly to C-reactive proteins). In terms of function, SAA are small lipoproteins, which during the acute phase of inflammation join the third fraction of high density lipoproteins (HDL3) and become a dominant apolipoprotein in such molecules. SAA inhibits thrombin-induced activation of platelets, as well as the activation of neutrophils to prevent oxidative tissue destruction during the course of inflammation. SAA is beneficial in acute inflammation, but is harmful in chronic inflammation (causing amyloidosis).

Severe combined immunodeficiency (SCID) This is a heterogeneous group of disorders caused by defects in the development of stem cells of the lymphoid line with the subsequent occurrence of serious disturbances in T- and B-lymphocyte functions. It is one of the most severe immunodeficiencies as there is almost complete absence of humoral and cellular immunities. Children with SCID have very severe lymphopenia (decreased peripheral lymphocyte count) with blood lymphocytes being functionally inactive. A severe agammaglobulinaemia develops within the first months of life. The thymus is either missing or present only in remnants localised in untraditional anatomic sites. There are also numerous disturbances observed in phagocytosis. Severe recurrent infections, including pneumonias, chronic otitis media, chronic diarrhoea and sepsis begin soon after birth. The body rapidly becomes overwhelmed by recurrent infections and children with SCID usually do not live to see the second year of life. The development of infection can only be prevented by a sterile birth and complete isolation of the child in a sterile environment for its whole life. SCID has several forms depending to the type of cells affected and the molecular defects, especially in the activity of various enzymes. Treatment is possible via bone marrow transplantation or gene therapy (supplementing missing or defective genes).

Sexually acquired reactive arthritis (SARA) Reactive arthritis secondary to sexually-acquired infection with chlamydia being the most frequent pathogen.

Sharp score → see Total Sharp score

Shock A systemic reaction of the body to sudden and intensive non-physiological impulses from the external or internal environment. It is manifested particularly by hypotension and respiratory distress. Depend-

ing on the underlying cause, shock can be subdivided into traumatic, haemorrhagic, cardiogenic, anaphylactic or endotoxic (septic) shock. Reduced tissue perfusion and insufficient oxygen delivery were considered as the typical cause. Lately, impaired mitochondrial function (defect of oxidative phosphorylation) has been included. At present, defects of certain mitochondrial enzymes, increased synthesis of nitric oxide and reactive oxygen intermediates, increased adhesion of neutrophils on endothelium and activation of proinflammatory cytokines are considered the main causes of hypotension. The condition of shock is thus the result of an imbalance between NO, superoxide and their metabolites.

Shoulder–hand syndrome → see Algodystrophic syndrome (ADS)

Shulman's syndrome → see Eosinophilic fasciitis (Shulman's Syndrome)

Sickness impact profile (SIP) → see Instruments of assessing (health status measurements, outcome measurement)

Signals of functional impairment (SOFI) → see Instruments of assessing (health status measurements, outcome measurement)

Silicone synovitis Develops as a reaction to a foreign body or to certain components of silicone arthroplasties (silicone elastomer, dimethylpolysiloxane). Clinical symptoms include pain, stiffness and swelling of the joint with the implanted silicone prosthesis. Silicone synovitis most frequently affects carpal and metacarpal implants and radial prostheses.

The diagnosis is confirmed on histological (inflammatory reaction to foreign body, large cell infiltration, silicone particles) or radiological findings (intramedullary destruction, erosion, destruction of surrounding bone). Ultrasound and magnetic resonance imaging significantly contribute to the diagnosis of silicone synovitis. Treatment consists of removal of the implant.

Sjögren's syndrome (SjS) A chronic inflammatory disease characterised by diminished function of salivary and lacrimal exocrine glands (Henrik Sjögren, Swedish eye doctor, 1899–1986). Lymphocytes infiltrate the functional component of the epithelium, which leads to glandular and ductal atrophy. Dry mucosa, particularly of mouth and conjunctiva, is a typical symptom. The disease can be primary or secondary. Secondary SjS is associated with other autoimmune diseases, such as rheumatoid arthritis, systemic lupus erythematosus or primary biliary cirrhosis. Antibodies directed against small ribonucleoprotein antigens SSA/Ro and SSB/La are of diagnostic significance. Positive associations between HLA-DR3 and primary SjS, as well as between HLA-DR4 and secondary SjS, accompanied by rheumatoid arthritis have been found. Approximately 90% of patients are women 40 to 60 years old.

Clinical symptoms: Dry mouth (xerostomia) and dry eyes (xerophthalmia) develop. Glands of the gastrointestinal system, the respiratory system, skin and vaginal mucosa, may also be affected. Skin symptoms, vasculitis, Raynaud's phenomenon, renal impairment, neuropathy and arthritis belong to the most frequent extraglandular symptoms of Sjögren's syndrome.

Skin test A test in which a test substance (usually antigen) is injected into the skin or is administered to the skin surface in order to assess the immune response of the host. Tuberculin test or determination test of host sensitivity to various allergens are the most frequently used methods.

SLE → see Systemic lupus erythematosus (SLE)

Sly's disease → see Mucopolysaccharidosis (MPS)

Sm antigen → see Antibodies against U1RNP and Sm antigen

Snapping hip syndrome → see Coxa saltans (snapping hip syndrome)

Somatic pain → see Types of pain

SOST → see Sclerostin (SOST)

Spasticity Increased muscle tension with increasing resistance during passive stretching. The trigger point is a painful point in the muscle, which is formed by spastic fibres of skeletal muscle. Its irritation causes referred pain in the periphery.

Specific features of rheumatological rehabilitation Exercise according to:
- Buerger-Allan – to improve circulation of the lower extremities,
- McIntry – to improve acral circulation of the upper extremities,
- Codmann – to relax the articular sheath,
- Kohlrausche – exercise in sitting up position without backrest used in ankylosing spondylitis (AS) and osteoarthrosis (OA),
- Kaltenborn – exercise for the back,
- Vale – spinal exercises,
- Guymans, Michel and Lewit (PIR) – facilitation-mobility techniques,
- Nordemar, Harcom and Ekdahl – aerobic exercise used in rheumatoid arthritis, OA and AS,
- Kubat – exercise for flatfoot and other foot deformities.

Spinal Canal Stenosis The narrowing of the central spinal canal, lateral recesses and neuronal foramen. The defect is either congenital, evolutionary conditioned or due to degenerative, inflammatory, traumatic, metabolic and endocrine changes of the vertebral column.

Clinical symptoms: Narrowing of the spinal canal manifests itself after reaching a critical point – when compression of nerve and vascular structures of the spinal canal occurs. Neurogenic claudication causing pain located in the thigh and calf are among typical symptoms of spinal stenosis. The claudication is associated with weakness of the lower extremity muscles and paraesthesiae evoked when the patient walks or stands. A typical sign of the disease is for symptoms to disappear when the patient sits down, lies

S

down or leans forward. Long-term lumbago frequently appears before the development of claudication. Spontaneous erection of the penis during walking or impotence is among less frequent symptoms. Initial neurological symptoms appear only during exercise or during extension of the spine, and tend to disappear during relaxation or spinal flexion. Progression of spinal canal stenosis increases mechanical pressure on intraspinal structures and symptoms can then occur as postural claudication or as nocturnal claudication.

Spondyloarthitis → see Seronegative spondyloarthritis

SRS-A Slow reacting substance of anaphylaxis – the mixture of the leukotrienes LTC_4, LTD_4 and LTE_4 causing slow contractions of smooth muscle of bronchi and are involved in the bronchospasm of bronchial asthma.

SSA → see Serum amyloid A (SAA)

SSc → see Systemic sclerosis (SSc)

Statins on bone metabolism Statins may inhibit the production and functional ability of osteoclasts interfering with the mevalonate pathway in synthesis of cholesterol. A reduction in fracture risk has been documented in a number of observations on patients taking statins longterm.

Still's disease → see Juvenile idiopathic arthritis (JIA)

Streptolysin O Bacterial cytolysin released by group A beta-haemolytic streptococci. They belong to perforins because after binding to the surface of target cells, the streptolysin O in the course of polymerization forms spiral tubes, which forms holes in the cytoplasm, leading to lysis of the affected cell (particularly the erythrocytes and leukocytes of the host). The detection of antibodies against streptolysin O (antistreptolysin O, ASO) is a test used to detect infection caused by these streptococci, which may lead to the development of rheumatic fever affecting ap-

proximately 2 to 3% of infected patients with a genetic predisposition to RF.

Stress proteins Intracellular proteins, the synthesis of which increases when the cell is exposed to stressful conditions. Most information is known about heat shock proteins, which are immediately produced by cells (from bacterium to mammals, including humans) when exposed to a higher than optimal temperature, and glucose regulated proteins, the production of which is induced by a lack of glucose and by certain other factors.

Strontium ranelate This drug contains 2 atoms of strontium and has a unique dual mechanism of action. It stimulates proliferation of the preosteoblasts (osteoanabolic effect) and at the same time inhibits differentiation of osteoclasts (antiresorptive effect). Strontium ranelate has a documented effect on the reduction of vertebral and nonvertebral fractures. This effect is highlighted in the most-at-risk groups of postmenopausal women with osteoporosis. It is administered in a dose of 2 g/day in the form of granules, mixed with water, preferably at bedtime.

Structural components of joints Tenuous connective tissue, adipose tissue, dense connective tissue, cartilage and bone belong to the group of tissues referred to as connective tissue. Certain connective tissues (bone and dentine) are mineralised. All forms of connective tissue are derived from embryonic tissue referred to as mesenchyme. The cells of mesenchyme are pluripotent cells, which differentiate into specialised fibrocytes, chondrocytes, osteocytes and adipocytes. Haematopoietic cells also originate from mesenchyme.

The presence of intercellular matter, which is located between particular cells or groups of cells, is a typical feature of connective tissue. The intercellular matter consists of fibres (collagen, elastic and reticular) and amorphous material referred to as matrix. The intercellular matter is a non-living supportive matter. Only certain types of connective tissue cells are able to produce intercellular matter. Such cells (e.g. fibroblasts, chondroblasts, osteoblasts) produce fibrous components and amorphous matrix. Amorphous matrix consists of macromolecules, which used to be referred to as acid mucopolysaccharides, but currently are referred to as glycosaminoglycans. Such a nomenclature better defines the chemical structure of their polysaccharide (glycan) chains.

The part of the nomenclature – glycosamino – suggests that the linear polysaccharide chain consists of repeated disaccharides; each containing uronic acid bound to a hexosamine (aminosaccharide) residue. Certain glycosaminoglycans (e.g. sulphonated glycosaminoglycans) are covalently bound to proteins, whereby they are a component of large macromolecules referred to as proteoglycans. For example, heparan sulphate, chondroitin sulphate and keratan sulphate belong to sulphonated glycosaminoglycans. Hyaluronan represents non-sulphonated glycosaminoglycans. Large glycoprotein laminin is present in basal membranes. Chondronectin, which mediates adhesion of chondrocytes on type II collagen, is present in cartilage. The intercellular matter localised between cells provides connective tissue with supportive and protective functions.

Substance P
A neuropeptide containing 11 amino acid units. It is present particularly in the nervous system of vertebrates. It may have a supportive function as a neurotransmitter and neuromodulator in the central nervous system, whereas in the peripheral nervous system and other tissues, it acts as a local hormone (tachykinin). Substance P causes hypotension and vasodilatation and may cause contraction of smooth muscles. Apart from the above, it is involved in a number of immune mechanisms, including stimulation of phagocytosis of professional phagocytes in a similar manner to tuftsin, stimulation of inflammatory cytokines (TNF-α, IL-1, IL-6) and prostaglandin production in cells of the inflammatory reaction, particularly in cells of the mononuclear line. Substance P acts through specific receptors (neurokinin 1 receptor).

Sudeck's atrophy
→ see Algodystrophic syndrome (ADS)

Sulfasalazine (SSZ)
At present it is the second most commonly used disease-modifying drug (DMARD) in the treatment of rheumatoid arthritis. It is also successfully used in the treatment of spondyloarthropathies, particularly in peripheral joint disease. The most favourable features of the drug include:
- Rapid onset of action within 3 to 4 days
- Absence of serious late adverse effects (e.g. malignancies)
- Favourable application in combination with other DMARDs.

Pharmacokinetics: Approximately 30% of SSZ is absorbed in the small intestine. As SSZ is subject to entero-hepatic circulation, its biological availability is only around 10%. Intact SSZ reaches the large intestine, where by the action of intestinal microorganisms, the double nitric bond of SSZ is broken, leading to the formation of 5-aminosalicylic acid (PAS) and sulfapyridine. PAS is poorly absorbed (around 30%), is subject to acetylation before excretion, and the remainder is excreted via the stool. Sulfasalazine is well absorbed and its metabolites appear in the blood 3 to 6 hours after drug administration. It is metabolised in the liver and excreted in urine in conjugated or unconjugated form. Different types of acetylation phenotype of patients exist – so called 'rapid' and 'slow' acetylators. The relationship between such a phenotype and the presence of adverse effects has not been confirmed. SSZ has a high affinity towards plasma proteins (>95%), the peak plasma concentration is achieved 3 to 5 hours after drug administration, and the plasma elimination half-life is 6 to 7 hours. A steady state is reached in 4 to 5 days.

Mechanism of action Not clearly understood, as the effective component of the drug is unknown. It is suggested that the whole molecule is the most effective anti-rheumatic agent. SSZ, similarly to methotrexate, blocks dihydrofolate reductase and other folate dependent enzymes. This may lead to adenosine accumulation and to increased levels of pro-inflammatory interleukins.

Adverse effects:

- Gastrointestinal,
- Skin reactions,
- Haematological,
- Hepatic.

Frequent adverse effects:

- *Gastrointestinal* – nausea, vomiting, anorexia, abdominal pain, dyspepsia,
- *Central nervous system* – headache, pyrexia, mild vertigo, tinnitus.

Less frequent adverse effects:

- *Systemic* – hypersensitivity reactions,
- *Skin* – exanthema (macular, papular, pruritus), alopecia (1 to 5%), Stevens-Johnson syndrome,
- *Ocular* – yellow staining of the lens/cornea,
- *Hepatic* – elevation of liver enzymes, acute hepatic reaction including serious damage,
- *Pulmonary* – rare reversible pulmonary infiltrations with eosinophilia, fibrosing alveolitis,
- *Haematological* – leukopenia, neutropenia thrombocytopenia, aplastic anaemia, agranulocytosis,
- *Nervous system* – irreversible changes to central nervous system (very rare),
- *Kidneys* – serious damage (very rare), orange-coloured urine (from excreted metabolite),
- *Autoimmune symptoms* – drug induced systemic lupus erythematosus.

Interactions:

- Cimetidine has often been used to treat NSAID-gastropathy and its interaction with SSZ is very important. Cimetidine increases the levels of sulfapyridine and thereby the risk of nausea and vomiting. N-hydroxymetabolite of cimetidine may increase the haematological toxicity of SAS.
- Corticosteroids were studied in patients treated with SSZ and receiving corticosteroids or a placebo in Great Britain. In spite of the fact that 20 patients were followed up for a period of one year, the supplement of corticosteroids was of no clinical benefit and the authors suggest that this may be due to biological interaction. This fact has not been confirmed by a Norwegian study; fewer adverse effects occurred in the group of patients receiving both SSZ and corticosteroids.

Sulphasalazine → see Sulfasalazine (SSZ)

Superantibodies A group of antibodies, which apart from their ability to bind an antigen, also possess other activities. They usually bind to insert the preserved (constant) parts of the variable domains and are able to bind nucleotides and superantigens, mediate mutual interactions and catalyse certain chemical reactions. Similarly to superantigens of B lymphocytes that can bind a number of antibodies with different specificity, superantibodies are able to bind various ligands to parts of their molecule other than the standard binding site for antigens.

Superantigens These can, like ordinary antigens, be divided into two groups: thymus dependent and thymus independent. The common feature of superantigens is their ability to non-specifically stimulate a number of T or B lymphocyte clones. Thymus dependent antigens do not require modification in antigen presenting cells, they stimulate 5 to 25% of all T helper lymphocyte clones that are present in the body by non-specific binding to the β-chain of the antigenic receptor (TCR) and concurrently to the α-chain of the class II MHC antigens (major histocompatibility complex). As a consequence of the binding, activated T_H-lymphocytes release large amounts of cytokines, which have a negative influence on the host causing systemic toxicity and suppression of the specific immune response. Another type of superantigens is the B cell type of superantigens.

As well as exogenous superantigens of B lymphocytes, endogenous superantigens can stimulate B cells to continuous expansion. It is suggested that superantigens play a key role in the pathogenesis of certain neurodegenerative (multiple sclerosis) and autoimmune diseases (rheumatoid arthritis, insulin dependent diabetes mellitus and psoriasis).

Superoxide radical Often referred to as superoxide anion or as superoxide ($\cdot O_2^-$), it

develops by single-electron reduction of molecular oxygen by virtue of the enzyme
NADPH oxidase. This enzyme is present
mainly in professional phagocytes but also in
the mitochondrial respiratory chain and so is
involved in certain other reactions. Hydrogen
peroxide and other reactive forms of oxygen
that are involved in antimicrobial and cytotoxic reactions originate during these reactions.

Sural nerve tunnel syndrome → see
Tunnel syndromes of foot

Sweet's syndrome → see Acute febrile
neutrophilic dermatoses

Synapse A functional connection between
two neurons (in the central nervous system),
or between a neuron and its effector cell in
muscles (referred to as myoneural or neuromuscular connection) or glands. Most synapses function by the nerve impulse arriving
at the afferent neuron releasing a neurotransmitter which then rapidly triggers the efferent neuron. A lack of neurotransmitter leads
to diseases such as myasthenia gravis.

**Syndrome RS3PE (remitting seroneg-
ative symmetrical synovitis with pitting oedema)** A rare disease of unknown
origin that predominantly affects older Caucasian individuals. The disease is characterised by acute symmetrical polysynovitis particularly affecting the radiocarpal joints and
small joints of the hand, as well as the talocrural joints and small joints of the foot.
Rheumatoid factors are not detected in the
serum, and there are no joint erosions on X-
ray. The disease has a good prognosis. The
synovitis subsides after low doses of glucocorticoids or antimalarial agents. The drug-induced remission is long-term, even after withdrawal of treatment. Such a fact distinguishes
RS3PE from rheumatoid arthritis and polymyalgia rheumatica. The RS3PE syndrome may
be present as a paraneoplastic symptom. Malignancy should always be considered. The
diagnostic criteria of RS3PE suggested in
1994 are as follows:

- Aged over 65, absence of IgM RF in the serum
- Symmetrical polysynovitis affecting the
wrist, CMC (carpometacarpal), MCP
(metacarpophalangeal) and PIP (proximal
interphalangeal) joints, TC (talocrural)
and MTP (metatarsophalangeal) joints,
tenosynovitis of hand flexors and extensors,
- Pitting oedema of hands and feet,
- Morning stiffness,
- Good response to glucocorticoids treatment,
- Exclusion of other pathological diseases.

Synovectomy A surgical procedure to remove inflamed synovial tissue by open joint
surgery or arthroscopy. It is rarely fully successful, as total synovectomy is difficult to
achieve. It is most effective if performed at an
early stage, before articular cartilage is damaged and allows regression of the inflammatory process and improvement in joint function. Indications are rheumatoid arthritis,
ankylosing spondylitis, monoarthritis.

Synovial chondromatosis The principle
of the disease is cartilaginous tissue formation in the process of synovial membrane
metaplasia. Pain and limitation in the range
of joint movement predominate the clinical
picture. Multiple shadows are visible on X-
ray. Malignant transformation is very rare.

Synovial fluid (SF) The volume of synovial
fluid in a healthy joint is only about 0.1 to 0.4
ml. SF forms a very thin layer (approx. 26
μm) in the articular cavity of a healthy joint.
Intraarticular pressure is subatmospheric
(negative) or slightly atmospheric (from −4 to
1 mm Hg), so the intraarticular cavity is only
a potential space and capillaries of synovial
membrane are in very close proximity to the
avascular articular cartilage. Furthermore, the
structure of the synovial membrane causes
synovial fluid to communicate directly with
the interstitial fluid of the synovial membrane.

SF is formed in the synovial membrane by
secretion of blood plasma and is then en-

riched by hyaluronan and other macromolecules. The synovial matrix can be considered as a special form of extracellular matrix with a high content of water, electrolytes and hyaluronan. The content of synovial fluid reflects the condition of the synovial membrane and avascular articular cartilage. The number of cells in a healthy joint is low. Gardner suggests the following number of cells in normal synovial fluid: cells with nucleus are less than 750 in 1 μL; neutrophil granulocytes are found around 200 in 1 μL; lymphocytes in small amount; mononuclear phagocytes only a few and synovial cells very few.

SF represents a liquid medium that is responsible for hydrodynamic changes in the course of joint movement. SF is of high viscosity; however, the physical properties of SF cause its viscosity to decrease during increased loading. Such properties enable SF to act as a unique lubricant of the cartilage, to transfer nutrients towards avascular articular cartilages, fibrous cartilages, discs and meniscus and also carry metabolites away.

SF is a clear, viscous, yellow fluid, which is present in all diarthrodial joints. It maintains lubrication of the cartilages of articulating bones. Healthy synovial membrane (SM) transmits only substances of small molecular weight (e.g. glucose); pathologically changed SM can transmit substances of higher molecular weight, e.g. proteins, complexes of oxygen radicals, cytokines etc. Hyaluronic acid, which is synthesised by B cells of the synovial lining, is a component of SF. Depending on the numbers of leukocytes, their differential picture and bacteriological assessment, SF can be subdivided into four groups: non-inflammatory, inflammatory, septic and haemorrhagic (table 14).

Table 14. Findings in synovial fluid classified according to particular groups (Hüttl 1970, 1971)

Parameter	Normal SF	Group I (non-inflammatory)	Group II (inflammatory)	Group III (septic)
Volume (mL)	< 3,0	> 3,0	> 3,0	> 3,0
Viscosity	High	Higher	Low	Variable
Colour	Clear/Straw	Amber	Yellow	Purulent
Turbidity	No	No	Present	Significant
Leukocytes	< 200	200–2000	2000–50 000	> 50 000
Neutrophils/ Granulocytes	< 25%	< 25%	> 50%	> 85%
Cultivations	Negative	Negative	Negative	Frequently positive
Total proteins (g/L)	11–22	Normal value	> 40	30–60
Uric acid (μmol/L)	180–116	Normal value	Normal value	Normal value
Glucose (mmol/L)	3.3–5,2	Normal value	Low in RA	1.1–1.6
Lactate (mmol/L)	0.9–1,8	Up to 4.2	Up to 6.9	Up to 28.0 (except for gonococcal arthritis)
LDH (U/L)	< 333	Normal value	> 333	> 501
Rheumatoid factors	Negative	Negative	Positive/ negative	Negative
Immunoglobulins	Approximately ½ of plasma concentration	Approximately ½ of plasma concentration	Increased	Increased

Synovial fluid analysis This is a comprehensive histopathological, microscopic, biochemical, immunological and bacteriological assessment of synovial fluid, which provides diagnostic information and assistance for appropriate therapeutic management. A less comprehensive analysis consists of macroscopic examination (colour, turbidity and viscosity of SF), cytological assessment with an emphasis on the number of nucleated cells and the leukocyte differential count, microscopic assessment focused on the presence or absence of microcrystals, and depending on need, a bacteriological examination.

Synovial joints These joints provide a very effective mechanical system and allow a wide range of movement. They are approximately 10^6 times exposed to load during the first year (each load is approximately three- to fourfold body weight) and remain effective for the remainder of life (approximately 70 years).

The bone terminals of synovial joints are covered by cartilage, which is referred to as articular cartilage. The main mechanical properties of synovial joints are due to the presence of such cartilage. The articular cartilage can be considered as hydrated gel strengthened by fibres, composed of a fibrous microskeleton of collagen. The gel consists of proteoglycans, which is capable of retaining huge amounts of water, and thereby act as a shock absorber. Articular cartilage reduces the load applied to subchondral bone, and provides contact areas with low friction that are resistant to attrition. Articular cartilage does not possess perichondrium. Synovial fluid as a component of the articular cavity is present between articular planes. The articular cavity is surrounded by the articular capsule, which consists of two layers (external and internal). The external layer (fibrous membrane) consists of dense fibrous tissue and is adherent with the bone through collagen fibres. Dense fibrous tissue of the layer is substituted by tenuous fibrous tissue of the synovial membrane. The synovial membrane possesses plicae or digitiform villi, which protrude into the articular cavity.

Synovial lining cells The surface of the synovial membrane is composed of synovial lining cells, which do not form a consistent layer, but have wide intercellular spaces between them, filled by intercellular matter and interstitial fluid. No intercellular connections of desmosomal type exist between particular lining cells, and there is no basement membrane under the synovial lining cells. The superficial layer of the synovial membrane is referred to as the synovial intima or the layer of synovial lining cells (consists of two to three layers of cells in various types of membrane). The underlying subintimal or subsynovial layer of synovial membrane consists of fibrous, loosely areolar or fatty tissues. Three major types of synovial membrane are distinguished according to the structure of subsynovial tissue: areolar, adipose and fibrous. Synovial membrane forms stratum synoviale, which is continuously substituted by stratum fibrosum of the articular sheath.

Two morphologically different types of synovial lining cells can be recognized in the intima: type A and type B cells. Such knowledge was first published in 1962 by Barland et al. The ultrastructure of type A cells suggest that they are phagocytosing cells with an abundance of vacuoles, pinocytic vesicles, mitochondria and lysosomes. Type A cells belong to the monocytomacrophage system and play an important role in the homeostasis of the synovial environment. A typical feature of type B cells is their well developed granular endoplasmic reticulum and Golgi apparatus. Histochemical studies and tissue cultures indicate that these cells produce hyaluronan (Worrall et al. 1991, Momberger et al. 2005).

Capillaries are present in close proximity to the surface of the synovial membrane, directly under the synovial lining cells. The large number and superficial location of capillaries explains the frequency of haemorrhages into the articular cavity, as even a simple puncture of the joint cavity can cause translocation of erythrocytes into synovial fluid. There are two types of capillaries in synovial membrane: continual and fenestrated. The walls of fenestrated capillaries are very thin, endothelial fenestrations are locat-

S

ed in those parts of capillaries that are closest to the joint cavity. It is suggested that such vessels are specialised for the rapid exchange of fluids and nutrients. Fenestrated venules have also been described in synovial membrane. It was found that dense corpuscular material (comparable to macromolecules of antigen-antibody complexes) leaks from the blood circulation into the interstitium of the synovial membrane and the joint cavity through the walls of fenestrated venules. It is suggested that the permeability of fenestrated capillaries is not under the control of endothelium but the surrounding tissue.

Lymphatic vessels of the synovial membrane are not as numerous nor superficially located as blood capillaries. Lymphatic capillaries accompany postcapillary venules and form a system in the subintimal layer of the synovial membrane. They continue along the flexor aspect of the limb and communicate with the lymphatic plexus in the periosteum. The system of lymphatic vessels plays a significant role in the homeostasis of the interstitial connective tissue of the whole body. Currently, it is well known that the lymphatic circulation significantly regulates the volume of the extravascular fluid and proteins in the tissues and forms pathways for the migration and circulation of lymphocytes, and thereby contributes to optimisation of the immune response. The lymphatic system plays an important role in metabolism of components of the connective tissue intercellular matter, especially hyaluronan (Rovenská et al. 2003).

Synovial sarcoma (synovioma) Synovi-

oma does not have a clear histology as epithelioid elements, spindle cellular particles, hyalinised fibrosis and calcifications can be present in this tumour. It occurs in the proximity of joints, particularly in the soft tissue, in the bursa of tendons, and rarely in continuity with the synovial membrane. It occurs in adolescents and young adults, more frequently in men.

Clinical picture: The tumour of soft elastic consistency is found in the proximity of joints, articular ends of bones or on tendon sheaths. Growth of the tumour is relatively

slow. The X-ray shows a picture of shadows of soft tissues with calcification. As nearby joints can react with secondary synovitis, synovitis due to rheumatoid arthritis, degenerative arthrosis, benign fibroma, fibrosarcoma, lipoma and liposarcoma must be ruled out.

Treatment: Radical excision followed by radiotherapy. The tumour is very malignant leading to development of metastases in lymph nodes and lungs in 50 to 70% of patients.

Synovioma → see Synovial sarcoma

Synovitis Inflammation affecting the synovial membrane of a synovial joint. Acute synovitis is accompanied by the typical symptoms and signs of inflammation, i.e. pain, tenderness, heat, swelling, erythema and impaired function. It is associated with an increased volume of synovial fluid. The microscopic picture is characterised by the presence of polymorphonuclear leukocytes and macrophages in the interstitium of the synovial membrane, as well as in the SF. Chronic synovitis is characterised by thickening of the synovial tissue without or only a small amount of fluid. Lymphoid follicles and multi-nucleated large cells and later also numerous mast cells occur in the synovium. Signs of hypertrophy and hyperplasia of the synovial tissue develop following repeated exacerbations of inflammation. The final outcome of this inflammatory process may be the development of fibrosis.

Syringomyelic arthropathy of shoulder Syringomyelia can lead to a neuropathic osteoarthropathy with a progressive destructive disease of the joints associated with loss of sensation, a decreased pain perception and characteristic destructive changes on X-ray. It is characterised by soft tissue swelling, mild pain and rapid destruction of the shoulder joint. The disease is more frequent in men between 20 and 40 years. Anaesthesia for pain, warm and cold sensations with no defect in the sensory function of deep sensations is present. Syringomyelic arthropathy should be considered if the large joint of the upper extremity is affected in a young patient, especially if the patient complains of little pain despite severe destructive disease.

SYSADOA; symptomatic slow acting drugs of OA
Symptomatic rapid acting drugs are used in the treatment of osteoarthrosis (SYRADOA, symptomatic rapid acting drugs of OA) in the form of analgesics. Slow acting drugs belong to the second group. Some of these drugs seem to be disease modifying drugs (DMOAD, disease modifying OA drugs) or more lately, structure disease modifying drugs (SMOAD, structure disease modifying OA drugs). Though their effects have been disputed in many experimental trials, there are two studies of glucosamine sulphate and one study on chondroitin sulphate indicating a structure modifying effect (Uebelhardt et al. 1998, Reginster et al. 2001, Pavelka et al. 2002). SYSADOA are slow acting drugs, but the effect lasts for up to two months after their withdrawal. It is supposed that they inhibit synthesis of lysosomal proteases, decrease the formation of oxygen and nitrous radicals and have a protective effect on cartilage against the impact of pro-inflammatory cytokines.

Systemic enzyme therapy (SET)
A therapeutic management consisting of the administration of a combination of enzyme agents (e.g. Wobenzym), usually by mouth. All preparations are in the form of tablets coated with an acid resistant cover to protect the contents from gastric acid. The tablet dissolves in the small intestine where the enzymes are partially absorbed and act systemically in the body. Enzymes of SET preparations belong to hydrolases and their major representatives are proteolytic enzymes of animal and vegetable origin. They help in the degradation of immune complexes, the optimisation of phagocytosis and the inflammatory reaction, which determine their immunonormalising effects. At present, SET is used particularly in surgical specialties, sport medicine (injury treatment), vascular diseases, the treatment of lymphoedema, and inflammatory and immunopathological processes. SET is also a component of complex oncology treatment. SET is different from thrombolysis, in which an intravenous thrombolytic agent (tissue plasminogen activator) is infused as a clot buster in acute coronary thrombosis.

Systemic lupus erythematosus (SLE)
An autoimmune disease affecting most of the important organs; however, particularly the skin, joints, cardiovascular system, kidneys, central nervous system and lungs. The disease is characterised by hyperactivity of B lymphocytes leading to the formation of auto-antibodies directed against organ non-specific antigens. It is still not clear whether SLE is a syndrome whose common feature is represented by the below mentioned symptoms.

Clinical symptoms:
- Clinical symptoms of the disease can be either systemic or they can be due to inflammation of a particular organ or system, such as skin, mucosa, joints, kidneys, brain, serous membranes, lungs, heart and sometimes the digestive system,
- The organs can be affected either individually or in combination,
- Impairment of vital organs, particularly the kidneys and the central nervous system, must be considered a significant feature influencing morbidity and the associated mortality,
- The morbidity and associated mortality may be caused by the distribution and severity of organ involvement by the underlying disease process or due to its treatment.

Diagnostic (classification) criteria: The variability of clinical symptoms, signs and laboratory findings and the need to monitor medical observations internationally led to the establishment of specific diagnostic criteria. The original proposals, on which specialists had been working since 1972, were finally reviewed and released in 1982. The original group of 14 signs was reduced to a final 11 (table 15).

The above classification is based on the presence of 11 criteria. In clinical trials, the

Table 15. ARA Diagnostic criteria of SLE

Criteria	Definition
1. Facial erythema (malar)	permanent, flat or raised, over the malar areas sparing the nasolabial folds
2. Discoid erythema	erythematous raised patches on facial skin with adherent keratotic scaling and follicular plugging, atrophic scars develop in older lesions
3. Photosensitivity	erythema as a consequence of increased reaction to sunlight in patient's history or observed by a physician
4. Mouth ulcers	oral or nasolaryngeal ulceration, usually painless, observed by a physician
5. Arthritis	non-erosive arthritis affecting two or more peripheral joints characterised by tenderness, swelling or effusion
6. Serositis	a. pleuritis – typical pleural pain in the history or friction murmur, or pleural effusion, confirmed by a physician, or b. pericarditis – confirmed by ECG, rub or pericardial effusion
7. Kidney impairment	a. proteinuria greater than 0.5 g/day, or greater than 3+ if quantitative evaluation has not been performed, or b. cellular casts, may be erythrocytes, haemoglobin, granular, tubular or mixed
8. Neurological disorder	a. convulsions – if not due to an offending drug or known metabolic disorder, i.e. uraemia, ketoacidosis or electrolyte disturbance, or b. psychosis – if not due to an offending drug or known metabolic disorder, i.e. uraemia, ketoacidosis or electrolyte disturbance
9. Haematological disorder defects	a. haemolytic anaemia – with reticulocytosis, or b. leukopenia (systemic) – less than $4.0 \times 10^9/l$, proved by at least two consequent examinations, or c. lymphopenia – less than $1.5 \times 10^9/l$, proved by at least two consequent examinations, or d. thrombocytopenia – less than $100 \times 10^9/l$, if not due to an offending drug
10. Immunological defects	a. anti-DNA –presence of elevated levels of circulating antibodies against native DNA, or b. anti-Sm – the presence of circulating antibodies against nuclear Sm antigen, or c. antiphospholipid antibodies – present in the serum, based on: – elevated serum concentrations of IgG or IgM anticardiolipin antibodies – positive test for lupus anticoagulant using standard method, or – false positive serological test for syphilis (Bordet-Wassermann reaction), proved positive for at least six months and confirmed by *Treponema pallidum* immobilization test or fluorescent treponemal antibody absorption test
11. Antinuclear antibodies	abnormal titre of antinuclear antibodies proved by immunofluorescent test or by an equivalent method at any period of time and with no drug treatment which can induce lupus erythematosus

S

diagnosis of SLE is confirmed when at least four of these criteria are present, either simultaneously or serially over the time of monitoring of the patient.

Deposits of immune complexes in target tissues (glomerulus, choroidal plexus etc.), along with cytokines and adhesive molecules, are involved in the pathogenesis of damaging inflammation. Proof of double-stranded DNA (anti-dsDNA) antibodies, anti-Sm antibodies, ribosomal ribonucleoprotein (anti-U1 RNP) antibodies (overlap syndrome), antibodies to Ro (SSA) or La (SSB), antiribosomal P protein antibodies (cerebritis) or antiphospholipid antibodies is crucial to the diagnosis of SLE. Many however are also present in other connective tissue diseases (ie SSA/SSB antibodies in Sjögren's syndrome).

Systemic lupus erythematosus disease activity index (SLEDAI) → see Instruments of assessing (health status measurements, outcome measurement)

Systemic sclerosis (SSc) Previously known as diffuse scleroderma or progressive systemic sclerosis is a chronic systemic disease affecting the skin, locomotor system and internal organs. It is characterised by fibroproductive changes of connective tissue, collagen overproduction, microvascular abnormalities and defects of humoral and cellular immunity. The disease affects women four times more commonly than men. It most frequently manifests itself between the ages of 45 to 65 years. Annually, there are 5 to 10 newly diagnosed cases in a population of one million individuals.

The first symptom of SSc is usually Raynaud's phenomenon. Arthralgias, joint stiffness, arthritis, myalgia and myositis occur in about half the patients. In most cases, systemic symptoms, such as loss of appetite, weight loss, subfebrile fevers and general fatigue occur.

The clinical signs are characterised by sclerosis of the skin, Raynaud's phenomenon, and gastrointestinal, lung and heart abnormalities. Antibodies against DNA-topoisomerase I (anti-Scl-70) are present in half the patients, more frequently in patients with lung fibrosis, the diffuse form of SSc, heart abnormalities, joint contractures and progressive disease. Anticentromere antibodies are present in approximately 20% of patients with SSc, a half of whom suffer from a limited form; the antibodies are most frequently present in CREST syndrome (in 90% of patients). The course of the disease is more favourable in patients with anticentromere antibodies; damage to the lungs and kidneys is less frequent and severe. Prognosis is worse in patients with progressive lung fibrosis, pulmonary hypertension and renal disease with malignant hypertension.

The principal subsets of SSc are:
- Diffuse cutaneous SSc (dcSSc)
- Limited cutaneous SSc (lcSSc)
- SSc sine scleroderma in which patients have only internal organ involvement
- Environmentally-induced scleroderma
- Overlap syndromes in which features of SSc coexist with elements of other rheumatic disorders

The use of disease modifying drugs is not well established, but those that influence the metabolism of collagen (D-penicillamine) and suppress the immune response, are often used in treatment, particularly cyclophosphamide, methotrexate and cyclosporin. Indications for corticosteroids include the early oedematous cutaneous stage, in patients with myositis, arthritis and serositis. Vasoactive drugs, ACE inhibitors and prostaglandins E1 are also used in treatment. Physical therapy is a component of the multi-disciplinary management.

S

T

Tai-chi exercise This is an undemanding but effective type of exercise for older people aimed at improving movement coordination, increasing functional capacity and global well-being. It also helps prevent traumas, especially falls, because it leads to awareness of the body and its parts, as well as positions in which the body is situated.

Takayasu's arteritis (TA) A chronic inflammatory disease affecting large arteries, particularly the aorta and its main branches. The disease mainly affects young women.

Clinical symptoms: The phase of vessel obliteration, manifested by upper extremity claudication, headaches, postural syncope and visual defects follows the phase of systemic symptoms. Weak or absent pulsation and bruits over the large arteries are typical.

Taping The use of special adhesive tapes in order to fix the supportive the fibro-tendinous apparatus of joints. It is used particularly in sports medicine in cases of swelling, joint subluxation, tendinitis and tenosynovitis. Its application is short term only, e.g. before overloading the joint or during various phases of rehabilitation, after trauma or operations in the area of the locomotor system. Taping requires an appropriate application technique in order to produce beneficial outcomes and avoid problems (callosities, pustules, defects of circulation). The main areas of application include the tibial area and the fingers. Taping in rheumatology is also applied in knee pain when the patella is shifted medially by the use of tape, which leads to significant pain relief.

Tarsal tunnel syndromes

Anterior tarsal syndrome
The deep peroneal nerve is compressed by the cruciform ligament on the anterior tarsal side. The patient complains of a sharp burning pain of the first and second toe of the foot. Hypo or hyper aesthesia is present on the medial side of the first and second toe. The strength of the extensor digitorum brevis muscle is weakened.

Medial tarsal syndrome
The tibial nerve is compressed by the flexor reticulatum behind the medial malleolus near the heel bone. Pain radiates either to the whole foot or only to one half of the foot and rarely just to the area of the heel. Hypo or hyper aesthesia is present over the whole foot or only on medial or lateral side.

Treatment: Glucocorticoids are administered locally or the nerve is released surgically in both syndromes.

Temporal Arteritis (TA) (Giant Cell Arteritis)

Vasculitis of unknown aetiology which affects both the external and internal carotid arteries (and other intracranial arteries) of individuals over the age of 50. It can lead to sudden blindness if not recognised and treated with high dose corticosteroids.

Clinical symptoms: The main clinical symptoms include fatigue, unilateral fronto-temporal headache, jaw claudication, visual disturbances, scalp tenderness, polymyalgia rheumatica and aortic arch syndrome.

Diagnosis: The clinical picture associated with a high erythrocyte sedimentation rate (ESR > 60mm/h) should give a strong suspicion. Temporal artery biopsy should be undertaken though may be normal in many patients, due the nature of the disease affecting the artery in skip lesions.

Treatment: Treatment with high dose prednisolone (40 to 60 mg daily) should be started as soon as the diagnosis is strongly suspected to avoid sudden blindness or stroke. The dose should be tapered slowly and treatment is often required for twelve months or longer.

Tendinopathy (tendonosis, tendoperiostosis, enthesopathy) A progressive degenerative change within the tendon insertions with gradual deposition of calcium. Causes include trauma, microtrauma and overloading. Genetic and metabolic factors also play an important role in their development. They can be diagnosed from the medical history, and palpation and movement of the affected muscle against resistance. Spontaneous pain is not usually present. Tendinopathies can also affect the spinous and lateral processes of vertebrae.

Tendinopathy of the rotator cuff A defect to the insertion area of the rotator cuff of the shoulder joint, most frequently affecting the tendons of the supraspinatus and infraspinatus muscles, and less frequently the subscapularis muscle. Impairment of a particular insertion can be distinguished by movement against resistance according to the movement pattern of the particular muscles (pain occurs), by palpation and frequently also by a typical painful arc.

Treatment: Physical therapy, non-steroidal anti-inflammatory drugs, local infiltration of corticoids.

Tendomyosis A frequent form of extra-articular rheumatism. Myalgia and pain of muscle and/or tendon insertions, which are worsened by various physical and psychological factors, such as changes in the weather, cold, fear, depression etc. are typical symptoms. Painful muscles show increased tone and areas of abnormal hardening of tissues – so called myogelosis – can be present. The causes include overloading and incorrect loading of the muscles during work and sporting activities, incorrect posture, incorrect movement habits, postural defects and others.

Tensilon test → see Myasthenia gravis

Teriparatide → see Parathormone – Teriparatide

Terraband (dynamoband) Terraband (rubber strap) is used to perform exercises, the difficulty of which can be adjusted by the elasticity and tonicity of the rubber strap. It is also used in patients with rheumatic diseases to exercise the long muscles of the extremities. Independent exercises at home after providing the patient with instructions is an advantage of this method.

Testosterone Does not have the same causal relation to osteoporosis in men as oestrogens have in women. In men, ageing is associated with changes in the hypothalamus-pituitary-gonadal axis with a consequent significant decrease in total as well as free testosterone. Testosterone has a direct stimulatory influence on the production and activity of the osteoblasts, shown by the finding of androgen receptors on their surface. Also, androgens act via growth factors. Testosterone deficiency reduces the secretion of calcitonin and synthesis of calcitriol. Testosterone deficiency is one of the commoner causes of osteoporosis in men. The administration of testosterone derivatives increases bone mineral density and reduces the risk of fractures.

Teufel's bandage A support to correct posture, which is used in Scheuermann's disease and cases of increased curvature of the vertebral column in the sagittal plane due to habitual incorrect posture, e.g. at work.

TGF (transforming growth factor) Two TGF's are well identified, TGF-α and TGF-β, though they are not related to each other structurally or genetically and act through different receptors. TGF-α is a small polypeptide growth factor, which affects cell division, wound healing and stimulates angiogenesis, and is upregulated in some forms of human cancer. TGF-β exists in three subtypes, TGF-β1, TGF-β2, and TGF-β3 and is commoner than TGF-α. The main feature of TGF-β is its involvement in the regulation of transformation of normal cells into malignant cells, regulation of embryonic development, wound healing, inflammatory and other immune responses, and is involved in cell apoptosis.

Thalassaemias → see Haemoglobinopathies and involvement of the locomotor organs

T

Thermal therapy The delivery of heat to the body for medical purposes. It can be referred to as positive (systemic application with warm bath, mud, sauna or local application with wax, infrared radiation, diathermy, ultrasound) or negative (referred to as cryotherapy using special bags, ice, cold air or gas) thermal therapy. Systemic cryotherapy is administered in special chambers at a temperature of −120°C for a few minutes only.

Positive thermal therapy is performed in three basic ways:
1. conduction (heated wax),
2. convection (hyperthermal bath),
3. conversion (infrared lamp – conversion of radiation energy into heat).

Heat is used in the treatment of the majority of rheumatic diseases, particularly for pain relief, muscle relaxation, improving circulation, increasing tissue metabolism, and to increase collagen fibre elasticity.

Thermographic index (TI) A frequently used index in rheumatology used for quantitative evaluation of thermal changes in the region of interest (ROI). It is described as the increase in the basal temperature over the monitored area and the temperature of isotherm multiplied by the surface of isotherm to total surface of ROI. The final TI is achieved by the sum of TI of particular isotherms. The normal TI value is 2, osteoarthrosis is 4, rheumatoid arthritis is >4; with acute gout giving the highest TI. TI is relevant for evaluating the efficiency of pharmacotherapy.

Thermography (TMG) A complementary imaging method by which the distribution of heat on the surface of subjects, including the human body, is detected. The principle is visualisation of infrared radiation with a thermographic camera. Two methods are used: contact TMG (liquid crystal encapsulated in foil), and non-contact (thermovision systems). In rheumatology, it is used to detect local hyperthermia (induced by inflammatory mediators), local hypothermia caused by nociceptive afferentation, or hypothermia due to vasospasm or obstruction of vessels. A relevant thermal picture can be obtained only

if strict standard conditions are adhered to. Thermography can also be utilised to evaluate thermal changes due to pharmacotherapy (temperature over affected joints) and physical medicine (local changes of micro- and macrocirculation). It is used in rheumatology, neurology, paediatrics, orthopaedics, gynaecology and reflexive therapy.

Thoracic outlet syndrome A compression syndrome due to compression of the neurovascular bundle as it passes from the thoracocervical region into the axilla. It can be caused by muscle hypertrophy, increased tone of the scalene muscles, weakness of the longissimus cervicis muscle and longus colli muscle or by bone or other fibrous surrounding structural abnormalities. The syndrome manifestation includes various sensory, motor, or vasomotor symptoms suggesting cervicobrachial syndrome.

Thymosins The group of approximately 30 polypeptide immunohormones released from the thymus. They regulate maturation and various activities of lymphocytes. They originate from the larger precursors prothymosins. The most common is thymosin α_1, whose molecule consists of 28 amino acid units. It stimulates activity of T helper lymphocytes, the humoral immune response, antiviral, antifungal and anticancer immunity. Its serum concentration decreases with age. It is suggested that loss of thymosins is one of many causes of ageing.

Thymulin A zinc-dependent peptide hormone (previously known as serum thymic factor) produced in the thymus from where it is released into the circulation. It increases the activity of certain T lymphocytes subpopulations (particularly suppressor and cytotoxic activities). Thymulin is able to renew the responsiveness of lymphocytes to mitogens in animals after thymectomy.

Thymus The endocrine gland producing thymosins, thymopoetins, thymulin and other immunohormones. It is the primary lymphatic organ where maturation and differentiation of T lymphocytes, which are able to detect antigens, occurs. Concurrently, elimination of the majority of autoreactive clones of T lymphocytes, which is one of the most important mechanisms of tolerance to autoantigens development, also occurs in the thymus. The thymus consists of a cortex and medulla. The cortex, which represents approximately 85% of gland weight, consists of thymocytes, epithelial cells and macrophages. The medulla comprises mainly of thymocytes. The gland reaches its maximum in adolescence (30 to 40 g), and decreases in size thereafter.

Thyroid disease → see Arthropathy in thyroid disease

Tietze's syndrome and costochondritis Tietze's syndrome is characterised by painful swelling of one or more costochondral joints.

Clinical picture: The course of the disease is benign, but relapses are frequent. The development of painful swelling may be acute or gradual. Pain may radiate to the shoulder, the arm, and is exacerbated by sneezing, coughing, deep inspiration and thoracic rotation. In approximately 70% of cases, the disease affects only a limited area, most frequently the second or third costochondral joints. Other joints – costosternal, manubriosternal and xiphisternal – are rarely affected.

Tinel's sign Palpation applied to the palmar aspect of the wrist (transverse carpal ligament) evokes pain or paraesthesiae of the first three fingers. It is positive in carpal tunnel syndrome.

T lymphocytes Lymphocytes are a subset of white blood cells, which after development from pluripotent haemopoietic stem cells in bone marrow, acquires immunocompetence within the thymus gland, i.e. typical morphological and functional properties. They are also referred to as T cells. The presence of specific antigen receptors, which are in the complex with differentiating determinant (antigen) CD3 molecule, is a fundamental feature of T lymphocytes.

T cells are a heterogenous population but consist mainly of two basic subpopulations: helper T lymphocytes (T_H) and cytotoxic T lymphocytes (T_C). The abbreviation of cytotoxic T lymphocytes is CTL. The differentiating determinants CD2 and CD3 are found on the surface of all T cells, but T_H lymphocytes also possess the CD4 determinant and CTL possess the CD8 determinant. The nomenclature 'helper' T lymphocytes is derived from their function, the fundamental of which is the help they provide for B lymphocytes during detection of the majority of antigens and induction of humoral immune response. Cytotoxic T lymphocytes are typical effector cells whose major task is to kill cells infected by viruses or other intracellular parasites, to kill malignant cells or cells with foreign histocompatibility antigens on their surface. Such target cells are detected by a specific manner in cooperation with class I HLA antigens (restriction of MHC). They are also involved in rejection after organ or tissue transplantation from non-identical donors. Contrary to this, exogenous antigens after transformation in antigen presenting cells (antigen presentation) are recognised by helper T lymphocytes in cooperation with class II HLA antigens. Apart from helper and cytotoxic T lymphocytes, the population of these cells also contain memory T lymphocytes, which are referred to as T_M-cells. A subpopulation of suppressor T lymphocytes (T_S cells) was considered in the past. According to contemporary opinions, suppressor T lymphocytes belong to the group of regulatory and cytotoxic T lymphocytes.

Neither subpopulation of T_H cells is homogenous, but is divided into four groups – T_H1, T_H2, T_H3 and T_R cells, which release various groups of cytokines. The precursors of T_H1 and T_H2 are naive (virgin) T_H0 cells, which have not yet come into contact with antigen and possess CD4 and CD45RA differentiating determinants. T_H cells, which have already been in contact with antigen, possess the differentiating determinants CD4 and CD45RO and are referred to as memory

T

Table 16. Production of cytokines and cytotoxins by the subpopulations of T_H-lymphocytes and T_C-lymphocytes, respectively

Cytokines	T_H1	T_H2	T_H3	T_H0	CTL
IL-2	++	–	–	+	+/–
IFN-γ	++	–	+/–	+	++
IL-3	++	++	+	+	+
GM-CSF	++	+	–	+	+
TNF-α	++	+/–	–	+/–	+
IL-4	–	++	–	+	–
IL-5	–	++	–	–	–
IL-6	–	++	–	–	–
IL-9	–	++	–	+	–
IL-10	–	++	+/–	+	–
IL-13	–	++	–	–	–
IL-17	+	–	–	–	–
TGF-β	–	+	++	–	–
Cytotoxins					
Lymphotoxin (TNF-β)	++	–	–	–	++
Perforins	–	–	–	–	++
Granzymes	–	–	–	–	++

cells. T_H3 cells produce transforming growth factor TGF-β and are involved in autotolerance.

T lymphocytes – activation The process by which clone expansion (proliferation of a particular clone) of naive T_H cells is initiated, and thereby their involvement in specific humoral or cellular immunity is enabled. For this purpose, the antigen receptor of a particular clone of cells in cooperation with class II MHC (major histocompatibility complex) antigens must recognise specific immunogenic peptide, which originates from the presentation of exogenous antigen via the antigen presenting cell. This primary stimulation signal must be confirmed at least by one other costimulating signal, which may be presented by certain molecules on the surface of antigen presenting cells and helper T lymphocytes.

T lymphocytes – cytotoxic A subpopulation of T lymphocytes with CD8 differentiating determinant on their surface. These cells are effector cells of specific cellular immunity.

They originate from precursors of cytotoxic T lymphocytes after recognising immunogenic peptide, which developed from endogenous antigen, originating from target cells infected by viruses, or from malignant cells, and after subsequent activation by IL-2. After contact with the target cell and activation, T lymphocytes release cytotoxic perforins and proteolytic enzymes (granzymes) onto the surface of the target cell. As a consequence, an influx of sodium ions and water and an outflux of potassium ions occur, leading to osmotic swelling and subsequent cell lysis.

T lymphocytes – suppressor A subpopulation of lymphocytes, whose function is to suppress the humoral immune response of T cells, as well as inhibit the specific cellular response carried out by T_H and T_C cells. At present, it is suggested that T_S lymphocytes do not exist as an independent subpopulation; however, natural regulator T_{reg} lymphocytes and inducer T_r1 and T_H3 lymphocytes carry out their function.

TNF receptor-associated factor 6 → see
TRAF6 – TNF receptor-associated factor 6

Toe swelling/deformity and associated diseases Oedema of one toe can be associated with gout, which manifests itself by acute inflammation, erythema and tenderness of the first metatarsophalangeal (MTP) joint (podagra).
  Treatment: See treatment of gout.
  Hallux valgus Develops mainly due to flatfoot and osteoarthrosis. The deformity is typical and the joint is painful during palpation. The X-ray picture is pathognomic. In long standing cases, treatment may require surgical intervention.
  Digitus rigidus Most frequently, stiffness of the first MTP joint occurs. Treatment consists of wearing good fitting shoes with specially shaped insoles.
  Hammer toe Caused by chronic diseases such as rheumatoid arthritis and other chronic inflammatory rheumatic diseases.
  Sausage toe Most frequently occurs in reactive arthritis or psoriatic arthritis.

Tomesa (balneophototherapy) The name for combined treatment with balneotherapy and selective UV radiation is deduced from the German words "TOtes MEer SAlz" meaning the use of Dead Sea salts in the bathing water. This modality imitates the microclimate of the Dead Sea. It is prepared as an 8 to 15% sodium chloride solution in a shallow bathtub, in which the patient turns around so the skin exposed to radiation is constantly wet. The dosage of radiation depends on the type of skin pigmentation and is gradually increased up to 30 minutes. It is used especially in the treatment of psoriasis and psoriatic arthropathy.

Tophus It is a deposit of sodium urate crystals. It is divided into bone tophus and tophus of soft tissues. The typical localisation of soft tissue tophi are the pinna of the ear (helix, less frequently antihelix), metatarsophalangeal joint of toe, ulnar margin of forearm, elbows (they may cause sack like dilatation of the olecranon bursa), above the extensor

planes of the small joints of hand, and Achilles tendon. Less frequently, tophi occur on the eyelids, the tongue, in the lungs, and rarely in the pericardium and on heart valves. Bone tophi occur in subchondral bone and can be seen on X-rays where they have a typical cystic structure in the form of significant transparency.

Total Sharp score (TSS) A scoring system used to quantify the radiological changes in patients with rheumatoid arthritis. The system describes erosions and narrowing of the joint space of 27 small joints of the hand, including the carpal bones. Van der Heide et al. modified the method in 1985 when feet joints, which in some patients are affected earlier than hand joints, were included in the scoring system. Sixteen areas for erosions and fifteen areas for joint space narrowing on each hand were established by the fusion of the Sharp and van der Heide scoring system. The erosion is evaluated from 0 to 5 points (1 = discrete changes, 2 to 3 = greater changes; score >3 includes the size of the erosions). The narrowing of the joint space is evaluated from 0 to 4 points (0 = normal space, 1 = suspect narrowing, 2 = global narrowing <50% of original space, 3 = global narrowing >50% of original space or subluxation and 4 = articular ankylosis or total luxation). The maximum score for hand joints erosions is 160 and for feet joints erosions 120; the maximum score for narrowing of hand joints' spaces is 120 and for feet joint spaces 48 (total maximum score is 448). The system is not universal, certain other scoring systems are also used, e.g. Raua score.

Toxic shock syndrome Caused by a bacterial toxin produced by *Staphylococcus aureus*. The toxin belongs to the superantigens (TSST-1 – toxic shock syndrome toxin). Symptoms include fever, arthralgias and exanthema accompanied by oedema of the hands, face and conjunctivae. Mouth ulcers and desquamation on the hands and feet occur in the second phase of the disease. TSST-1 affects many organs. Symptoms may include hypotension, arthralgias, nausea, vomiting, neurological

T

symptoms, and even adult respiratory distress syndrome. In certain cases, the symptoms are only mild, suggesting an influenza-like illness.

Toxin A poisonous substance of biological origin, which is usually immunogenic and therefore able to induce synthesis of antibodies. The antibodies are referred to as *antitoxins* and are able to neutralise the harmful effects of the toxin, against which the antibody is directed. Toxins can be the products of micro-organisms (tetanus toxin, diphtheria toxin, botulinum toxin etc.), herbs (e.g. ricin, abrin) or animals (snakes, scorpions, bees, wasps).

Toxoid A microbial toxin that has inactivated toxicity (harmful effects), but has maintained its immunogenicity. It is therefore used as an antigen to induce protective immunity against microbial exotoxins, such as tetanus or diphtheria toxoid.

Träbert currents Rectangular impulses lasting 2 ms with a 5 ms pause between single impulses, leading to a frequency of approximately 143 Hz. The intensity of the current is mediated depending on the patient's tolerance (increases up to the first perception of the current). Träbert currents mainly are suitable for pain relief in the area of the locomotor system.

Traction *Traction of cervical spine* Performed by staged traction using a Glisson loop. The traction can be continuous or intermittent, applied in a sitting or lying position, and performed manually, which is a safer and more effective technique.
Traction of lumbar spine Performed after a traction test on a traction table either in extension (with extended lower extremities) or in flexion (with flexed hip joints and knees at a 90° angle). This traction can also be performed manually, which is particularly suitable for painful conditions.
Traction of the spine in a vertical position is performed in baths; the patient wears a floating collar and a load is attached to the legs. The effect of such traction is increased by the warm environment of the water.

Traction test A test performed in the region of the cervical and lumbar spine before manual or device traction. The aim is to determine the most suitable direction of traction that provides patient with the best pain relief.

TRAF6 – TNF receptor-associated factor 6 RANK, as with other members of the family of TNF receptors, controls its intracellular signalling via a group of proteins known as TRAF – TNF receptor-associated factors. To date, 6 TRAF factors, mostly without specificity for a certain receptor, have been described. TRAF6 is an exception as it links only with RANK and CD40 and transmits signals from these receptors. Knockout mice for a gene coding for TRAF6 are characterised by severe osteopetrosis, which confirms that TRAF6 plays an essential role in osteoclastogenesis.

Tramadol A synthetic opioid, the structure of which is similar to codeine. Its analgesic effect is similar to pethidine and has 1/10 of the efficacy of morphine. The ratio between parenteral and oral efficacy is 1:3. It is one of the most widely used opioids for grade II analgesia and is suitable for the treatment of mild and moderately acute or chronic pain. Its metabolite mono-O-desmethyltramadol is pharmacologically active, with a higher affinity for receptors than tramadol itself. The analgesic effect is conditioned by activation of μ-1, δ and κ receptors, but it also influences pain by non-opioid mechanisms – stimulates serotonin release and inhibits the reuptake of serotonin and noradrenalin by nerve endings. This mechanism explains its greater efficiency in neuropathic pain. It is well tolerated at therapeutic doses, with milder and less frequent adverse effects. The risk of drug addiction is low. It can be administered parenterally, rectally or orally in conventional and slow release forms.

Transforming growth factors (TGF)
These are glycoproteins originally described as products of cells transformed by viruses that change (transform) the phenotype of normal cells to a neoplastic phenotype. They are found in normal as well as neoplastic cells and belong to two families: TGF-α and TGF-β. They are cytokines regulating tumorigenesis, embryonic development and the healing process of damaged tissues. TGF-β also participates significantly in the regulation of immune responses.

Transcription Transcription of genetic information from DNA into mRNA.

Transcutaneous Electrical Nerve Stimulator (TENS) Treatment with low frequency rectangle currents with impulses shorter than 1 ms, which are used for pain relief, particularly in extraarticular rheumatism and in radicular pain. Electrodes are placed in a position where the running current stimulates either the area of maximum pain (trigger points) or part of a specific nerve. Independent use by the patient after instruction is advantageous. The effect can be explained in two ways. Selective stimulation of type A nerve fibres, which conduct sensation, prevents the transfer of pain through thin type B fibres, which are designed to conduct pain (70 ms, 70 Hz). The second theory is based on the principle of selective stimulation of B fibres using longer lasting impulses (around 100 ms, with frequency of 10 Hz), which leads to increased synthesis of endorphins (with their generally accepted influence on pain perception).

Transdermal therapy with NSAIDs (non-steroidal anti-inflammatory drugs) Although NSAIDs are commonly given by mouth, they can also be administered locally in the form of creams, gels, sprays and patches. These latter methods are used with advantage in the treatment of the early stage of osteoarthrosis in order to achieve pain relief of painful areas, such as muscle insertions, tendons and ligaments. The concentration of the effective substance in the area of the activity is higher with local therapy than with systemic administration. Avoidance of the gastrointestinal system and the liver to major concentrations of the drug by the use of transdermal therapy is particularly beneficial to elderly patients.

Transduction The transfer of a specific part of the DNA chain (encoding a specific gene or its part) from a donor cell to a recipient cell by the use of a virus. This new genetic information will then alter the recipient cells phenotype.

Transient coxitis It may affect children and teenagers after upper airway infection, probably caused by a viral infection. Perthes' disease or slipped epiphysis should be taken into consideration as a differential diagnosis. Laboratory results are not diagnostic. The radiological picture is normal, but fluid accumulation in the joint can be proven by ultrasound.

Treatment: The disease recovers spontaneously; non-steroidal anti-inflammatory drugs can help to alleviate symptoms.

Translation Translation of genetic information encoded in the sequence of nucleotides of the mRNA molecule into the sequence of amino acids (primary structure) of the polypeptide protein chain.

Traumatic arthritis This can be caused by a hit, distortion or strain. Articular fluid can be sanguineous, but, this does not need to be due to intra-articular structure trauma (e.g. meniscus) but most frequently is caused by partial or total rupture of a cruciate ligament, or possibly by rupture of a joint bursa.

Treatment: Bed rest, splintage, non-steroidal anti-inflammatory drugs, joint aspiration as needed, glucocorticoids (intra-articularly), later mobilisation and physiotherapy.

Tremor An involuntary rhythmic muscle contraction of agonists and antagonists of certain parts of the body. Although the commonest tremor is not associated with pathology (essential tremor), most other tremors are related to underlying pathology (Parkin-

T

son's disease, dystonias, cerebellar disorders, etc) and can be diagnosed clinically.

Trendelenburg's test A positive Trendelenburg's test indicates weakness of the gluteus medius muscle on the side of the lifted leg. The patient stands on one leg with the examiner standing behind and observes whether the patient is able to hold the pelvis on the side of the lifted leg in the plane or whether the pelvis tilts downwards. This tilt indicates weakness of the gluteus medius muscle. A positive test signifies muscle imbalance of the pelvis and a possible pathological process in the hip of the standing leg.

Triamcinolone → see Glucocorticoids

Trigger points Hyperirritable areas in the skin, subcutaneous tissue, muscles or on the periosteum, which are asymptomatic at rest, but are activated by muscle and joint activity and evoke nociceptive reactions leading to limitation of movement and pain. The trigger points are sensitive to pressure and can be identified by the use of specific techniques, such as Kibler diagnostic fold, Dick-Leube technique or Vogler technique. The trigger points can be influenced by reflexive massage, acupuncture, acupressure, or by local anaesthetic injections.

T-score → see Osteoporosis – Diagnosis, Bone Mineral Density (BMD) Measurement – evaluation

Tuberculin Sterile solution of proteins obtained from the medium, in which *Mycobacterium tuberculosis* was cultivated. It is used for a tuberculin skin test.

Tuberculous arthritis A progressive chronic low grade monoarthritis, sometimes clinically intermittent, which if untreated leads to abscess and fistula formation in the established stages of the disease. It is usually due to lymphohaematogenous spread from a primary pulmonary or gastrointestinal focus.

Depending on the location of the initial focus, the primary synovial or bone disease can

be distinguished. The synovial form of joint tuberculosis has three stages. The initial synovitis, with insidious onset and mild pain only, usually without any symptoms of active inflammation affects one joint with swelling of its soft tissues and production of joint fluid. The next stage is characterised by granulating synovitis, hyperaemia, synovial hyperplasia, development of fibrocaseous changes and xanthochromic synovial fluid. In severe cases, the synovium is roughened and irregular layers of fibrin cover its surface. In the third stage, arthritis becomes prominent with the inflammatory process gradually affecting the cartilage and bony structures. This leads to chondral and subchondral destruction and dissection of cartilage, bone sequestration and fistula formation.

The primary bone form is associated with extravasation into the joint with the gradual development of arthritis. The secondary bone form originates from primary tenosynovitis and bursitis if the inflammation affects joint structures. It affects mainly weight-bearing joints. The X-ray picture shows little change in the early stages, but later cystic changes and marginal destruction in peri-articular bone due to the presence of granulation and caseous substances can be visible. Due to the absence of proteolytic enzymes in mycobacterial organisms, the joint configuration is preserved with little sclerosis of the adjacent bone for a relatively long period of time in the early active stage. Later sequestration and significant structural destruction can be seen. Diagnosis may be difficult without a good synovial biopsy and/or appropriate synovial fluid culture.

Clinical forms of tuberculous arthritis:
- Chronic synovitis,
- Chronic arthritis,
- Caries sicca (more commonly seen with syphilis),
- BCG arthritis.

Other forms of musculoskeletal tuberculosis:
- Spondylitis,
- Osteitis and osteomyelitis,
- Spina ventosa/dactylitis,
- Tenosynovitis/bursitis,
- Poncet's disease.

Tuftsin A Thr-Lys-Pro-Arg tetrapeptide produced by enzymatic cleavage of the Fc-domain of the heavy chain of immunoglobulin G (positions 289–292) in the spleen. It acts as a cytokine regulating the chemotaxis, phagocytosis and respiratory activation of neutrophils and macrophages. Deficiency develops after splenectomy.

Tumour necrosis factors (TNF) There are two TNFs: TNF-α (cachectin) and TNF-β (lymphotoxin). They have cytostatic and cytotoxic effects not only on neoplastic cells, but also on other biological activities. TNF-α is a typical cytokine acting as a trigger of the inflammatory reaction, as an endogenous pyrogen and endogenous mediator of the toxic effects of endotoxins of Gram-negative bacteria. It is able to induce pathological emaciation (cachexia). Lymphotoxin is a prototype of a new group of substances referred to as cytotoxins.

Tumoral calcinosis The main features of this hereditary disease are periarticular metastatic calcifications. Their appearance is in the soft tissue mass in the area of the large joints, particularly the hip and shoulder. Usually, the disease is autosomal recessive, but an autosomal dominant form is also possible.

Pathogenesis: The genetic background is still unclear, but appears to be due to a mutation leading to a disorder of phosphate metabolism regulation via FGF23 (fibroblast growth factor 23). One of the significant factors in the development of the disease is increased phosphate reabsorption in the kidney tubules, which is not associated with changes in parathormone levels. The disease can start as calcific bursitis, later spreading into surrounding the fascia. Trigger factors can include tissue damage with adipose necrosis. Increased local synthesis of calcitriol in granulomatous tissue leads to increased calcium absorption and decreased parathormone secretion.

Clinical picture: The disease affects children mainly of African and Afro-American descent. Initially, hyperplastic fibrous tissue with ectopic calcifications does not cause pain and grows at varying rates. With time, this creates a mechanical obstacle, causing nerve compression, joint movement limitation or skin ulcerations, which can become infected. Accompanying symptoms include anaemia, lymphadenopathy, increased body temperature, splenomegaly, and eventually amyloidosis. The disease is lifelong.

Tunnel syndromes of foot *Metatarsal tunnel syndrome (Morton's metatarsalgia)*

The common plantar digital nerve is compressed under the transverse metatarsal ligament. Clinical symptoms include a sharp burning pain, which most frequently radiates to the third and fourth toe. It does not cause hypo- or hyper-aesthesia or muscle weakness. Typical pain occurs when pressure is applied laterally to the metatarsophalangeal (MTP) joints (lateral pressure test).

Sural nerve tunnel syndrome

Causes pain radiating from the lateral aspect of the ankle distally to the little toe.

Treatment: Glucocorticoids are administered locally or the nerve is released surgically in both syndromes.

T

U1RNP → see Antibodies against U1RNP and Sm antigen

UCTD → see Undifferentiated connective tissue disease (UCTD)

Ultrasound The principle is the transformation of the electrical energy of a high frequency current into mechanical energy of longitudinal vibration of the physical environment with a frequency above the level of audibility (approximately 20,000 Hz). The vibration of all atoms and molecules, or of entire cells, occurs in the trajectory of the ultrasound ray leading to micro-massages with subsequent dispersal effects (the transformation of gel into fluidity, gel fluidisation) and the transformation of mechanical energy into thermal energy, and thereby to the heating up of deep tissues.

Ultrasound in rheumatology (arthrosonography) A diagnostic method using ultrasound to measure the varying degree of its reflection when passing through tissues of the body and produces two- or three-dimensional reconstruction images of the examined area. It is a promising non-invasive method, which is easily available, reproducible and economically advantageous, but is dependent on a well trained operator. It is particularly used in the detection of joint effusions, changes in muscles, periarticular structures, ligaments, tendons, bursae, cartilage and the bone surface. High frequency probes (above 10 to 15 MHz) can detect the early erosive changes around joints. Doppler mode enables assessment of blood flow.

Undifferentiated connective tissue disease (UCTD) The term undifferentiated connective tissue disease applies to the complex of symptoms that occur in patients with a systemic connective tissue disease which does not meet diagnostic criteria for any of the recognised systemic connective tissue diseases, i.e. MCTD (mixed connective tissue disease).

Clinical symptoms: The following symptoms may occur in UCTD:
- Non-specific clinical symptoms (arthralgia, myalgia, photosensitivity, overall weakness, subfebrile body temperatures, Raynaud's phenomenon),
- Symptoms relatively specific for systemic connective tissue diseases (arthritis, myositis, Raynaud's phenomenon with finger ulceration, morning stiffness, erythema and exanthema of face and extremities, serositis).

Urticarial vasculitis (URV) A disease manifesting itself by recurrent rashes with the histological finding of leukocytoclastic vasculitis. Apart from the skin, the disease may affect many organ systems. It occurs mainly in women in the fourth decade of life.

Clinical symptoms: The main symptoms include urticaria and papular exanthema, pruritus, arthralgia and systemic diseases such as glomerulonephritis, gastrointestinal and bronchopulmonary diseases.

V

Vaccine Active, but attenuated or dead pathogenic microorganisms or viruses, vaccine particles or products, which contain antigens able to stimulate a specific humoral or T cell immune response, producing immunity against these microorganisms or viruses.

Vasculitis Vasculitis is an inflammatory disease of blood vessels leading to thickening and/or fibrosis of the wall, with subsequent obliteration of its lumen.

Clinical symptoms: Clinical syndromes are the consequence of ischaemia of tissues supplied by the affected vessels associated with systemic symptoms (fever, weight loss, anorexia).

Classification: Most frequently done on the basis of the size of blood vessels affected.

Large: Giant cell arteritis, Takayasu arteritis.

Medium: Polyarteritis nodosa, Kawasaki disease, isolated CNS vasculitis.

Small: Wegener's granulomatosis, microscopic polyarteritis, Churg-Strauss syndrome, Henoch-Schönlein purpura, essential cryoglobulinaemic vasculitis, hypersensitivity vasculitis, vasculitis associated with connective tissue diseases, vasculitis due to viral infection.

Diagnosis is established by the clinical picture, blood tests including serum ANCA, and biopsy of relevant tissues.

Vertebrogenic algic syndrome This represents a common diagnostic and therapeutic problem in neurology, rheumatology, orthopaedics and rehabilitation therapy. Two types of disease should be distinguished, namely those with morphological defects (with symptoms and signs of locomotor system disease on X-ray or in laboratory findings) and those with functional defects without morphological and laboratory changes.

Vertebrogenic algic syndrome is a common term used for all painful conditions that originate from the vertebral column or from its surrounding soft structures (muscles, ligaments, fascia, and insertions). Nociceptive stimulation evokes a pathological process in the affected spinal segment with radiating pain, muscle spasm and the development of hyperalgic skin and muscle zones which are referred to as vertebrogenic algic syndrome. Contrary to radicular vertebrogenic algic syndrome, there are no signs of spinal nerve palsy.

Common symptoms are present in both types of syndrome:
- Algic syndrome with reflex symptoms in muscles, skin and subcutaneous tissue (muscle spasm, painful trigger points, hyperalgic zones, vegetative defects)
- Impairment of static and kinetic functions of the vertebral column (changes of curvature in the sagittal and frontal planes, reduced mobility) in morphological defects which frequently attack nerve roots, impairment of motor and sensory functions, trophic changes of muscles and reduced muscle tone in the affected segment; positive stretch tests are almost obligatory signs of nerve root compression.

Viral arthritis An inflammatory arthritis or tenderness of the soft structures of the locomotor system may occur in the course of a viral disease, which is usually short lived and has a good prognosis.

Clinical picture: Most cases of viral arthritis are usually acute short lived arthritis with a good prognosis, often associated with increased body temperature, skin symptoms and haematological abnormalities. Chronic polyarthritis suggestive of rheumatoid arthritis is rare (usually due to parvovirus B19). Exanthema is a typical accompanying sign of togavirus infections (rubella); however, it can also occur in arthritis associated with hepatitis B (urticarial rash).

Virulence Refers to the quantitative degree of pathogenicity of a microbe or virus to cause disease in certain animal species.

Virus An infective particle which consists of a single or double chain of DNA or RNA and is covered by a protein coat known as capsid. Viruses do not possess a proteosynthetic apparatus, and therefore can only undergo replication inside animal or plant cells which they have invaded through specific receptors. They cause a number of human, animal and plant diseases.

Vitamin D This vitamin influences bone metabolism in a complex way and has an essential role in the normal development of the skeleton. Small stature and development of rickets are the consequences of its deficiency in childhood. In adults, vitamin D deficiency leads to the development of secondary hyperparathyroidism with a resulting mobilisation of calcium from bone and the development of osteoporosis or osteomalacia or their combination. Several studies have confirmed a high prevalence of hypovitaminosis D in the European population, especially in the elderly (MacFarlane et al. 2004, Hirani and Primatesta 2005). Chronic hepatic, renal disorders and several drugs influence vitamin D metabolism or its clearance leading to 1,25-dihydroxy vitamin D3 deficiency.

Vitamin D deficiency develops predominantly in the following conditions:
- increased demands (children, pregnancy, menopause),
- low dietary intake,
- inadequate exposure to sunlight (UVB radiation),
- disturbances of intestinal absorption (disturbance of lipid absorption, disturbance of secretion of bile and pancreatic enzymes, post-resection conditions, etc.),
- disturbances of vitamin D metabolism (disorders of the liver and kidneys, treatment with anticonvulsants)
- resistance to vitamin D.

As well as the dietary intake, the synthesis of vitamin D3 (cholecalciferol) in skin by sunlight is the main source of vitamin D in humans. Following hydroxylation in the liver, it is transformed into 25-hydroxy (25-OH) vitamin D3 (disturbance of hydroxylation in hepatic diseases) and then, in the kidneys, 1,25-dihydroxy vitamin D3 and 24,25-dihydroxy vitamin D (disturbance of hydroxylation in renal disorders) are synthesised via relevant hydroxylases. The bone and intestines are the main target organs of calcitriol. It stimulates the absorption of calcium and phosphate in enterocytes, and stimulates the reuptake of calcium in the kidneys. Calcitriol increases the mineralisation as well as osteoresorption of bone. 24,25-dihydroxy vitamin D on the contrary inhibits osteoresorption induced by PTH. Vitamin D plays an important role in calcium homeostasis. A number of cells possess receptors for vitamin D. The concentration of 25(OH) vitamin D3 is a relevant indicator of the total vitamin D status in the body as it represents the amount of vitamin D synthesised and ingested.

The recommended daily intake of vitamin D is approximately 800 I.U. and over 1000 I.U for treatment. Some authors recommend even higher doses. A daily intake up to 2000 I.U. is generally considered safe.

It is possible to give cumulative doses of vitamin D up to 15000–20000 I.U. per week. A supplementation of medium-level doses of vitamin D appears to be safe and effective in patients at risk of vitamin D deficiency and is also effective in patients with mild-to-moderate renal insufficiency due to age or a renal disease. The beneficial effect of administration of vitamin D on reducing the incidence of fractures has been unambiguously shown in the elderly, where a deficit in exposure to sunlight, nutritional deficiency and disturbance of renal hydroxylation of vitamin D is hypothesised. Vitamin D supplementation is indicated in all cases where deficiency may be assumed or determined (for example winter months).

V region of immunoglobulins The variable region of polypeptide chains of immunoglobulin molecules, which form a variable domain. The sequence of amino acids of this region is not constant but variable, as various antibodies have different amino acids in particular positions of the region. This is the essence of the enormous variability of antibody specificity of immunoglobulin molecules.

Weber-Christian disease → see Panniculitis

Wegener's granulomatosis A necrotising systemic vasculitis which primarily affects the upper and lower respiratory systems and kidneys. It is more frequent in men, usually between 50 and 60 years of age.

Systemic symptoms, such as tiredness, weight loss and subfebrile temperatures, are frequent. Upper airways involvement includes epistaxis, chronic rhinitis and sinusitis. Otitis media and conductive hearing impairment are also frequent. Symptoms from the lower airways include cough, haemoptysis or chest pain. Renal damage (glomerulonephritis) is frequent and may lead to renal impairment. Ocular diseases include conjunctivitis, episcleritis, corneal ulcers, retinal vasculitis, optic nerve neuropathy and exophthalmos. Mononeuritis multiplex is the most frequent form of peripheral nerve involvement. Gastrointestinal symptoms include diarrhoea, haemorrhage, abdominal pain, and rarely bowel perforation.

Anaemia, leukocytosis and thrombocytosis are often present in laboratory findings. Other findings include increased erythrocyte sedimentation rate, elevated levels of C-reactive protein and hypergammaglobulinaemia, mainly IgA. The presence of ANCA (anti-neutrophil cytoplasmic antibodies) either c-ANCA (anti-PR3 antibodies) or p-ANCA (anti-MPO antibodies) is found in 90% of patients, however, anti-proteinase 3 (PR3) activity is more frequent.

Treatment consists of a combination of corticoids and cyclophosphamide, often initially active disease must be treated by the use of corticoids pulse therapy and cyclophosphamide. High doses of intravenous immunoglobulins or plasmapheresis are indicated in patients who are resistant to cyclophosphamide.

Western Ontario and McMaster universities osteoarthritis index (WOMAC) → see Instruments of assessing (health status measurements, outcome measurement)

Williams-Beuren syndrome The original description of children with supravalvular aortic stenosis and 'troll face' has been completed by the presence of transient hypercalcaemia during the first year of life. At present, it is suggested that a number of abnormalities exist within the syndrome; however, they need not necessarily all be fully expressed. Approximately 2/3 of children suffer from low birth weight and many are born after term. Small and defective dentition, large lower lip, long philtrum, short nose, epicanthus, skull asymmetry with temporal depression and microcephaly are present in children with 'troll face' abnormality. The voice of the children is squeaky. The children suffer from hypotonia and retardation of motor development. They are very friendly to strangers. Apart from a heart defect, they can also suffer from stenosis of peripheral organ arteries and hypertension is diagnosed in some of them at breastfeeding age. Hypercalcaemia, if present, spontaneously recovers towards the end of the first year of life. Hypercalciuria is relatively frequent. Approximately 1/3 of patients have radioulnar synostosis, which is the reason for inadequate development of the upper extremity. Genetic studies have localised the defect causing the syndrome to the q11.2 region of chromosome 7. The exact pathogenesis of the disease still remains unclear (Joyce et al. 1996).

Wiskott-Aldrich syndrome A rare recessive immunodeficiency linked to the short arm of the X chromosome. Affected boys suffer from suppressed T cell immunity, late sensitivity reaction and decreased synthesis of antibodies against polysaccharide antigens.

The number of B lymphocytes in the peripheral blood is normal. Serum IgM levels are significantly decreased, whereas IgA and IgE levels are increased, and the IgG level is usually normal. The syndrome manifests during the first year of life by severe thrombocytopenia leading to haemorrhagic symptomatology, recurrent infections and eczema. Sialophorin (CD43) a membrane glycoprotein involved in activating and regulating processes is missing on the surface of lymphocytes. The disease frequently leads to malignancies, particularly of the lymphatic system and epithelial tumours. The patient's condition may improve after transplantation of bone marrow. However, the overall prognosis is unfavourable.

W

Xenogenous (Xenogenic) An adjective referring to the different genetic relationship between individuals of two different animal species. It is used particularly in transplantation terminology. Skin graft or organ transplant, which has been donated by a donor of a different animal species, is referred to as a xenograft or xenotransplant. It possesses xenoantigens against which xenoantibodies are formed.

X-ray → see Radiography

Z

Zidovudine A 3'-azido-3'-deoxythymidine, inhibitor of reverse transcriptase, the enzyme that is necessary for transcription of genetic information from viral RNA to host DNA. It is used in the treatment of AIDS.

Zinc This element plays a significant role in the normal functioning of the immune system. It is complementary to many enzymes and other substances involved in the synthesis of nucleic acids and proteins. Reversible dysfunction of T lymphocytes, thymus atrophy, selective decrease in the number of circulating T helper lymphocytes, decreased synthesis of antibodies, as well as functional defects of macrophages and granulocytes develop in cases of zinc deficiency. All this leads to an increased risk of infections and to poor wound healing.

Zoledronate A bisphosphonate with a unique administration in the form of once a year intravenously. Currently, it is indicated for the treatment of the Paget's disease and bony metastases. Its effect in the treatment of osteoporosis has been completed in clinical trials. A single intravenous infusion of 5 mg of zoledronate is administered in the treatment of Paget's disease.

Z-score → see Osteoporosis – Diagnosis, Bone Mineral Density (BMD) Measurement – evaluation

Zymosan A complex polysaccharide isolated from the cellular wall of the *Saccharomyces cerevisiae* yeast. It contains mainly β-D-glucans and mannans. It activates the complement by the alternative pathway and binds to the receptors for C3b fragment of complement.

References

ANDERSON K, BRADLEY LA, MCDANIEL LK et al (1987) The assessment of pain in rheumatoid arthritis: disease differentiation and temporal stability of a behavioral observation method. J Rheumatol 14:700–704

BATHON JM, MARTIN RW, FLEISCHMANN RM et al (2000) A comparison of etanercept and methotrexate in patients with early rheumatoid arthritis. N Engl J Med 343:1586–1593

BELLAMY N (2008) Principles of outcome assessment. In: Hochberg MC, Silman AJ, Smolen JS (eds) Rheumatology, 4th edn. Mosby Elsevier, Philadelphia

BELLAMY N, BUCHANAN WW, GOLDSMITH CH et al (1988) Validation study of WOMAC: a health status instrument for measuring clinically important patient relevant outcomes to antirheumatic drug therapy in patients with osteoarthritis of the hip or knee. J Rheumatol 15:1833–1840

BENSEN WG, FIECHTNER JJ, MCMILLEN JI et al (1999) Treatment of osteoarthritis with celecoxib, a cyclooxygenase-2 inhibitor: a randomized controlled trial. Mayo Clin Proc 74:1095–1105

BERGNER L., HALLSTROM AP, BERGNER M (1985) Health status of survivors of cardiac arrest and of myocardial infarction controls. Am J Public Health 75:1321–1323

BOMBARDIER C, GLADMAN DD, UROWITZ MB et al (1992) Derivation of the SLEDAI. A disease activity index for lupus patients. The committee on prognosis studies in SLE. Arthritis Rheum 35:630–640

BURCKHARDT CS, CLARK SR, BENNETT RM (1991) The fibromyalgia impact questionnaire: development and validation. J Rheumatol 18:728–733

CALIN A (1994) Ankylosing spondylitis: defining disease status and the relationship between radiology, metrology, disease activity, function, and outcome. J Rheumatol 22:740–744

DELLA ROSSA A, TAVONI A, BOMBARDIERI S (2008) Cryoglobulinemia. In: Hochberg MC, Silman AJ, Smolen JS (eds) Rheumatology, 4th edn. Mosby Elsevier, Philadelphia

DOUGADOS M, GUEGUEN A, NAKACHE JP (1988) Evaluation of a functional index and an articular index in ankylosing spondylitis. J Rheumatol 15:302–307

EBERHARDT KB, SVENSSON B, MORTIZ U (1988) Functional assessment of early rheumatoid arthritis. Br J Rheumatol 27:364–371

EMERY P, BREEDVELD FC, HALL S et al (2008) Comparison of methotrexate monotherapy with a combination of methotrexate and etanercept in active, early, moderate to severe rheumatoid arthritis (COMET): a randomized, double-blind, parallel treatment trial. Lancet 372:375–382

EMERY P, FURST DE, KEYSTONE EC et al (2008) Certolizumab pegol remains equally efficacious in the treatment of rheumatoid arthritis over a range of background methotrexate regimens (10–30 mg/wk): analysis of the rapid 1 trial. Ann Rheum Dis 67(Suppl II):180

FERRACCIOLI GF, BAMBARA LM, FERRARIS M et al (1997) Effects of cyclosporin on joint damage in rheumatoid arthritis. Clin Exp Rheum 15(Suppl 17):83–89

FORRE O, NORWEGIAN ARTHRITIS STUDY GROUP (1994) Radiologic evidence of disease modification in rheumatoid arthritis patients treated with cyclosporine: result of a 48 week multicenter study comparing low dose cyclosporine and placebo. Arthritis Rheum 37:1506–1512

FRIES JF, SPITZ P, GUY KRAINES R et al (1980) Measurement of patient outcome in arthritis. Arthritis Rheum 23:137–145

FURST DE, BREEDVELD FC, KALDEN JR et al (2007) Updated consensus statement on biological agents for the treatment of rheumatic diseases, 2007. Ann Rheum Dis 66(Suppl III):iii2–iii22

HAAS M, NYIENDO J (1992) Diagnostic utility of the McGill Pain Questionnaire and the Oswestry Disability Questionnaire for classification of low back pain syndromes. J Manipulative Physiol Ther 15:90–98

HIRANI V, PRIMATESTA P (2005) Vitamind D concentrations among people aged 65 years and over living in private households and institutions in England: population survey. Age Ageing 34:485–491

HUNT SM, MCEWEN J, MCKENNA SP (1985) Social inequalities and perceived health. Eff Health Care 2:151–160

HURST NP, JOBANPUTRA P, HUNTER M et al (1994) Validity of Euroqol–a generic health status instrument–in patients with rheumatoid arthritis. Economic and Health Outcomes Research Group. Br J Rheumatol 33:655–662

HÜTTL S (ed) (1970) Synovial effusion I. Acta rheumatologica et balneologica Pistinina Československé štátne kúpele, Piešťany

HÜTTL S (ed) (1971) Synovial effusion II. Acta rheumatologica et balneologica Pistinina Československé štátne kúpele, Piešťany

JOHNSON R, CHARNLEY J (1979) Hydroxychloroquine in prophylaxis of pulmonary embolism following hip arthroplasty. Clin Orthop Relat Res 144:174–177

JOHNSON R, GREEN JR, CHARNLEY J (1977) Pulmonary embolism and its prophylaxis following the Charnley total hip replacement. Clin Orthop Relat Res 127:123–132

JOYCE CA, ZORICH B, PIKE SJ et al (1996) Williams-Beuren syndrome: phenotypic variability and deletions of chromosomes 7, 11, and 22 in a series of 52 patients. J Med Genet 33:986–992

KLARESKOG L, VAN DER HEIDE D, JAGER JP et al (2004) Therapeutic effect of combination of etanercept and MTX compared with each treatment alone in patients with rheumatoid arthritis: double blind randomised trial. Lancet 363:675–685

LANDEWÉ R, SMOLEN J, KEYSTONE EC et al (2008) Radiographic inhibition of progression of structural damage: results from the rapid 2 trial. Ann Rheum Dis 67(Suppl II):321

LANE N, LEBOFF MS (2005) Metabolic bone disease. In: Harris ED Jr, Budd RC, Genovese MC (eds) Kelley´s textbook of rheumatology, Elsevier Saunders, Philadelphia

LEQUESNE MG, MERY C, SAMSON M et al (1987) Indexes of severity for osteoarthritis of the hip and knee. Validation–value in comparison with other assessment tests. Scand J Rheumatol 65(Suppl):85–89

MACFARLANE GD, SACKRISON JL JR, BODY JJ et al (2004) Hypovitaminosis D in a normal, apparently healthy urban European population. J Steroid Biochem Mol Biol 89–90:621–522

MARCUS R, FELDMAN D, NELSON DA (eds) (2008) Osteoporosis. 3rd edn. Elsevier Academic Press, London

MASON JH, ANDERSON JJ, MEENAN RF (1992a) The rapid assessment of disease activity in rheumatology (radar) questionnaire. Validity and sensitivity to change of a patient self-report measure of joint count and clinical status. Arthritis Rheum 35:156–162

MASON JH, MEENAN RF, ANDERSON JJ (1992b) Do self-reported arthritis symptom (RADAR) and health status (AIMS2) data provide duplicative or complementary information? Arthritis Care Res 5:163–172

MEENAN RF, GERTMAN PM, MASON JH (1980) Measuring health status in arthritis. Arthritis Rheum 23:146–152

MILLER FW (1993) Myositis-specific autoantibodies. Touchstones for understanding the inflammatory myopathies. JAMA 270:1846–1849

MOMBERGER TS, LEVICK JR, MASON RM (2005) Hyaluronan secretion by synoviocytes is mechanosensitive. Matrix Biol 24:510–519

MORELAND LW (ed) (2004) Rheumatology and immunology therapy. Springer, Berlin

OLIVIERI I, PADULA A, PALAZZI C (2006) Pharmacological management of SAPHO syndrome. Expert Opin Investig Drugs 15:1229–1233

OLSSON KS (2008) Hemochromatosis. In: Hochberg MC, Silman AJ, Smolen JS (eds) Rheumatology, 4th edn. Mosby Elsevier, Philadelphia

OVESEN L, ANDERSEN R, JAKOBSEN J (2003) Geographical differences in vitamin D status, with particular reference to European countries. Proc Nutr Soc 62:813–821

PAVELKA K, GATTEROVÁ J, OLEJÁROVÁ M et al (2002) Glucosamine sulphate use and delay of progression of knee osteoathritis: a 3 year, randomised, place-controlled, double-blind study. Arch Intern Med 162:2113–2123

PAVELKA K, ŠTOLFA J (2005) Systémová nesteroidní antirevmatika. In: Pavelka K (ed) Farmakoterapie revmatických onemocnění. Grada Publishing, Praha

PAYER J, ROVENSKÝ J, KILLINGER Z (eds) (2007) Lexikón osteoporózy. Slovak Academic Press, Bratislava

PETRI M, HOCHBERG M, HELLMAN D et al (1992) Incidence of and predictors of thrombotic events in SLE. Protective role of hydroxychloroquine. Arthritis Rheum 35:S54

PETRI M, LAKATTA C, MAGDER L et al (1994) Effect of prednisone and hydroxychloroquine on coronary artery disease risk factors in systemic lupus erythematosus: A longitudinal data analysis. Am J Med 96:254

PIPER BF (1990) Piper fatique scale available for clinical testing. Oncol Nurs Forum 17:661–662

PLANT MJ, SCHLATVALN J, BORG AA et al (1994) Measurement and prediction of radiological progression in early rheumatoid arthritis. J Rheumatol 21:1808–1813

REGINSTER JY, DEROISY R, ROVATI LS et al (2001) Long-term effects of glucosamine sulphate on osteoarthritis progression: a randomised, placebo-controlled trial. Lancet 357:251–256

ROVATI LC (1997) The clinical profile of glucosamine sulfate as a selective symptom modifying drug in osteoarthritis current data and perspectives. Osteoarthritis Cartilage 5(Suppl. A):72

ROVENSKÁ E, ROVENSKÁ E, NEUMÜLLER J (2003) Structure of synovial lymphatic capillaries in rheumatoid arthritis and juvenile idiopathic arthritis. Int J Tissue React 25:29–39

ROVENSKÝ J, PAVELKA K, SZILASIOVÁ A et al (2000) Reumatoidná artritída. In: Rovenský J, Pavelka K (eds) Klinická reumatológia. Osveta, Martin

SCHILLING F, ECKARDT A, KESSLER S (2000) Chronic recurrent multifocal osteomyelitis. Z Orthop Ihre Grenzgeb 138:530–539

SCOTT DL (2000) Prognostic factors in early rheumatoid arthritis. Rheumatology (Oxford) 39(Suppl 1):24–29

SELDIN MF, AMOS C1, WARD R et al (1999) The genetics revolution and the assault on rheumatoid arthritis. Arthritis Rheum 42:1071–1079

SHARP GC, IRVIN WS, TAN EM et al (1972) Mixed connective tissue disease: an apparently distinct rheumatic disease syndrome associated with a specific antibody to an extractable nuclear antigen. Am J Med 52:148–159

SILMAN AJ (1997) Problems complicating the genetic epidemiology of rheumatoid arthritis. J Rheumatol 24:194–196

SMOLEN JS, KADLEN JR, SCOTT DL et al (1999) Efficacy and safety of leflunomide compared with placebo and sulphasalazine in active rheumatoid arthritis: a double blind, randomized, multicenter study. Lancet 353:259–266

STRAND V, COHEN S, SCHIFF M et al (1999) Treatment of active rheumatoid arthritis with leflunomide compared with placebo and methotrexate. Arch Intern Med 159:2542–2550

STUCKI G, LIANG MH, STUCKI S et al (1995) A self-administered rheumatoid arthritis disease activity index (RADAI) for epidemiologic research. Psychometric properties and correlation with parameters of disease activity. Arthritis Rheum 38:795–798

SYMMONS DP, HASSELL AB, GUNATILLAKA KA et al (1995) Development and preliminary assessment of a simple measure of overall status in rheumatoid arthritis (OSRA) for routine clinical use. Q J Med 88:429–437

SZUMLANSKI CL, HONCHEL R, SCOTT MC et al (1992) Human liver thiopurine methyltransferase pharmacogenetics: biochemical properties, liver-erythrocyte correlation and presence of isozymes. Pharmacogenetics 2:148–159

TUGWELL P, BOMBARDIER C, BUCHANAN WW et al (1987) The MACTAR Patient Preference Disability Questionnaire–an individualized functional priority approach for assessing improvement in physical disability in clinical trials in rheumatoid arthritis. J Rheumatol 14:446–451

UEBELHARDT D, THOMAN JMA, DELMAS D et al (1998) Effects of chondroitin sulfate on the progression of knee osteoarthritis: a pilot study. Osteoarthritis Cartilage 6(Suppl. A):39–46

WALLACE JD, METZGER AL, STECHER VJ et al (1990) Cholesterol-lowering effect of hydroxychloroquine (Plaquenil) in rheumatoid disease patients: Reversal of deleterious effects of steroids on lipids. Am J Med 89:322

WEINBLATT ME, KREMER JM, BANKHURST AD et al (1999) A trial of etanercept, a recombinant tumor necrosis factor receptor: Fc fusion protein, in patients with rheumatoid arthritis receiving methotrexate. N Engl J Med 340:253–259

WHO SCIENTIFIC GROUP TECHNICAL RE-PORT (2007) Assessment of osteoporosis at the primary health care level. University of Sheffield

WILES N, SYMMONS DP, HARRISON B et al (1999) Estimating the incidence of rheumatoid arthritis: trying to hit a moving target? Arthritis Rheum 42:1339–1346

WORRALL JG, BAYLISS MT, EDWARDS JC (1991) Morphological localization of hyaluronan in normal and diseased synovium. J Rheumatol 18:1466–1472

ZEIDLER KH, KVIEN TK, HANNONEN P et al (1998) Progression of joint damage in early active severe rheumatoid arthritis during 18 month of treatment: comparison of low-dose cyclosporin and parenteral gold. Br J Rheumatol 37:874–882

ŽITŇAN D, PAVELKA K (2000) Artropatie indukované kryštálmi. In: Rovenský J, Pavelka K (eds) Klinická reumatológia. Osveta, Martin

SpringerMedizin

Miroslav Ferencik, Jozef Rovensky,
Vladimir Matha, Manfred Herold

Kompendium der Immunologie

Grundlagen und Klinik

2006. XII, 319 Seiten. 55 Abb. in Farbe.
Gebunden **EUR 44,95**, sFr 70,–*
ISBN 978-3-211-25536-0

Die Standardlehrbücher zur Immunologie bieten meist sehr komplexe
und detaillierte Informationen, die beim Leser bestimmte Kenntnisse
über Biochemie, Physiologie und Mikrobiologie voraussetzen.

Dieses Kompendium wurde für den „Erstkontakt" mit dieser kom-
plexen Thematik konzipiert. Wichtige Basisinformationen über die
Struktur und Funktion von Zellen des Immunsystems, über Anti-
körper, Zytokine und andere regulatorischen Moleküle, sowie über
Abwehrmechanismen gegen Infektionserreger und spontan entste-
hende Tumore werden ebenso beschrieben wie unspezifische und
spezifische Immunantworten und Störungen des Immunsystems
durch Autoimmerkrankungen oder Allergien.
Aufgrund der didaktischen Aufbereitung und den zahlreichen
anschaulichen Abbildungen ist dieses Werk bestens als Nach-
schlagewerk und Lehrbuch für Studenten der Medizin und
Naturwissenschaften geeignet.

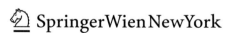 Springer Wien New York

P.O.Box 89, Sachsenplatz 4–6, 1201 Wien, Österreich, Fax +43.1.330 24 26, books@springer.at, **springer.at**
Haberstraße 7, 69126 Heidelberg, Deutschland, Fax +49.6221.345-4229, SDC-bookorder@springer.com, springer.com
P.O. Box 2485, Secaucus, NJ 07096-2485, USA, Fax +1.201.348-4505, service@springer-ny.com, springer.com
Preisänderungen und Irrtümer vorbehalten. *Unverbindliche Preisempfehlung

SpringerMedizin

Miroslav Ferencik, Jozef Rovensky,
Vladimir Matha, Erika Jensen-Jarolim

Wörterbuch Allergologie und Immunologie

Fachbegriffe, Personen und klinische Daten von A-Z

2005. IX, 349 Seiten. 77 Abbildungen. Mit CD-ROM
Gebunden **EUR 54,95**, sFr 85,50*
ISBN 978-3-211-20151-0

Die Immunologie und Allergologie zählen zu den am schnellsten
wachsenden Bereichen der Wissenschaft, vor allem in Hinblick
auf experimentelle und klinische Forschung. Um diesem Wachstum
gerecht zu werden, ist es notwendig, über gesicherte Grundlagen
Bescheid zu wissen. Mit diesem Werk können auf einfache Art und
Weise wichtige allergologische und immunologische Fachbegriffe,
wie auch klinisch relevante Themen nachgeschlagen werden.
Auch aktuelle Themen, wie etwa Anthrax, Hühnergrippe, DNS-
Vakzine, Prionosen, SARS werden umfassend und praxisnah dar-
gestellt. Das Spektrum der präsentierten Themen umfasst daher
unterschiedliche Fachdisziplinen, wie Molekularbiologie, Mikrobiologie, Biotechnologie und Klinische Medizin. Aufgrund der
didaktischen Aufbereitung und den zahlreichen anschaulichen
Abbildungen ist dieses Werk auch als Lehrbuch für Studenten der
Naturwissenschaften bestens geeignet. Die Farbabbildungen auf
der beigelegten CD-ROM eignen sich gut für Vorträge, Präsen-
tationen und Lehrzwecke.

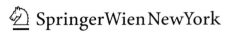 Springer Wien NewYork

P.O.Box 89, Sachsenplatz 4–6, 1201 Wien, Österreich, Fax +43.1.330 24 26, books@springer.at, **springer.at**
Haberstraße 7, 69126 Heidelberg, Deutschland, Fax +49.6221.345-4229, SDC-bookorder@springer.com, springer.com
P.O. Box 2485, Secaucus, NJ 07096-2485, USA, Fax +1.201.348-4505, service@springer-ny.com, springer.com
Preisänderungen und Irrtümer vorbehalten. *Unverbindliche Preisempfehlung

SpringerMedicine

Gerhard Nahler

Dictionary of Pharmaceutical Medicine

With contributions by A. Mollet.
2nd edition.
2009. Approx. 350 pages.
Softcover approx. **EUR 39,95**
Recommended retail price. Net price subject to local VAT.
ISBN 978-3-211-89835-2. Due March 2009

The dictionary contains various terms typically used in pharmaceutical medicine. The 2nd edition reflects the increasing importance of this science and the changing regulatory environment in particular on research and development of new therapies as well as on the conduct of clinical trials, marketing authorisation of new medicinal products and safety aspects including pharmacovigilance.
The number of key words has been considerably enlarged and increased to over 1.600 terms; it includes new scientific areas such as gene therapy and proteomics. Furthermore, given the importance of the internet, the new edition contains a list of most important web sites. Similar to the 1st edition, also the book explains about 1.000 abbreviations most commonly used in pharmaceutical medicine.
This book will be a valuable tool for professionals in the area of the pharmaceutical industry, medical and pre-clinical research, regulatory affairs, marketing and marketing authorisation of pharmaceuticals.

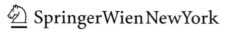

SpringerWienNewYork

P.O.Box 89, Sachsenplatz 4–6, 1201 Vienna, Austria, Fax +43.1.330 24 26, books@springer.at, **springer.at**
Haberstraße 7, 69126 Heidelberg, Germany, Fax +49.6221.345-4229, SDC-bookorder@springer.com, springer.com
P.O. Box 2485, Secaucus, NJ 07096-2485, USA, Fax +1.201.348-4505, service@springer-ny.com, springer.com
Prices are subject to change without notice. All errors and omissions excepted.